Introduction to the
FINANCIAL
MANAGEMENT
of Healthcare Organizations

Introduction to the
FINANCIAL
MANAGEMENT
of Healthcare Organizations

MICHAEL NOWICKI

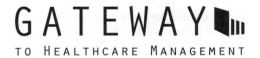

GATEWAY

TO HEALTHCARE MANAGEMENT

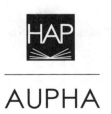

HAP

AUPHA

Health Administration Press, Chicago, Illinois
Association of University Programs in Health Administration, Arlington, Virginia

Your board, staff, or clients may also benefit from this book's insight. For more information on quantity discounts, contact the Health Administration Press Marketing Manager at (312) 424-9470.

19   18   17   16   5   4   3

Library of Congress Cataloging-in-Publication Data

Nowicki, Michael, 1952–

   Introduction to the financial management of healthcare organizations / Michael Nowicki. — Sixth edition.
      pages cm
   ISBN 978-1-56793-669-8 (alk. paper)
   1. Hospitals—Business management. 2. Hospitals—Finance. 3. Health facilities—Business management. 4. Health facilities—Finance. I. Title. II. Title: Financial management of healthcare organizations.
   RA971.3.N69 2015
   362.11068'1—dc23

              2014005161

The paper used in this publication meets the minimum requirements of American National Standard for Information Sciences—Permanence of Paper for Printed Library Materials, ANSI Z39.48-1984. ∞ ™

Acquisitions editor: Janet Davis; Project manager: Amy Carlton; Cover designer: Mark Oberkrom; Layout: Cepheus Edmondson

Found an error or typo? We want to know! Please e-mail it to hapbooks@ache.org, and put "Book Error" in the subject line.

For photocopying and copyright information, please contact Copyright Clearance Center at www.copyright.com or (978) 750-8400.

Health Administration Press
A division of the Foundation
   of the American College of
   Healthcare Executives
One North Franklin Street
Suite 1700
Chicago, IL 60606-3529
(312) 424-2800

Association of University Programs
   in Health Administration
2000 North 14th Street
Suite 780
Arlington, VA 22201
(703) 894-0940

I dedicate this book to my parents who, by their actions more than their words, instilled in me the value for lifelong learning. From my mother, I learned that effort is a reward in itself. From my father, I learned that correct answers count, always.

BRIEF CONTENTS

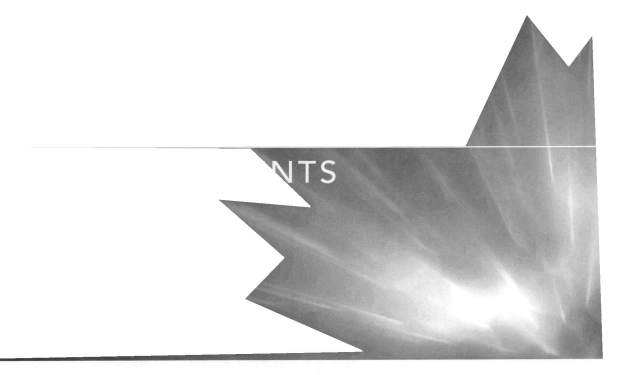

NTS

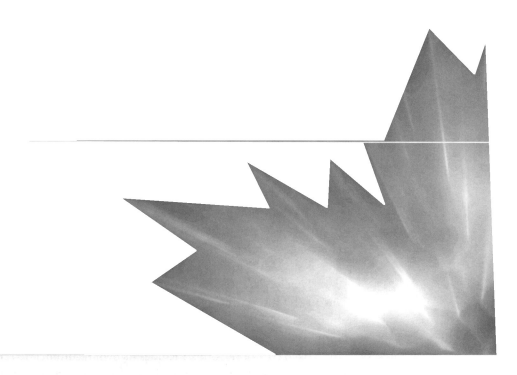

Introduction to the Financial Management of Healthcare Organizations is intended to be the primary textbook in introductory courses in healthcare financial management at both the undergraduate and graduate levels as well as a reference book for program graduates and other practicing healthcare managers. The purpose of this book is to introduce nonfinancial students and managers to the fundamental concepts and skills necessary to succeed as managers in an increasingly competitive employment environment.

For instance, program graduates find employment in a variety of healthcare settings. Therefore, the focus of this book—as well as the title of the book—extends beyond the hospital. Program graduates consistently report a deficiency in quantitative skills; this book includes problems representing key concepts. Traditional-age students report a need to apply the quantitative skills introduced in financial management. To address both of these concerns, this book includes mini-cases within chapters, practice problems at the ends of many chapters, and a comprehensive case at the end of the book.

Introduction to the Financial Management of Healthcare Organizations is part of Health Administration Press's Gateway to Healthcare Management series. The textbooks in this series are geared specifically for students new to healthcare management.

In this edition, Part I includes an overview of financial management; the organization of financial management, including updated information on job responsibilities and salaries; and the tax status of healthcare organizations, including the most recent court cases differentiating for-profit and not-for-profit hospitals.

Part II includes information about third-party payers and payment methodologies, Medicare, and Medicaid, including updated laws pertaining to these public programs, federal government settlements with providers on fraud and abuse allegations, cost accounting and analysis, and rate setting.

Part III covers the management and financing of working capital, materials management, and accounts receivable management.

Part IV includes strategic, strategic financial, and operational planning; budgeting; and capital budgeting.

Part V covers financial analyses and describes a new set of financial statements and management reporting, including the latest changes to generally accepted accounting principles (GAAP) for healthcare entities.

Finally, Part VI provides an analysis of trends that will affect healthcare organizations in the future, including healthcare cost projections and the need for entitlement reform. The Affordable Care Act (ACA) of 2010, commonly referred to as healthcare reform, is discussed throughout the book but more prominently in Parts II and VI.

Each part of the book includes its own recommended reading list. A running glossary of important terms accompanies each chapter and is compiled at the end of the book; a list of acronyms used in the text is also included at the end of the book. At the end of every chapter, important points and discussion questions encourage students to summarize what they are learning and put it into their own words. The chapters are modular to allow instructors to either delete specific chapters or assign the chapters in an order based on individual preference or classroom requirements.

Instructor resources, including a test bank, PowerPoints, and answer guides for the in-book discussion questions, are available online. Instructors who adopt this book for use in their class may request access to the instructor's resources by e-mailing hapbooks@ache.org.

I hope you find *Introduction to the Financial Management of Healthcare Organizations* relevant, current, and easy to understand.

ACKNOWLEDGMENTS

I would like to gratefully acknowledge those who assisted me in this sixth edition: my wife, Tracey, and our kids, Hannah and David, who have often sacrificed time with Dad so that I could write; my many students over the years, who have challenged me to find a better way to explain, teach, and evaluate the understanding of difficult concepts; Texas State University for continuing to support faculty research efforts; and Dick Clarke, president emeritus of HFMA, who in ways too numerous to mention has always supported my academic career. Finally, special thanks to those at Health Administration Press who have made this sixth edition what it is.

—Michael Nowicki

PART I

FINANCIAL MANAGEMENT

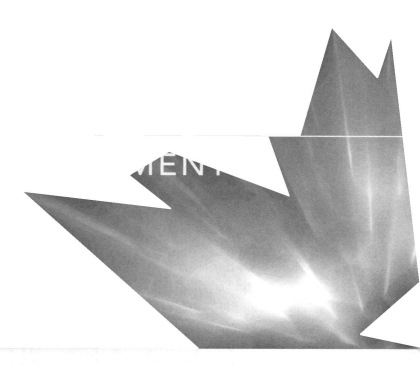

No matter where you are in the healthcare finance arena, there are opportunities to move things forward, to act, to resist complacency, to refuse to allow yourself to think that things won't ever change. As finance professionals we all have strengths that will serve our organizations well in these times of change.

Debora Kuchka-Craig, 2011 chair of the Healthcare
Financial Management Association

LEARNING OBJECTIVES

After completing this chapter, you should be able to do the following:

➤ Understand the purpose of healthcare organizations

➤ Relate the purpose of healthcare financial management to the purpose of the organization

➤ Understand the objectives of healthcare financial management

➤ Apply quality assessment to healthcare financial management

➤ Apply organizational ethics to healthcare financial management

➤ Examine the value of healthcare financial management to the management functions and the changing face of healthcare

➤ Review background accounting, economics, and statistics information (Appendices 1.1, 1.2, and 1.3)

INTRODUCTION

Successful organizations, whether for-profit, not-for-profit, or governmental, have two things in common: a congruent and well-understood organizational purpose, and a functional management team. The purpose of this introductory chapter is to describe financial management in healthcare organizations within the context of organizational purpose and a competent management team.

ORGANIZATIONAL PURPOSE

Organizational purpose is often determined by the owner. While a community-owned, not-for-profit healthcare organization's purpose is to provide healthcare services to the community, a corporate-owned (via stockholders), for-profit healthcare organization's purpose is to provide profit for the owner.

By necessity, most organizations have more than one organizational purpose. For instance, even though a not-for-profit healthcare organization's purpose is to provide healthcare services to the community, the organization must survive economically—meaning that it must generate sufficient revenue to offset expenses and allow for growth. A for-profit healthcare organization's purpose is to provide profit for the owner; however, the organization must meet the customer's needs—meaning it must keep the physicians, patients, employers, and insurance companies satisfied.

Most healthcare organizations also have secondary purposes—for example, many government-owned healthcare organizations provide large-scale medical education programs.

To maintain congruence, the management team must communicate the organizational purpose or purposes not only to the employees, but also to owners, customers, and other important constituents. When multiple purposes are present, the management team must prioritize the purposes.

HEALTHCARE MANAGEMENT

In its broadest context, the objective of healthcare management is to accomplish the organizational purposes. Doing so is not as simple as it sounds, especially if the healthcare organization's purposes are "to provide the community with the services it needs, at a clinically acceptable level of quality, at a publicly responsive level of amenity, at the least possible cost" (Berman, Kukla, and Weeks 1994, 5). Healthcare managers must identify, prioritize, and often resolve these sometimes contradictory purposes in a political environment that involves the organization's governing board and medical staff; in a regulatory environment that involves licensing and accrediting agencies; and in an economic environment that involves increasing competition, resulting in demands for lower prices and higher quality.

Competent healthcare managers attempt to accomplish the organizational purposes by planning, organizing, staffing, directing, and controlling (called the **management**

management functions
The key functions of a manager, including planning, organizing, staffing, directing, and controlling.

functions) and by communicating, coordinating, and decision making (called the **management connective processes**). For more information on the management functions and connective processes, see *Dunn and Haimann's Healthcare Management* (2010).

With the exception of nursing home administrators, no licensure requirements are needed to be a practicing healthcare manager. However, facility-accrediting organizations such as **The Joint Commission** require healthcare managers to possess such education and experience as required by the position. Moreover, formal educational programs for healthcare management do exist at both the undergraduate and graduate levels. Undergraduate programs can seek program review and approval from the Association of University Programs in Health Administration. Graduate programs can seek program review and accreditation from the Commission on Accreditation of Healthcare Management Education. Furthermore, healthcare managers can seek membership and certification in professional associations, including the American College of Healthcare Executives (ACHE), which has more than 36,000 members, more than 9,000 of whom are certified as Fellows of the American College of Healthcare Executives (FACHE) (ACHE 2013).

PURPOSE OF HEALTHCARE FINANCIAL MANAGEMENT

The purpose of healthcare financial management is to provide accounting and finance information that helps healthcare managers accomplish the organization's purposes. No licensure requirements are needed to be a practicing healthcare financial manager. Facility-accrediting organizations such as The Joint Commission rarely provide requirements for healthcare financial managers; they often hold the organization's chief executive officer (CEO) responsible for financial management.

Formal educational programs for healthcare financial management are not common and usually exist as postgraduate certificate programs. The chief financial officers of most large healthcare organizations possess a master's degree in business administration, a bachelor's degree in accounting, and a certificate in public accounting and have healthcare experience. For formal continuing education and certification in healthcare financial management, healthcare financial managers can seek membership and certification in healthcare professional associations, including the **Healthcare Financial Management Association (HFMA)**. HFMA has more than 40,000 affiliates, including 1,034 certified healthcare financial professionals (CHFPs) and 1,845 certified as fellows of the Healthcare Financial Management Association (FHFMA) (HFMA 2014).

ACCOUNTING

Accounting is generally divided into two major areas: financial accounting and managerial accounting. The purpose of financial accounting is to provide accounting information, generally historic in nature, to external users, including owners, lenders, suppliers, the government, and insurers.

management connective processes
Management functions that connect elements of the healthcare organization, including communicating, coordinating, and decision making.

The Joint Commission
The primary accrediting body for healthcare organizations.

Healthcare Financial Management Association (HFMA)
Association of healthcare financial managers; confers four certifications: certified revenue cycle representative, certified technical specialist, certified healthcare financial professional, and fellow of the Healthcare Financial Management Association.

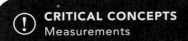

CRITICAL CONCEPTS
Measurements

Healthcare financial managers monitor many measurements. Among the most common are:

- Admissions, which is the number of patients, excluding newborns, accepted for inpatient service

- Average daily census, which is the average number of inpatients, excluding newborns, receiving care each day during the reporting period

- Average length of stay (ALOS), which is derived by dividing the number of inpatient days by the number of admissions

- Occupancy rate, which is the ratio of average daily census to the average number of statistical (set up and staffed for use) beds

Accounting information prepared for external use must follow formats established by the American Institute of Certified Public Accountants (AICPA) and other, similar organizations and must follow generally accepted accounting principles used for standardization. The 1996 *AICPA Audit and Accounting Guide for Health Care Organizations* (AICPA 1996) established four basic financial statements that hospitals should prepare for external users:

1. A consolidated balance sheet

2. A statement of operations

3. A statement of changes in equity

4. A statement of cash flows

The purpose of managerial accounting is to provide accounting information, generally current or prospective in nature, to internal users, including managers. Such accounting information supports the planning and control management functions. In this way, managerial accounting is the link between financial accounting and the manager. Managerial accounting, or accounting information prepared for internal use, requires no prescribed format and therefore varies greatly among organizations. Managerial accounting topics like budgeting and inventory control require knowledge of economics, statistics, and operations research.

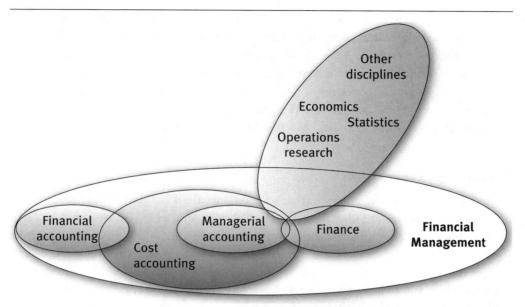

Exhibit 1.1
Financial
Management
Relationships

Many managerial accountants believe that cost accounting—which is the study of costs, including methods for classifying, allocating, and identifying costs—is either synonymous with or a subset of managerial accounting. Others argue that cost accounting includes all managerial accounting and also requires some financial accounting. Cost accounting and managerial accounting also include topics that could be considered finance.

FINANCE

Historically, the purpose of finance has been to borrow and invest the funds necessary for the organization to accomplish its purpose. Today, the purpose of finance is to analyze the information provided by managerial accounting to evaluate past decisions and make sound assessments regarding the future of the organization (Finkler 2003). Finance uses techniques such as **ratio analysis** and **capital analysis** and requires knowledge of financial and managerial accounting (see Appendix 1.1), economics (see Appendix 1.2), statistics (see Appendix 1.3), and operations research. Exhibit 1.1 shows the relationship of finance to the aforementioned supporting disciplines.

MAJOR OBJECTIVES OF HEALTHCARE FINANCIAL MANAGEMENT

GENERATE INCOME

While the purpose of healthcare financial management is to provide accounting and finance information that assists healthcare management in accomplishing the organization's

ratio analysis
Evaluation of an organization's performance by computing the relationships of important line items in the financial statements.

capital analysis
A process to determine how much a capital expenditure will cost and what return it will generate.

objectives, all organizations have at least one objective in common: to survive and grow. Organizations in other industries might refer to this as maximizing owners' wealth; healthcare organizations typically refer to this as maintaining community services. In either event, the organization will be of little use if it cannot afford to continue to operate.

Therefore, the most important objective of healthcare financial management is to generate a reasonable net income (i.e., the difference between collected revenue and expenses) by investing in assets and putting the assets to work.

RESPOND TO REGULATIONS

Although financial management in healthcare organizations has similar objectives to that of organizations in other industries, different objectives also exist. The government regulates healthcare to a significant degree because healthcare organizations are in a position to take advantage of the sick and the elderly; regulation protects individuals who cannot protect themselves. Federal, state, and local governments pay more than 53 percent of all healthcare bills and therefore have a vested interest in ensuring that government money is well spent (Martin et al. 2014). Healthcare organizations must also be accredited or certified to qualify for reimbursement from many third-party payers and to qualify for loans from certain lenders. Therefore, the second objective of healthcare financial management is to respond to the myriad of regulations in a timely and cost-effective manner.

third-party payer
An agent of the patient (the first party) who contracts with providers (the second party) to pay all or a portion of the bill to the patient.

FACILITATE RELATIONSHIPS WITH THIRD-PARTY PAYERS

The third objective of healthcare financial management is to facilitate the organization's relationship with **third-party payers**, such as insurance companies, who pay all or a portion of the bill. Major third-party payers account for more than 79 percent of a healthcare organization's operating revenue (CMS 2014). Financial management must be responsive to third-party payers and in many ways must treat third-party payers as customers because the third party pays the bill. At the same time, financial management must be attentive to the patient because the patient has influence over the third-party payer and in some cases may be partially responsible for the bill.

prospective payment
A payment system in which a healthcare organization accepts a fixed, predetermined amount to treat a patient, regardless of the true ultimate cost of that treatment. Diagnosis-related groups (DRGs) are one type of prospective payment; Medicare pays hospitals a fixed amount for an episode of treatment based on that treatment's DRG.

INFLUENCE METHOD AND AMOUNT OF PAYMENT

The fourth objective of healthcare financial management is to influence the method and amount of payment chosen by third-party payers. Third-party payers are becoming increasingly aggressive in asking healthcare organizations for discounts if they provide large numbers of patients. In certain cases, healthcare organizations are discounting prices below costs to maintain market share. Some third-party payers, such as Medicare, are asking healthcare organizations to assume part of the financial risk for the patient by agreeing to a **prospective payment** or, in other words, agreeing in advance to a price for providing care to a patient. Healthcare organizations lose money if they provide care that costs more than the prospective payment. Some third-party payers are asking healthcare organizations to assume risk by agreeing to a **capitated price** (i.e., a price per head or subscriber) before the subscriber actually needs care. Capitated prices put healthcare organizations at risk for the cost of care, if needed.

MONITOR PHYSICIANS

The fifth objective of healthcare financial management is to monitor physicians and their potential financial liability to the organization. In 2012, physicians and clinical services accounted for 31.9 percent of all healthcare spending (Martin et al. 2014). However, physicians influence much of the healthcare spending that is not directly attributed to them. For example, physicians order the patient admission, the diagnostic testing and treatment for the patient, and the patient discharge. Healthcare financial management must ensure through the utilization review process that physician ordering patterns are consistent with what the patient needs. In addition, healthcare financial management must ensure through the credentialing process and the risk management process that the healthcare organization has minimized its exposure to legal liability for a physician's possible negligent actions.

PROTECT TAX STATUS

The sixth major objective of healthcare financial management is to protect the organization's tax status. For-profit healthcare organizations seek ways to reduce their tax liability, and not-for-profit healthcare organizations try to protect their tax-exempt status. Protecting tax-exempt status has become more difficult as state and local governments seek new revenue sources, and tax-exempt status has come under judicial and public scrutiny (see Chapter 3).

QUALITY ASSESSMENT AND HEALTHCARE FINANCIAL MANAGEMENT

"Quality . . . you know what it is, yet you don't know what it is. But that's self-contradictory. But some things are better than others. That is they have more quality. But when you try to say what that quality is, apart from the things that have it, it all goes poof! There's nothing to talk about. But if you can't say what quality is, then for all practical purposes, it doesn't exist at all. But for all practical purposes it does exist. What else are

capitated price, capitation

A healthcare payment system in which an organization accepts a monthly payment from a third-party payer for each individual covered by that payer's plan, regardless of whether a given individual is treated in a given month. Capitation provides a financial incentive to a healthcare organization to keep its population from using more healthcare services than necessary because the organization only profits if the total cost of treating the specified population falls below the total capitation provided by the third-party payer.

You were recently hired to manage a new primary care physician's office. The physician's office will be located downtown in a major metropolitan area with significant competition. You need to establish the organization's purpose and financial objectives. What items should you consider in establishing the organization's purpose? What organizational purpose should you suggest to the physician owners? What should the financial objectives of the organization be?

the grades based upon? Why else would people pay fortunes for some things and throw others in the trash pile? Obviously, some things are better than others . . . but what's the 'betterness?' . . . So round and round you go, spinning mental wheels and nowhere finding any place to get traction" (Pirsig 1974, 179).

During the past 40 years, healthcare organizations have responded to serious pressure to define quality. In the early 1970s, accrediting agencies and third-party payers applied this pressure. In the late 1970s and early 1980s, the consumer movement added pressure. In the late 1980s through the present, competition has added pressure. Economists predict that the pressure will continue as competition drives prices to their lowest, and relatively equal, point, and the market will force healthcare organizations that survive to compete on quality in addition to price. Healthcare organizations have responded to this pressure with two different strategies: a proactive strategy that attempts to adopt a comprehensive view of quality, and a reactive strategy that attempts to limit views of quality to views developed by others.

PROACTIVE STRATEGY

Healthcare organizations that have adopted a proactive strategy have developed multiple measures of quality, including direct and indirect measures that go beyond the minimum measures required by accrediting organizations (Conrad and Blackburn 1985). Direct measures of quality assume that the organization can define and measure quality itself. These measures include the following:

1. *Goal-based measures* assess quality by the progress made toward the goals of the strategic and operating plans. The key advantage of goal-based measures is that they focus attention on success or failure.

2. *Responsive measures* assess quality by customer opinion. The key advantage of responsive measures is that they understand quality from the customer's point of view.

3. *Decision-making measures* assess quality by evaluating decisions. The key advantage of decision-making measures is that they direct accountability to the decision maker.

4. *Connoisseurship measures* allow quality to be assessed by expert opinion, such as accreditation. The key advantage of connoisseurship measures is that they inspire high credibility.

Indirect measures of quality assume that the organization cannot define and measure quality itself but can define and measure the results of quality. These measures include the following:

1. *Resource measures* assume that price reflects quality. The key advantage of resource measures is that they provide quantitative data that are readily available.

2. *Outcome measures* assume that results reflect quality. The key advantage of outcome measures is the emphasis on results.

3. *Reputational measures* assume that public perception reflects quality. The key advantage of reputational measures is that they produce ratings for the public.

4. *Value-added measures* assume that process reflects quality. The key advantage of value-added measures is that, after adjusting for input and output, they focus on process, which the organization can control.

REACTIVE STRATEGY

Healthcare organizations that have adopted a reactive strategy have responded in several ways to accrediting agencies and quality consultants, including

◆   ensuring quality by centralizing quality efforts in a quality assurance department, then decentralizing quality efforts to clinical departments, and then further decentralizing quality efforts to all departments;

◆   ensuring quality by studying clinical outcomes, then studying clinical processes, then studying all outcomes and all processes, and finally studying key outcomes and key processes;

◆   improving quality by continuous attention and total management; and

◆   assessing quality by identifying key processes and desired outcomes.

Since 1986 The Joint Commission has focused on quality, the customer, work processes, measurements, and improvements. To its primary goal of accrediting healthcare organizations, The Joint Commission added the goal of developing and implementing a national performance measurement database. The standard related to quality reads, "the [healthcare organization] has a planned, systematic, [organization]-wide approach to process design and performance measurement, assessment, and improvement" (Joint Commission 1996, 134).

The following is a summary of the standard. Starting with each department's goals and objectives, the manager and employees should discuss desired outcomes and their indicators. Desired indicators should be both sentinel and rate based. A **sentinel indicator** measures a process so important that every time the indicators occur, the manager initiates an individual case review. A **rate-based indicator** measures a process of lesser importance

sentinel indicator
Measures a process so important that every time the indicator occurs, the manager initiates an individual case review. For example, an ICU manager would initiate a review for each patient that dies in ICU.

rate-based indicator
Measures a process of lesser importance; a manager initiates an individual case review only after a certain rate is exceeded. For example, a pharmacy manager might initiate case reviews if the expected medication error rate of 5 percent is exceeded.

and allows for an error rate; the manager initiates case reviews only if the error rate is exceeded. For instance, an objective of a patient accounts department may be to collect patient bills as rapidly as possible. Desired outcomes may be no lost bills and no more than 5 percent of the total bills going to a collection agency. A sentinel indicator would be a lost bill, initiating a case review on why the bill was lost. The rate-based indicator would be the percentage of total bills going to a collection agency. Reviews would be necessary only if the rate exceeded a predetermined rate—in this example, 5 percent. Reviews should result in recommendations to improve the key processes necessary to meet the desired outcomes. Exhibit 1.2 reflects these steps.

In response to the Institute of Medicine's (IOM) 1999 report that as many as 98,000 Americans die each year as a result of errors in hospitals, The Joint Commission announced a new set of patient safety and medical error reduction standards that took effect July 1, 2001 (Joint Commission 2001). The IOM report was reinforced by three 2006 studies that measured not only deaths caused by hospital-acquired infections, but also the increased costs associated with the preventable hospital errors (Conn 2006). The Joint Commission standards require accredited hospitals (Lovern 2001) to

- ◆ make their doctors tell patients when they receive substandard care or care that differs significantly from anticipated outcomes;

- ◆ implement an organization-wide patient safety program with procedures for immediate response to medical errors;

- ◆ report to the hospital's governing body at least once annually on the occurrence of medical errors; and

- ◆ revise patient satisfaction surveys to ask patients how the organization can improve patient safety.

EXHIBIT 1.2
Simplified Quality
Improvement
Process

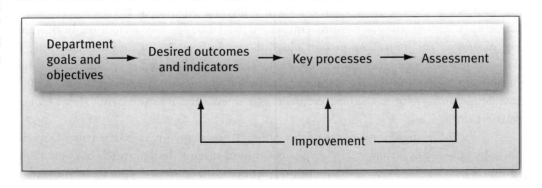

In the 2009 hospital accreditation standards, The Joint Commission separated five chapters from the previous edition to further emphasize those issues. The new chapters include (Joint Commission 2009):

◆ Emergency Management

◆ Life Safety

◆ Record of Care, Treatment, and Services

◆ Transplant Safety

◆ Waived Testing

In July 2002, The Joint Commission approved the first **National Patient Safety Goals** (NPSGs) for hospitals. The NPSGs help accredited organizations address specific areas of concern regarding patient safety. Each goal includes no more than two evidence- or expert-based requirements. Each year the goals are reevaluated, and the goals may be continued or replaced based on new patient safety priorities. The 2014 Joint Commission NPSGs for hospitals include (Joint Commission 2014):

National Patient Safety Goals
A set of goals established by The Joint Commission to address safety areas of special concern for hospitals.

◆ Improve the accuracy of patient identification.

◆ Improve the effectiveness of communication among caregivers.

◆ Improve the safety of using medications.

◆ Reduce the risk of healthcare-associated infections.

◆ Identify safety risks inherent in the hospital's patient population.

◆ Improve the safety of clinical alarm systems.

National Patient Safety Goals for other types of healthcare providers can be viewed at www.jointcommission.org/standards_information/npsgs.aspx.

EFFECTS OF QUALITY ON PROFITABILITY

Significant evidence shows that improved quality has led to improved profitability in healthcare. Solucient, a healthcare information company, each year ranks the nation's top 100 hospitals using clinical measures. In 2003, *Modern Healthcare* for the first time reported financial data for the top 100 hospitals. These hospitals consistently outperformed their peer group hospitals on both the clinical and financial measures, as indicated in Exhibit 1.3.

EXHIBIT **1.3**

National
Performance
Comparisons

Measures	100 Top Hospitals	Peer Hospitals	100 Top to Peer Hospitals
Mortality index	0.82	0.97	15.5% lower mortality
Complications index	0.84	0.94	10.6% fewer complications
Average length of stay (LOS)	3.60	3.94	8.6% shorter LOS
Average expense/ discharge	$3,795	$4,677	18.9% lower expenses
Profitability (margin)	6.90%	2.13%	223.9% higher margins

Source: Modern Healthcare. 2003. "They 'Just Do It Better.'" Solucient 100 Top Hospitals. Supplement to *Modern Healthcare* 33 (39): 6–12.

ORGANIZATIONAL ETHICS AND HEALTHCARE FINANCIAL MANAGEMENT

The Joint Commission and healthcare professional associations such as ACHE and HFMA have emphasized organizational ethics over the past two decades. Several Joint Commission standards require healthcare organizations to have mechanisms in place to address ethical issues related to such topics as patient rights and management responsibilities. Ethical issues concerning patient rights include informed consent, do-not-resuscitate orders, and patient confidentiality. Ethical issues concerning management responsibilities include resource allocation, conflicts of interest, and patient billing practices.

Resource allocation decisions by managers often conflict with the decisions made by physicians and other clinicians. Managers typically represent a utilitarian view of ethics, best represented by the phrase "the greatest good for the greatest number." This view allows managers to sacrifice the use of resources for one patient to maintain resources for other patients, given the assumption that resources for the healthcare organization are limited. Clinicians typically represent a deontological view of ethics, which means their decisions are governed by their duties to patients, which take precedence over the ends-based decision making of the manager. This continuous conflict seems to keep resource allocation decisions somewhat balanced.

You are the administrator of a nursing home owned by a for-profit parent corporation that owns 30 nursing homes. You have been asked by the board of directors of the parent corporation to explain how your quality initiatives will improve profitability. What is your presentation?

Conflicts of interest occur when an individual owes duties to two or more persons or organizations and when meeting a duty to one somehow harms the other (Darr 2011). Perhaps the worst examples of conflict of interest involve the conflict between a manager's duties to the organization and a manager's duties to self, such as when managers use their positions of authority for personal gain. Even the perception of impropriety may cause a loss of credibility (Nowicki and Summers 2001). This is especially true in financial management, where contracts for services and products are awarded to vendors who may attempt to buy influence with a lunch or a gift.

For the most part, patient billing practices are covered by law; however, even certain legal practices have ethical ramifications. For instance, how long should a healthcare organization hold a patient's deposit after the insurance company pays in full? While a healthcare organization may be under no legal obligation to refund overpayments by insurance companies (Sturn 1995), is keeping someone else's money ethical? What is the organization's obligation to generate a bill free of errors? What is the organization's obligation to release prices to patients and otherwise assist patients in the buying decision?

Many healthcare organizations use ethics committees to provide answers to these and other billing questions. Although healthcare organizations are not required to organize ethics committees, committees are a useful way to solicit community input on billing issues.

Value of Healthcare Financial Management

Healthcare financial management provides accounting information and financial techniques that allow managers to perform the management functions and the management connective processes and therefore accomplish the organizational objectives. In addition, healthcare financial management also has direct value to these functions, as explained in the following list of management functions (Dunn 2010).

◆ Planning: After the governing body completes the strategic plan and senior management completes the operating plan, financial management is often responsible for completing the operating budget and capital budget. The operating budget often provides the incentives to plan properly.

◆ Organizing: Financial management provides a chart of accounts based on the organizational chart that identifies revenue centers and cost

You manage a four-physician office practice in a competitive neighborhood. Vendors often bring lunches and gifts for your staff and samples of prescription medications that the physicians give to patients. Could this be a problem?

centers. Together with the organizational chart, this provides the basis for responsibility accounting, which is the ability to hold department managers responsible for their revenues and expenses.

◆ Staffing: Financial management often staffs a variety of departments and processes important to the healthcare organization. Departments such as medical records and information systems are currently being placed under the supervision of financial management, in addition to departments such as accounting, admitting, and materials management, which have been traditionally under financial management. The increasing importance of nontraditional departments in the billing process appears to justify this trend.

◆ Directing: Financial management provides rewards and penalties to motivate others to accomplish the organization's purposes.

◆ Controlling: Perhaps the responsibility closest to the overall function of financial management, the control of the budget, financial reports, financial policies and procedures, and financial audits allows financial management to monitor performance and take the appropriate corrective action when performance is unsatisfactory.

These management functions mean little without the management connective processes to integrate the functions.

MANAGEMENT CONNECTIVE PROCESSES

Communicating and coordinating are important to financial management for both reporting and advising. Also important is coordinating the relationships between, for example, revenue and expenses, capital budgets and operating budgets, and volumes and prices and collected revenues.

Decision making is important to financial management as a direct measure of quality. Governing boards, CEOs, and outside sources such as independent auditors often judge the quality of financial management on the basis of the decisions and recommendations made by financial management. The advantage of this view of quality is that it holds the decision maker accountable. The disadvantage is that it assumes rational decision making. Decisions made in healthcare financial management are often based on politics or other criteria that are unknown to the evaluator of the decision. Therefore, a decision may be evaluated as bad on the basis of the known facts, but it may be evaluated as good on the basis of other criteria unknown to the evaluator.

EFFECT OF FINANCIAL MANAGEMENT ON THE CHANGING FACE OF HEALTHCARE

Many say that financial management is the most important predictor of whether health-care organizations will survive in the current competitive climate and beyond. The recession that began in 2008 affected healthcare organizations as much as it affected many other industries, and the passage of healthcare reform is creating entirely new financial challenges. The implications of reform on healthcare finance will not be known for many years, but at least three elements of the legislation will profoundly affect the financial situation of healthcare organizations: the increase in the number of individuals with health insurance; the changing reimbursement structures; and the explicit linking of reimbursement with quality measures.

Clearly, only the well-managed healthcare organizations will survive this changing situation; financial management will be instrumental in their survival.

CHAPTER KEY POINTS

➤ The difference between the organizational purpose and the financial purpose of the organization is important.

➤ The major objectives of financial management, and which one is most important, is relevant to any healthcare manager.

➤ Quality is important, and understanding its impact on profitability makes good managers great managers.

➤ Sound ethical reasoning should affect every decision, even financial decision making.

DISCUSSION QUESTIONS

1. Why is financial management important to the organization?

2. Distinguish between the purpose of healthcare management and the purpose of healthcare financial management.

3. Prioritize the major objectives of healthcare financial management.

4. Describe the major ethical theories and how they apply to the role of a healthcare manager.

5. Describe why financial managers should be concerned with quality initiatives in the healthcare organization.

6. Predict how financial management and the management functions will be important as healthcare changes in the future.

Appendix 1.1
Financial Accounting Outline

I. Financial accounting is the science of preparing financial statements for use by individuals and organizations external to the organization.

II. Accounting equation

Total assets = Liabilities + Net assets

III. Objectives of financial accounting

A. Provide information that is useful to present and potential investors, creditors, and other decision makers.

B. Provide information about the economic resources of the healthcare organization, the claims to those resources, and the effects of transactions, events, and circumstances that change those resources.

C. Provide information about a healthcare organization's performance.

D. Provide information about how a healthcare organization generates and expends cash, about its loans and repayment of loans, and about its capital expenditures.

E. Provide information about how a healthcare organization has discharged its stewardship duties to its owners.

IV. Accounting concepts

A. Entity—The healthcare organization stands apart from all other organizations and is capable of taking on economic transactions.

B. Reliability—Accounting records must be based on information that is verifiable from an independent source.

C. Cost valuation—Assets and services are recorded at actual, historic cost.

D. Going concern—The entity will operate long enough to recover the cost of its assets.

E. Stable monetary unit—This is the basis for ignoring the effects of inflation in short-term transactions.

V. Accounting principles

A. Accrual accounting—Revenue is recorded when it is realized (i.e., billed), and expense is recorded when it contributes to operations.

B. Cash accounting—Revenue and expenses are recorded when cash is actually received or paid.

C. Accounting period—This is a defined fiscal year or month.

D. Matching—Related revenue and expense should be reported in the same accounting period.

E. Conservatism—Uncertainty dictates understating revenues and volumes that lead to revenues, and overstating expenses.

F. Full disclosure—All economic transactions should be recorded.

G. Industry practices—Accounting principles are relatively unique to the healthcare industry.

1. Fund accounting—This allows not-for-profit and governmental healthcare organizations to establish separate entities for specified activities. Typical funds include operating or general funds, specific-purpose funds, plant-replacement funds, and endowment funds. Each fund is self-balancing in that assets equal liabilities added to net fund balance.

2. Contractual allowances—This is the revenue account that records the difference between billed charges and the price a customer has agreed in advance to pay via contract.

3. Depreciation—This is the expense account that records the estimated cost of an expiring asset.

4. Funded depreciation—This is the amount saved to replace assets at the end of their useful life.

5. *AICPA Audit and Accounting Guide for Health Care Organizations*

   a. There were major changes in the 1990 edition.

      1) On the statement of revenues and expenses, operating revenue is reported net of contractual allowances.

      2) On the statement of revenues and expenses, operating revenue is reported net of charity care; however, the healthcare organization's policy for charity care, in addition to the level of charity care, must be in the footnotes.

      3) On the statement of revenues and expenses, bad debt expense is reported as an expense based on price.

      4) On the statement of revenues and expenses, donated assets are reported at fair market value as of the date of the gift.

      5) On the statement of revenues and expenses, donated services are reported as an expense, and a corresponding amount is reported as a contribution, but only if the services are significant and measurable.

   b. There were major changes in the 1996 edition.

      1) Changes were made to the basic financial statements.

         a) Balance sheet (consolidated)

         b) Statement of operations

         c) Statement of changes in equity

         d) Statement of cash flows

      2) The balance sheet reports net assets.

         a) Unrestricted

         b) Temporarily restricted

         c) Permanently restricted

          3) Statement of operations reports performance indicator
            a) Revenues over expenses
            b) Earned income
            c) Performance earnings

  c. There were major changes in the 2010 edition.
      1) Update on the hierarchy of generally accepted accounting principles
      2) Omnibus change to the consolidation and equity method guidance for not-for-profit organizations
      3) Determining fair value when the volume and level of activity for the asset or liability have significantly decreased
      4) Interim disclosure about fair value of financial investments
      5) Recognition and presentation of other-than-temporary impairments
      6) The hierarchy of generally accepted accounting principles for state and local governments
      7) Land and other real estate investment by endowments
      8) Charity care remains a note to the financial statements but must be reported at full cost with the method used to determine cost.

  d. There were major changes in the 2011 edition.
      1) Conforming to changes resulting from the *ASB Clarity Project*
      2) Reporting relationships with other entities
      3) Reporting and measuring noncash gifts
      4) Expiring donor-imposed restrictions
      5) Reporting program-related investments and microfinance loans
      6) Reporting net assets and related disclosures
      7) Accounting for contributions and receivables
      8) Accounting for investments
      9) Auditing net asset classification and revenue and expense recognition
     10) Healthcare entities that recognize a significant amount of patient services revenue at the time the services are rendered, even though the entity does not assess the patient's ability to pay, shall present that portion of bad debt as a deduction of revenue and shall report its policy for assessing collectibility in determining the timing and amount of patient service revenue by payer.

VI. Sarbanes-Oxley Act of 2002
  A. Federal corporate accountability legislation passed in the aftermath of Enron's downfall and intended to improve governance and corporate practices. The legislation includes the following standards.

1. Accounting firms are prohibited from providing certain nonaudit services to a client contemporaneously with an audit.
2. Accounting firms are required to "timely report" to the board's audit committee material communications between the auditor and management.
3. Principal executive and financial officers are required to certify financial reports, subject to civil and criminal penalties.
4. Eligibility for audit committee membership, including no affiliation with the company or its subsidiaries, and specific duties of the audit committee are established.
5. The Securities and Exchange Commission (SEC) is directed to establish "minimum standards of professional conduct" for lawyers whose practice includes SEC matters.
6. Personal loans to directors and executive officers are prohibited.
7. Companies are required to maintain an internal control structure and procedures for financial reporting.
8. Companies are required to disclose whether they have a code of ethics for senior financial officers.
9. Disclosure of off–balance sheet transactions is required.
10. New record retention rules and penalties are established.

B. The act applies only to public companies, though many states are considering adopting similar legislation for nonprofits (e.g., New York).
C. Some nonprofits are holding themselves voluntarily to Sarbanes-Oxley standards.

Appendix 1.2
Economics Outline

I.   Economics is the science of producing, distributing, and consuming material goods and services to make better decisions in a world of limited resources.

II. Economic systems
  A. Capitalism is based on private property rights with distribution decisions made by the free market based on ability.
      1. Adam Smith's theory was that an "invisible hand" guides the free market economy. Individuals who pursue their own self-interests actually produce economic results beneficial to society as a whole (Smith 1766).
      2. The government's role
          a. National defense
          b. Administration of justice
          c. Facilitation of commerce
          d. Provision of certain public works
  B. Socialism is based on private and government property rights with distribution decisions made by the government based on effort.
      1. Karl Marx defined socialism as a transitory stage between capitalism and communism. Socialism is classified by government ownership of all important property, and means of distribution of surplus by the government based on the formula: "from each according to ability, to each according to labor" (Marx 1848).
      2. The government's role: "dictatorship of the proletariat" during an economic class struggle.
  C. Communism is based on public property rights with distribution decisions made by the public based on need.
      1. Karl Marx classified communism as the final and perfect goal of historic development characterized by (1) a classless society in which all people live by earning and no person lives by owning; and (2) the abolition of the wage system so that all citizens live and work based on the formula: "from each according to ability, to each according to need."
      2. The government's role: no government.

III. Free markets under capitalism
  A. Characteristics of free market
      1. There is a large number of buyers and sellers, each with a small share of the total business so that no single participant can affect market price.
      2. Buyers and sellers are unencumbered by economic or institutional restrictions, and they possess full knowledge of market prices and alternatives. As a result, they enter or leave markets whenever they wish.

B. Functions of free market
   1. Competitive prices through the law of supply and demand are established.
   2. Efficient use of resources is encouraged.
C. Theories of free market
   1. Classical—At market equilibrium (supply equals demand therefore price remains constant), the economy attains full employment; supply creates its own demand; flexibility exists in wages, prices, and interest rates; and savings are invested.
   2. Demand side—At market equilibrium, the economy does not attain full employment, demand creates its own supply, wages and prices are "sticky," and savers and investors are different people with different motivations.
   3. Supply side—At market equilibrium, the economy does not attain full employment; supply creates its own demand; flexibility exists in wages, prices, and interest rates; and savings are invested.
D. Policy implications of free market theories
   1. Classical—Market is self-correcting; no policies are needed.
   2. Demand side—Market self-correction is possible; however, it may take a long time. Therefore, government intervention is necessary to stimulate the economy by regulating demand through large-scale government spending programs supported by increased taxes or increased money supply.
   3. Supply side—Market self-correction is possible; however, it may take a long time. Therefore, government intervention is necessary to stimulate the economy by stimulating supply (production) through tax reductions, nonmonetization of government deficits, and deregulation of certain industries.
E. Supply side economics—Did it work during the 1980s?
   1. Efficiency
      a. The inflation rate fell from an annual average of 10.3 percent under President Carter to 3.9 percent under President Reagan.
      b. The unemployment rate fell from an annual average of 7.5 percent under Carter to 5.3 percent under Reagan.
      c. Per capita disposable income rose from $9,800 under Carter to $11,000 under Reagan.
      d. Interest rates declined from 12.5 percent under Carter to 8.5 percent under Reagan.
   2. Growth—The gross national product rose from an annual average of 2.7 percent under Carter to 3.0 percent under Reagan.

3. Deregulation—Modest gains were achieved under Reagan; most notable was the airline industry.
4. Equity—Families living in poverty increased from 11.9 percent under Carter to 13.7 percent under Reagan.
5. Stability—Deficits increased from an annual average of $60 billion under Carter to $190 billion under Reagan.

F. Regulation in the free market
   1. Costs of regulation (Weidenbaum and DeFina 1981)
      a. Direct costs = $10 billion per year
      b. Indirect costs, or compliance costs = $200 billion per year
   2. Economic justifications for regulation
      a. Public interest theory—to protect the public
      b. Industry interest theory—to protect the industry
      c. Public choice theory—to protect government

IV. Healthcare economics
   A. External effects on healthcare economics
      1. Federal debt (in billions) and as a percent of GDP
         1965 = $317.2, 37.9 percent
         1975 = $533.1, 25.3 percent
         1985 = $1,823.1, 36.4 percent
         1995 = $4,973.9, 49.1 percent
         2005 = $7,933.0, 36.9 percent
         2006 = $8,507.0, 36.6 percent
         2007 = $9,007.6, 36.3 percent
         2008 = $10,024.7, 40.5 percent
         2009 = $11,909.8, 54.1 percent
         2010 = $13,500.0, 62.9 percent
         2011 = $14,800, 67.8 percent
         2012 = $16,100, 72.6 percent
         2013 = $17,200, 75.1 percent
      2. Federal budget surpluses (in billions)
         1965 = ($2)
         1975 = ($55)
         1985 = ($222)
         1995 = ($226)
         2005 = ($494)
         2006 = ($435)
         2007 = ($342)
         2008 = ($455)
         2009 = ($1,587)

2010 = ($1,342)

2011 = ($1,300)

2012 = ($1,087)

2013 = ($973)

3. Aging population

1960 = 9.3 percent over 65 years old

1995 = 13.0 percent over 65 years old

2030* = 20.7 percent over 65 years old

*projected

B. Internal effects on healthcare economics

1. Health expenditures by population over 65 years

1960 = 23.6 percent

1995 = 33.0 percent

2030* = 52.5 percent

*projected

2. Health expenditures (in billions) and as a percentage of the gross domestic product

1960 = $27.4, 5.3 percent

1970 = $74.9, 7.2 percent

1980 = $255.8, 9.1 percent

1990 = $724.3, 12.3 percent

2000 = $1,377.2, 13.6 percent

2005 = $2,030.5, 15.7 percent

2006 = $2,163.3, 15.8 percent

2007 = $2,302.9, 15.9 percent

2008 = $2,411.7, 16.4 percent

2009 = $2,504.2, 17.4 percent

2010 = $2,599.0, 17.4 percent

2011 = $2,692.8, 17.3 percent

2012= $2,793.4, 17.2 percent

2013*= $2,915.0, 18.0 percent

2014* = $3,093.0, 18.3 percent

2015* = $3,273.0, 18.4 percent

*projected

3. Health expenditures per person

1960 = $146

1970 = $356

1980 = $1,100

1990 = $2,814

2000 = $4,789

2005 = $6,701
2006 = $7,071
2007 = $7,649
2008 = $7,936
2009 = $8,170
2010 = $8,411
2011 = $8,658
2012 = $8,915
2013* = $9,216
2014* = $9,697
2015* = $10,172
*projected

4. Personal health expenditures by type of service, 2012
    Hospital care, 37.4 percent
    Professional service, 31.9 percent
    Prescription drugs, 11.2 percent
    Nursing homes, 6.4 percent
    Medical equipment and supplies, 4.0 percent
    Home health, 3.3 percent
    Other personal care, 5.8 percent

5. Personal health expenditures by source of funds, 2012
    Private health insurance, 32.8 percent
    Medicare, 20.5 percent
    Private out of pocket, 11.7 percent
    Medicaid, federal, 8.5 percent
    Medicaid, state, 6.6 percent
    CHIP, DOD, VA, 3.8 percent
    Other third party, 10.4 percent
    Investment, 5.7 percent

6. Health expenditures by percentage increase from previous year
    1990 = 11.7 percent
    1991 = 9.5 percent
    1992 = 8.6 percent
    1993 = 7.3 percent
    1994 = 5.5 percent
    1995 = 5.4 percent
    1996 = 5.2 percent
    1997 = 5.4 percent
    1998 = 4.8 percent
    1999 = 5.6 percent

2000 = 6.3 percent
2001 = 8.5 percent
2002 = 6.4 percent
2003 = 8.2 percent
2004 = 7.9 percent
2005 = 7.4 percent
2006 = 6.7 percent
2007 = 6.3 percent
2008 = 4.7 percent
2009 = 3.8 percent
2010 = 3.8 percent
2011 = 3.6 percent
2012 = 3.7 percent
2013* = 4.0 percent
2014* = 6.1 percent
2015* = 5.8 percent

* projected

Appendix 1.3
Statistics Outline

I. Statistics is the science of collecting, organizing, presenting, analyzing, and interpreting numbers to make better decisions in a world of uncertainty.
II. Descriptive statistics
    A. Descriptive statistics are used to describe various features of a data set.
    B. Measures of central tendency
        1. Mean, or average, is derived by summing the observations and dividing by the number of observations.
        2. Median is derived by arranging the observations from smallest to largest and selecting the midpoint observation.
        3. Mode is derived by selecting the observation that occurs most often.
        4. Modified mean is derived by deleting the smallest and the largest observations.
        5. Weighted mean is derived by multiplying each observation by a volume, summing the results, and then dividing by the total volume.
    C. Measures of dispersion and shape
        1. Range is the difference between the largest and smallest observation.
        2. Variance is the average of the squared differences between each observation and the mean.
        3. Standard deviation is the square root of the variance.
        4. Shape
            a. Symmetrical—Mean and median are the same.
            b. Right or positive skewed—Mean exceeds the median.
            c. Left or negative skewed—Median exceeds the mean.
    D. The index number is derived by calculating the number in current year divided by the number in base year times 100.
III. Inferential statistics
    A. Inferential statistics are used to infer the characteristics of a sample to the characteristics of the population.
    B. Probability
    C. Hypothesis testing
    D. Linear regression and correlation are used to predict future events and the strength of the association between variables.
    E. Tests of significance
        1. The t-test is used to determine how likely it is that two mean scores differ by chance.
        2. Analysis of variance is used to determine whether a significant difference exists between two or more means.

3. Analysis of covariance is used to determine whether there is a significant difference between two or more means for groups that are initially unequal.

IV. Healthcare statistics

A. Adjusted average daily census is derived by dividing the number of inpatient day equivalents (also called adjusted inpatient days) by the number of days in the reporting period.

B. Adjusted expenses per admission is derived by removing expenses incurred for the provision of outpatient care from total expenses and then dividing by the total admissions in the reporting period.

C. Adjusted expenses per inpatient day is derived by dividing total expenses by inpatient day equivalents (also called adjusted inpatient days).

D. Adjusted inpatient days—See inpatient day equivalents.

E. Admissions include number of patients, excluding newborns, accepted for inpatient service.

F. Average daily census is the average number of inpatients, excluding newborns, receiving care each day during the reporting period.

G. Average length of stay is derived by dividing the number of inpatient days by the number of admissions.

H. Expenses includes all expenses for the reporting period.

1. Payroll expenses includes all salaries and wages.

2. All professional fees and those salary expenditures excluded from payroll are defined as nonpayroll expenses and are included in total expenses. Labor-related expenses is defined as payroll expenses plus employee benefits. Nonlabor-related expenses is all other nonpayroll expenses. In accordance with the AICPA Audit and Accounting Guide for Health Care Organizations (AICPA 1996), bad debt has been reclassified from a "deduction from revenue" to an expense. However, for historic consistency purposes, expense totals may not actually include bad debt expense.

I. Full-time equivalent personnel is derived by adding the number of full-time personnel to one-half the number of part-time personnel.

J. Inpatient day equivalents is derived by multiplying the number of outpatient visits by the ratio of outpatient revenue per outpatient visit to inpatient revenue per inpatient day, and adding the product (which represents the number of patient days attributable to outpatient services) to the number of inpatient days (can also be used to adjust patient days for skilled nursing facilities, rehab, home care, etc.).

K. Occupancy rate is the ratio of average daily census to the average number of statistical (set up and staffed for use) beds (AHA 1985).

L. Revenue—Gross patient revenue (inpatient and outpatient) is revenue from services rendered to patients, including payments received from or on behalf of individual patients. Net patient revenue is derived by subtracting contractual adjustments and charity care from gross patient revenue. Net patient revenue represents what the organization actually intends to collect. Net total revenue is net patient revenue plus all other revenue, including contributions, endowment revenue, government grants, and all other revenue not made on behalf of patients.

CHAPTER 2

ORGANIZATION OF FINANCIAL MANAGEMENT

One of the signs of excellence in a manager is the ability to anticipate problems, not just react to them.

Sir Liam Donaldson, former chief medical officer of
National Health Service, England

LEARNING OBJECTIVES

After completing this chapter, you should be able to do the following:

➤ Understand how healthcare organizations are organized
➤ Understand how chief financial officers receive their authority regarding the financial matters of the organization
➤ Identify the roles and responsibilities of the key financial managers
➤ Examine the alternative corporate structures available to healthcare organizations

INTRODUCTION

The successful accomplishment of organizational purposes requires a sound organizational structure. After the governing body has established a healthcare organization's purposes, management must determine the best way to accomplish them. To do this, management must identify and assign tasks to employees, departments, and divisions. In other words, management must organize. According to Dunn (2010), organizing includes

◆ specialization: dividing tasks into manageable categories and assigning the categories to employees with the appropriate skills;

◆ departmentalization: dividing employees into groups or teams that have similar responsibilities;

◆ defining the span of management: determining the optimum number of employees that a manager can manage based on the nature of the tasks and the background of the employees;

◆ defining authority: determining the amount of authority to delegate to employees so that they can perform their assigned tasks;

◆ defining responsibility: determining the obligation necessary to perform assigned tasks;

◆ establishing a unity of command: appointing one manager to be responsible for a group of employees; and

◆ defining the nature of relationships: determining whether managers and employees have a line or staff relationship in the organization. In a line relationship, the manager or employee is directly responsible for resources, such as employees and supplies. In a staff relationship, the manager or employee acts in an advisory capacity without direct control over resources.

Most healthcare organizations are organized as legal entities called *corporations.* Corporate status is granted by the state and provides advantages for the healthcare organization. Corporate status provides limited liability, meaning that the owners of the corporation are seldom found to be personally liable for the contracts or negligence of the corporation. Another advantage of corporate status is its continuity of existence, meaning that the corporation continues even after the death of an owner. The third advantage of corporate status is the increased ability to raise capital, because the risk of investing in a corporation is only financial. In the case of for-profit corporations, a fourth advantage of corporate status is that shareholders are free to sell their shares at any time. For further discussion of these advantages, refer to *The Law of Healthcare Administration* (Showalter 2011).

This chapter provides a comprehensive description of the organization of financial management in healthcare organizations.

Governing Body

The governing body of a healthcare organization is responsible for the proper development, utilization, and maintenance of all resources in the organization. The governing body typically delegates the authority for accomplishing this duty to the organization's CEO. However, the governing body maintains legal responsibility for the organization. Because of this fact, courts continue to stress the importance of the governing body's duty of responsibility in selecting a competent CEO.

The governing body uses organized committees to monitor the CEO's performance. Although committee structures vary from organization to organization, an **executive committee** of the governing body typically monitors all committees and includes the chairs of all the committees as members. The **finance committee** monitors the CEO's performance in financial affairs. This committee includes governing body members with a financial interest or occupation. In smaller organizations, the duties of the finance committee also include audit responsibilities; in larger organizations, audit responsibilities may be monitored by an audit committee. Generally, the CEO and/or the chief operating officer (COO) and chief financial officer (CFO) attend finance committee meetings ex officio and also serve as staff support to those committees. Exhibit 2.1 identifies these relationships.

The governing bodies of healthcare organizations with corporate status cannot be held personally liable for either the contracts of the corporation or the negligence of the corporation's employees or agents (i.e., physicians). However, the governing body can be held collectively liable for a breach of its duty to act as a **fiduciary**, which means its duty to act as a person in a position of great trust and confidence. The legal duties of a fiduciary include loyalty and responsibility. Loyalty requires fiduciaries to act in the best interests of the healthcare organization and to subordinate their personal interests to those of the organization. Responsibility requires fiduciaries to act with reasonable care, skill, and diligence in accomplishing their duties as members of the governing body (Showalter 2011).

executive committee
A committee of the governing body of an organization that monitors all the other committees.

finance committee
A committee of the governing body of an organization that monitors the CEO's performance in financial affairs.

fiduciary
A person, or governing body, in a position of great trust and confidence. The term is typically used to describe the duty of an entity to be loyal and responsible.

> **⚠ CRITICAL CONCEPTS**
> The Trustees' Responsibility
>
> The governing body of a healthcare organization is responsible for hiring a competent CEO. Of course, that does not always happen. When a board fails in the regard, it can be in legal trouble. In *Reserve Life Insurance Company v. Salter* (1957), one of the first cases establishing this duty, the court was severe in its finding.
>
> "Failing to appreciate their duties and responsibilities led these trustees to feel, according to their testimony, that they had discharged their duties by picking as administrator, Salter, a former school teacher, apparently as ignorant of operating a hospital as they themselves were."

EXHIBIT 2.1

Financial
Organization

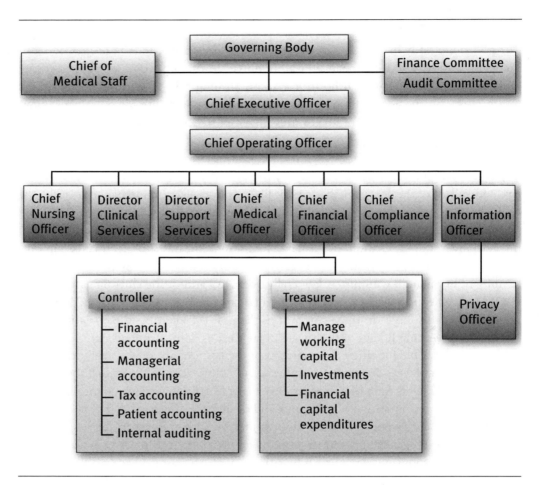

After the Enron bankruptcy, the federal government passed strict corporate accountability standards known as the Sarbanes-Oxley Act of 2002 (see Appendix 1.1 in Chapter 1). While the standards only apply to publicly held, for-profit organizations, many not-for-profit organizations are attempting to comply with the standards. New York and California passed Sarbanes-Oxley–like state legislation in 2005, and in those states it applies to not-for-profits.

FINANCIAL ORGANIZATION

In November 2003, Richard Scrushy, founder and former chairman of for-profit Health-South, was indicted for 85 counts of conspiracy, fraud, and money laundering. The indictment alleged that Scrushy was the mastermind of a wide-ranging scheme to inflate the rehabilitation and outpatient-care company's earnings to meet Wall Street expectations.

The indictment further alleged that Scrushy added at least $2.7 billion in fictitious income to HealthSouth's books during a multiyear conspiracy dating back to 1996. Scrushy became the first CEO (and as a result, healthcare became the first industry) indicted under Sarbanes-Oxley, which holds the CEO personally liable for financial misreporting. In what was characterized as healthcare's trial of the century, the jury in the five-month Scrushy trial acquitted Scrushy of all federal charges after 21 days of deliberation. Even though five of HealthSouth's CFOs testified against Scrushy, the jury chose to favor the defense's portrayal of Scrushy's character. Legal analysts also criticized the prosecution's strategy to prove 85 counts over a six-month trial.

Both federal regulatory agencies and bond rating firms are paying special attention to the healthcare industry since the HealthSouth trial (Piotrowski 2003a). In 2013 (through November), Moody's reported 30 hospital downgrades and 18 hospital upgrades (Herman 2013).

CHIEF FINANCIAL OFFICER

In larger healthcare organizations, the CEO delegates the authority for accomplishing the duties related to financial management to the CFO. However, the CEO has become increasingly involved in financial matters in recent years. In fact, in a 2012 survey conducted by the American College of Healthcare Executives (ACHE), CEOs ranked financial concerns as their top concern for the eleventh consecutive year (ACHE 2013).

The Committee on Ethics and Eligibility Standards of the Financial Executives Institute has defined the CFO duties as follows (Berman, Kukla, and Weeks 1994):

1. Establish, coordinate, and maintain, through authorized management, an integrated plan for the control of operations. Such a plan would provide cost standards, expense budgets, sales forecasts, profit planning, and programs for capital investments/financing to the extent required in the business.

2. Measure performance against approved operating plans and standards, and report and interpret the results of operations to all levels of management. This function includes the design, installation, and maintenance of accounting policy and the compilation of statistical records as required.

3. Measure and report on the validity of the objectives of the business and on the effectiveness of its policies, organization structure, and procedures in attaining those objectives. This includes consulting with all segments of management responsible for policy or action concerning any phase of the operation of the business as it relates to the performance of this function.

4. Report to government agencies as required and supervise all matters relating to taxes.

5. Interpret and report on the effect of external influences on the attainment of the objectives of the business. This function includes the continuous appraisal of economic and social forces and of government influences as they affect the operations of the business.

6. Provide protection for the assets of the business. This function includes establishing and maintaining adequate internal control and auditing and ensuring proper insurance coverage.

A profile of the average hospital and system CFO, according to information provided by the Healthcare Financial Management Association (HFMA), is shown in Exhibit 2.2.

All six surveys that make up Exhibit 2.2 include compensation comparisons by gender. The percentage of women CFOs responding to the survey was consistent in 2009 and 2001: 71 percent. In 2011, women CFOs earned an average of $62,400 less than men, up from a difference of $42,900 reported in 2009. After adjusting for other determining factors, such as job tenure, total number of reporting employees, net patient revenue of the organization, the area's wage index, possession of a certificate in public accounting (CPA), eligibility for bonus or profit sharing, and bed count, regression analysis finds that gender is still a significant determinant of compensation, accounting for $15,000 of the reported difference in 2003 and $14,000 of the reported difference in 2001. Since 2005, the regression model did not assign any of the difference to gender, indicating that the differences in salary can be explained by variables other than gender.

EXHIBIT 2.2
Hospital CFO
Profile

	2005	2007	2009	2011	2013
Annual compensation	$172,000	$196,000	$209,800	$224,500	$236,600
Average age	48	49	50	51	53
Percent male	77	78	71	71	72
Percent with master's degree	46	46	50	51	51
Percent with CPA	47	43	47	50	47
Percent with HFMA certification	19	15	24	27	28

Source: HFMA (2013).

At an average age of 53, hospital and system CFOs are relatively young. This means that organizations and associations like HFMA will need to find new ways to motivate CFOs who have reached the top of their career ladder at a young age (the 1995 CFO profiles reported that only 8 percent of the surveyed CFOs aspired to be the CEO). Although only 16 percent of the CFOs were women in 1995, that percentage has increased steadily over the years, and it will continue to increase as women who graduated from business schools in the 1970s and 1980s gain the prerequisite experience to be CFOs. Fifty-one percent of the CFOs have advanced degrees, usually in business administration. Most CFOs have undergraduate degrees in accounting, and 47 percent are certified in public accounting.

Many CFOs with multiple certifications would argue that certification in HFMA is the most meaningful certification for CFOs in the healthcare industry. However, many CFOs received their public accounting certification shortly after graduation and feel additional certification in HFMA is unnecessary. Currently, 28 percent of the CFOs in the 2013 survey are HFMA certified. Certification in HFMA requires a person to

◆ be a current and active regular member or advanced member (not student member) and

◆ successfully complete a comprehensive certification exam over a core body of knowledge in revenue cycle, budgeting and forecasting, financial reporting, internal controls, disbursements, and contracting.

Certified members must remain active HFMA members in good standing and complete 60 contact hours of eligible education every three years.

Fellowship (FHFMA) requires a certified member to

◆ complete five years as a regular or advanced member;

◆ have a bachelor's degree or 120 semester hours from an accredited college or university;

◆ complete volunteer activity in healthcare finance within three years of applying for fellowship; and

◆ submit an FHFMA application.

At the 2003 CFO Exchange sponsored by HFMA's CFO Forum, HFMA President Dick Clarke introduced a healthcare financial competency model that demands new, more complex roles for healthcare CFOs in addition to more traditional roles as identified in Exhibit 2.3.

> ## ⚠ CRITICAL CONCEPTS
> ### Who Makes a Good CFO?
>
> Successful CFOs require a broad range of traits and skills. One survey of healthcare CFOs (Doody 2000) identified five traits possessed by born leaders that CFOs must nurture:
>
> 1. Strategic thinking
> 2. Ability to adjust to change
> 3. Personal integrity
> 4. Vision
> 5. Ability to be a team player
>
> The CFO survey also identified six acquired leadership skills:
>
> 1. Communicate clearly
> 2. Provide leadership in day-to-day operations
> 3. Manage resources and finances
> 4. Build coalitions
> 5. Create a positive organizational culture
> 6. Maintain strong physician relationship
>
> Accompanying the 2005 HFMA Compensation Survey is a list of characteristics necessary for CFOs to be successful in the future. The following characteristics were added to the characteristics already discussed (HFMA 2005):
>
> - *Case management*: Fixed reimbursements will drive CFOs into operations to lower costs via case management.
> - *Sales*: Lowering costs will necessitate CFOs selling new ways of doing things to the hospital and medical staffs.
> - *Education:* New ways of doing things will mean CFOs must educate the nonfinancial managers on how their operations affect the financial position of the organization.
>
> The old way of getting things done was transactional, which means that CFOs exert their authority—they tell people what to do. As organizations get larger and more bureaucratic, CFOs are going to have to become transformational managers: They're going to have to get things done by winning people over (HFMA 2005, CS2).

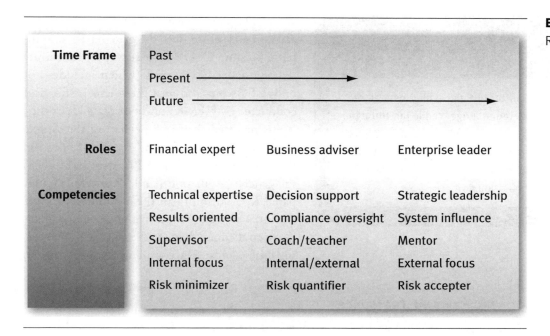

EXHIBIT 2.3
Roles of the CFO

Time Frame	Past		
	Present ———————————➤		
	Future ——————————————➤		
Roles	Financial expert	Business adviser	Enterprise leader
Competencies	Technical expertise	Decision support	Strategic leadership
	Results oriented	Compliance oversight	System influence
	Supervisor	Coach/teacher	Mentor
	Internal focus	Internal/external	External focus
	Risk minimizer	Risk quantifier	Risk accepter

Do CFOs and accountants have personalities conducive to these expanded roles demanding new competencies? Using Myers-Briggs personality typing, several studies have shown that the predominant personality types of accountants are

◆ introversion (I) (versus extroversion),

◆ sensing (S) (versus intuitive),

◆ thinking (T) (versus feeling), and

◆ judging (J) (versus perceiving).

Laribee (1994) reported that 37.3 percent of the study sample were STJs (significant compared to 20.5 percent found in the general population), and 56.0 percent were Is (significant compared to 40.1 percent found in the general population). The consistency among the findings of the personality studies on accountants is remarkable considering when the studies were conducted (from 1980 to 1997) and where the studies were conducted (United States, United Kingdom, and the Netherlands).

ISTJs represent 7 to 10 percent of the American population and are serious, responsible, sensible, and trustworthy, and they honor their commitments. Practical and realistic, they are matter-of-fact and thorough. They are painstakingly accurate and methodical and have great powers of concentration. They value and use logical and impersonal analysis and are organized and systematic in getting things done on time (Tieger and Barron-Tieger 2001).

You are the chief financial officer of Smithsville Hospital, and you have recently implemented a budget reduction throughout the hospital. You want to ensure your actions are accepted among the hospital department managers. What would be the best way to communicate with these department managers? If there is resistance, what should you do?

Do CFOs have the same personalities as accountants, or do only the extroverted accountants become CFOs? In a survey of healthcare senior financial executives (which includes not only CFOs but also vice presidents of finance) conducted by HFMA and Texas State University, it was reported that 37.8 percent of the sample were STJs (compared to 37.3 percent found in the accountant sample and 20.5 percent found in the general population), and 57.0 were Is (compared to 56.0 found in the accountant sample and 40.1 percent found in the general population), confirming that healthcare CFOs have personalities similar to accountants (Nowicki 2003).

CONTROLLER AND TREASURER

controller
The chief accounting officer of an organization.

Reporting to the CFO are the **controller** and the **treasurer**. The controller is the chief accounting officer of the healthcare organization and is usually responsible for financial accounting, managerial accounting, tax accounting, patient accounting, and internal auditing. The treasurer is responsible for managing working capital, the healthcare organization's investment portfolio, and the financing of capital expenditures. In smaller organizations, the controller function and the treasurer function may be combined into one position, or may be integrated with the CFO's responsibilities. According to the 2013 HFMA Compensation Survey (shown in Exhibit 2.4), average compensation for controllers was $111,300 (HFMA 2013).

treasurer
The person responsible for managing the capital of an organization.

CORPORATE COMPLIANCE OFFICER

Many organizations have corporate compliance officers (CCOs) in their senior management teams. The final compliance program guidelines for hospitals issued by the US Department of Health and Human Services (HHS) Office of Inspector General list the appointment of a CCO as a critical element of any corporate compliance plan (HHS 2000b). Healthcare compliance officers usually report directly to the CEO or board and are seen as peers of the CFO (Doody 1998). CCOs are typically responsible for conducting compliance reviews (to assess how well the organization complies with fraud and abuse laws), investigating potential fraud and abuse problems, and examining relationships and contracts for possible illegal provisions. In organizations that do not have a CCO, COOs, staff or retained attorneys, or CFOs perform these functions. Because no education, certification, or licensure is required for CCOs, CEOs seek individuals who understand the legal issues involved with compliance and exhibit the following personal characteristics that might support the compliance functions (Doody 1998):

	2005	2007	2009	2011	2013
Director/manager of finance	$98,800	$111,300	$114,600	$121,200	$122,200
Director/manager of managed care	$100,300	$110,800	$115,400	$122,300	$128,100
Director/manager of reimbursement	$98,200	$100,500	$109,500	$113,800	—
Controller	$95,400	$104,600	$109,000	$109,600	$111,300
Compliance officer	$96,600	$113,400	$117,500	$124,700	$130,300
Director/manager of patient financial services	$86,300	$92,200	$99,400	$105,700	$101,900
Director/manager of accounting	$73,200	$83,900	$88,000	$95,000	$100,400
Director/manager of decision support	—	—	$108,200	$113,700	—

EXHIBIT 2.4
Healthcare Middle Manager Compensation Trends

Source: Data from HFMA (2013).

- ◆ Analytical, inquisitive, persistent
- ◆ Detail-minded
- ◆ Skilled in dealing with people
- ◆ Dispassionate and objective
- ◆ Courageous
- ◆ Discreet
- ◆ Has a strong moral sense

In its 2013 survey of compliance officers, the Health Care Compliance Association found that more than 50 percent of compliance officers had a JD or MBA degree.

CHIEF INFORMATION OFFICER

Given the increasing importance of clinical information systems, the role of the chief information officer (CIO) is growing. Typically reporting directly to the CEO, the CIO is responsible not only for providing management oversight to all information processing and telecommunications systems in the organization, but also for assisting senior management in using information in management decision making (Glandon, Slovensky, and Smaltz 2008). The responsibilities of CIOs include e-commerce, e-health, and other web-based and multimedia technologies; business-service formats to respond tactically to strategic business initiatives; and outsourcing of all or a portion of the information technology departments. As CIOs become an accepted part of the executive team, leadership skills will become more important and technology skills will become less important. In fact, CIOs have delegated many of their technology responsibilities to chief technology officers.

PRIVACY OFFICER

Health Insurance Portability and Accountability Act of 1996 (HIPAA)
Legislation that mandated privacy and security regulations for the healthcare industry.

The Health Insurance Portability and Accountability Act of 1996 (HIPAA) mandated privacy and security regulations for the healthcare industry. HHS's final rule on privacy, issued in 2002 and effective in 2003, requires that an "entity must designate a privacy official who is responsible for the development and implementation of the privacy policies and procedures of the entity" (CMS 2004). HHS's final rule on security, issued in 2003 and effective in 2005, requires that the "security responsibility be assigned to a specific individual or organization . . . for the management and supervision of the use of security measures to protect data and of the conduct of personnel in relation to the protection of data" (CMS 2004). The American Health Information Management Association (AHIMA) makes a good case that health information management (HIM) professionals should have the training and experience to handle most of the skills required for privacy officers, and in 2002 AHIMA introduced a certification in healthcare privacy, which subsequently became a certification in healthcare privacy and security (CHPS).

HIM professionals should have the following traits (Dennis 2001):

◆ HIPAA competency

◆ Knowledge of how confidential information is used

◆ Knowledge of how confidential information is disclosed

◆ Knowledge of information technology

◆ Knowledge of state and federal laws on information

◆ The ability to promote unpopular positions

INTERNAL AUDITOR

Independent auditors are different from internal auditors. An independent auditor is typically a large accounting firm that has a contract with the healthcare organization. An internal auditor is an employee of the organization who usually reports to the controller. The independent auditor's primary concern is the financial reporting needs of external entities, and the internal auditor's primary concern is protecting the organization's assets from fraud, error, and loss. The independent auditor's responsibilities are limited primarily to financial matters; the internal auditor's responsibilities include both financial and operational matters. The independent auditor is only incidentally concerned with identifying fraud (i.e., the independent auditor is not looking for fraud, but is duty-bound to report any fraud found in the organization to the party that engaged the auditor's services); the internal auditor is directly concerned with identifying fraud.

INDEPENDENT AUDITOR

Independent auditors are retained by the healthcare organization to ensure that the financial reports sent to external agencies are in the correct accounting format. Examples of external agencies include the state and federal government, commercial insurance companies, and lenders. The correct accounting format means that the healthcare organization used generally accepted accounting principles (GAAP) in preparing the report. This does not guarantee that the healthcare organization is financially sound. The American Institute of Certified Public Accountants in 1997 issued Statement on Auditing Standards (SAS) No. 82, Consideration of Fraud in a Financial Statement Audit, which requires independent auditors to obtain reasonable assurance that financial statements are free of material misstatements caused by error or fraud. While SAS No. 82 provides guidelines for independent auditors to use to help detect and document risk factors related to potential fraud, it does not expand their detection responsibility. Therefore, healthcare organizations and independent auditors should discuss thoroughly the scope and focus of the audit as it relates to the organization's compliance efforts (Reinstein and Dery 1999).

Independent auditors typically audit the healthcare organization once each year. The duration of the audit partially depends on the size of the organization. At the end of the audit, the independent auditor produces an audit report made up of three paragraphs:

1. The introductory paragraph identifies the financial statements audited, management's responsibilities in preparing the financial statements, and the auditor's responsibilities in expressing the audit opinion.

2. The scope paragraph describes the criteria used in the audit (for instance, GAAP).

3. The opinion paragraph includes the auditor's statement about whether the financial statements are in the correct accounting format.

A fourth paragraph, the explanatory paragraph, is included only if GAAP were not used in preparing the financial statements or if any uncertainty exists regarding how the financial statements were prepared. The *AICPA Audit and Accounting Guide for Health Care Entities* (2010) provides examples of audit reports, including the four different types of opinions referenced next.

The opinion paragraph is the heart of the audit report. Independent auditors use four types of opinions in rendering their reports:

1. An unqualified opinion means that, in all material respects, the financial statements fairly present the financial position, results of operations, and cash flows of the organization in conformance with GAAP. An unqualified opinion may have an additional explanatory paragraph, but an explanatory paragraph does not affect the opinion. Auditors use an explanatory paragraph when they are basing their opinion in part on the work of a different external auditor, or when they need additional information to prevent the audit report from being misleading when uncertainties exist that they cannot reasonably resolve by the publication date of the audit report.

2. A qualified opinion means that the financial statements fairly present, in all material respects, the financial position, results of operations, and cash flows of the organization in conformance with GAAP, except for matters identified in additional paragraphs of the report. Auditors use a qualified opinion when there is insufficient evidentiary matter, when the organization has placed restrictions on the scope of the audit, or when the financial statements depart in a material, though not substantial, manner from GAAP.

3. An adverse opinion means that the financial statements do not fairly present the financial position, results of operations, and/or cash flows of the organization in conformance with GAAP. Auditors use additional paragraphs after the opinion to describe the reasons for an adverse opinion.

4. A disclaimer of opinion means that the auditor does not express an opinion on the financial statements, usually because the scope of the audit was insufficient for the auditor to render an opinion.

corporate restructuring
A legal strategy involving the establishment of subsidiaries or related corporations in order to maximize the economic position of a healthcare organization.

ALTERNATIVE CORPORATE STRUCTURES

As previously mentioned, healthcare organizations are chartered as corporations by the state. Prior to the late 1970s, most healthcare corporations consisted of one corporation or a limited number of corporations. Beginning in the late 1970s, a legal strategy called **corporate restructuring** became popular in response to increasing economic pressures on healthcare organizations. The purpose of corporate restructuring was to maximize the economic position of the healthcare organization by developing new corporations (see Stromberg 1982). Typically, healthcare organizations restructure for one or more of the following four reasons, which dictate the corporate restructuring model.

1. Healthcare organizations that need to facilitate the development of a new service may develop a wholly controlled subsidiary corporation. For example, a for-profit healthcare organization may develop a wholly controlled subsidiary not-for-profit corporation, called a **foundation**, to facilitate education and research. In addition to facilitating education and research, the foundation allows the for-profit healthcare organization to shelter some income from taxes by using the income for purposes that are tax-exempt.

2. Healthcare organizations that need to protect assets may develop a parent holding corporation. For example, for-profit healthcare organizations may develop several parent corporations to layer their liability in the event of malpractice suits. Courts allow only the assets of the organization, and not the assets of the parent corporation, to be introduced during deliberations regarding damage awards.

3. Healthcare organizations that need to maximize patient care and other operating revenues and even nonoperating revenues may develop a quasi-independent sister corporation. In this model, the healthcare organization can control no more than 49 percent of the governing body of the sister corporation. For example, a healthcare organization, either for-profit or not-for-profit, may develop a gift shop whose governing body usually uses the income to benefit the healthcare organization. The healthcare organization believes that the perception of independence on the part of customers, both in terms of who controls the governing body and who controls the employees or volunteers, gives the gift shop an advantage in generating revenue. Customers are more likely to buy gifts in an "independent" corporation than to buy gifts from the healthcare organization that sends them a bill.

4. Healthcare organizations that need to attract additional funds through philanthropy may develop a wholly independent corporation. In this model, the healthcare organization cannot control any of the governing body. For example, a healthcare organization may develop a foundation whose governing body raises money using relationships established by the healthcare organization. The governing body of the foundation usually uses the income to benefit the healthcare organization, much in the same way that university alumni associations, which are independent from the universities, use their income to benefit universities.

foundation
A not-for-profit corporation, usually a subsidiary of a for-profit organization, that facilitates education and research or otherwise undertakes charitable projects.

Mr. Jones, an 87-year-old widower who lives alone, was admitted to the hospital through the emergency room for shortness of breath and swollen ankles. After an extensive interview, the admitting physician discovered that Mr. Jones had been admitted two weeks earlier with the same symptoms and had been diagnosed with congestive heart failure. At that time he spent four days in the hospital, and then was transferred to a skilled nursing facility, where he spent three days before being discharged with a prescription for a diuretic to help reduce fluid buildup. The admitting physician discovered that no one at the hospital or the skilled nursing facility had explained to Mr. Jones the importance of maintaining a low-sodium diet (high-sodium diets cause fluid retention). Mr. Jones had attended a birthday party and eaten several hot dogs before his latest symptoms appeared. Who should be financially responsible for the costs related to Mr. Jones's latest admission? Should Medicare, or any insurer, pay for readmissions related to errors in discharge instructions? Would it be different had Mr. Jones received instructions for a low-sodium diet but chosen to ignore them?

Although corporate restructuring was popular in the late 1970s and 1980s, both Medicare and the Internal Revenue Service (IRS) have increased their interest in the resulting corporations. For instance, Medicare's position has been that a portion of the income generated by quasi-independent corporations like gift shops should be deducted from the amount Medicare owes the healthcare organization under cost-based reimbursement. Medicare reasons that a portion of the gift shop sales is attributable to Medicare patients and their visitors.

The IRS's position is that corporate restructuring that allows a corporation to avoid paying taxes should be reviewed to ensure that the primary purpose of the corporate restructuring is legitimate. Areas of concern include the unrelated business income generated by wholly controlled subsidiary corporations (e.g., parking garages, adjacent hotels, catering services). Chapter 3 provides an overview of the tax status of corporations and reviews in detail the tax-exempt organization.

ORGANIZATIONS DESIGNED TO INTEGRATE CARE

Physicians historically have not worked for hospitals. Rather, most are independent practitioners who use the hospital facilities to treat their patients. However, healthcare organizations have been attempting to integrate physicians into the organizational setting for decades. Many healthcare leaders and payers, such as Medicare and Medicaid, believe integrating the delivery and financing of care into one organization would result in higher quality healthcare delivered at a lower cost. However, many physicians and other professional providers are accustomed to practicing with a great deal of autonomy and have resisted efforts to coordinate and integrate their care.

integrated delivery system
A system of healthcare providers capable of accepting financial responsibility for and delivering a full range of clinical services.

Over 30 years ago, employers began seeking **integrated delivery systems**, systems of healthcare providers capable of accepting financial responsibility for and delivering a full range of clinical services. These systems promised higher quality at lower costs by reducing errors (one study found that the cost of medical errors in the United States reached

$19.5 billion in 2008, resulting in 2,500 preventable deaths and 10 million lost days of work [Society of Actuaries 2010]). The government spends an estimated $12 billion per year on potentially preventable hospital readmissions, according to the Medicare Payment Advisory Commission, or MedPAC (Winslow and Goldstein 2009).

In order to better coordinate care, many hospitals have initiated **physician–hospital organizations**, joint ventures capable of contracting with managed care organizations. Both integrative delivery systems and the more recent physician–hospital organizations have had limited success in coordinating and integrating healthcare.

In 2005, MedPAC reported that future government reimbursement for health services should be based on four criteria—one of which was high-quality, cost-effective care. In 2006, President Bush signed an executive order asking federally sponsored health plans, including Medicare, to adopt the four criteria. The concept of **accountable care organizations (ACOs)**, which emphasize coordinated care and mandate provider accountability, was born in 2007 (Fisher et al. 2007). The ACO concept includes financial incentives for organizations that take responsibility for the quality and cost of patient care to a defined population. In 2009, MedPAC recommended that Medicare encourage the development of ACOs, and Section 3022 of the Affordable Care Act of 2010 encouraged the voluntary development of ACOs (Tuma 2010).

physician–hospital organization
Joint venture between healthcare organizations and physicians that is capable of contracting with managed care organizations.

accountable care organization (ACO)
An organization that coordinates care among healthcare organizations and physicians. A key element of an ACO is that some portion of its reimbursement is tied to accountability.

CHAPTER KEY POINTS

➤ The governing body of a healthcare organization has several duties, including proper development of resources and monitoring of the CEO's performance.

➤ If a governing body breaches its duty, it may be legally liable.

➤ The CFO is responsible for financial management of the organization, requiring the skills of a supervisor and intrinsic traits.

➤ The CCO's duty is to ensure the organization supports compliance functions.

➤ Information processing and telecommunications systems of the organization are the responsibility of the CIO.

➤ Other management positions in an organization include the privacy officer, internal auditor, and independent auditor.

➤ Corporate structures include wholly controlled subsidiary, parent holding corporation, quasi-independent sister corporation, and wholly independent corporation.

➤ Organizations designed to integrate patient care include integrated delivery systems (IDSs), physician–hospital organizations (PHOs), and accountable care organizations (ACOs).

DISCUSSION QUESTIONS

1. Explain the meaning of corporate status in relation to healthcare organizations, and the advantages corporate status provides.

2. What is the role of the governing body? How does the governing body use organized committees to monitor the performance of the CEO?

3. What are the responsibilities of the CFO? Discuss the characteristics and traits of a successful CFO.

4. Both the corporate compliance officer and chief information officer report to the CEO but have very different positions. Explain the roles of the CCO and CIO.

5. Compare and contrast the roles of the internal auditor and the independent auditor. What must the independent auditor include in the audit report?

6. Compare and contrast organizational models that attempt to integrate patient care.

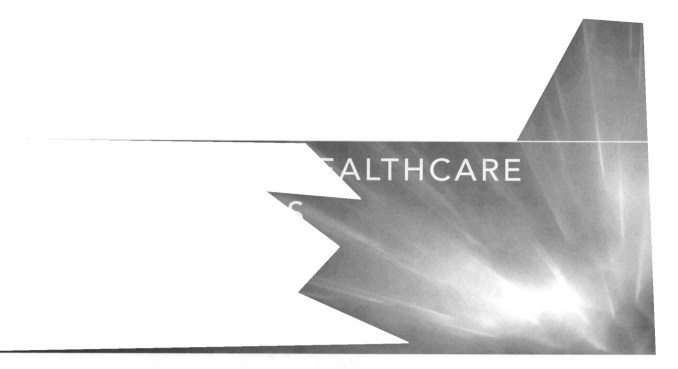

EALTHCARE

Nonprofit hospitals have historically played and continue to play a key role in the financing and delivery of healthcare in the United States because they are bound by their missions to do good for the benefit of the communities they serve.

Greg Pope, vice president of philanthropy for the Saint Thomas Health Services Foundation, Nashville, Tennessee

LEARNING OBJECTIVES

After completing this chapter, you should be able to do the following:

➤ Analyze the rationale for tax-exempt status and apply the rationale to healthcare

➤ Appreciate the value of tax-exempt status

➤ Identify the steps necessary to qualify for tax-exempt status

➤ Relate the importance of community benefits to tax-exempt status in healthcare

➤ Examine judicial challenges to tax-exempt status

➤ Examine legislative challenges to tax-exempt status

➤ Examine IRS challenges to tax-exempt status

INTRODUCTION

As discussed in Chapter 2, healthcare corporations are granted legal status as corporations by the state. Although the state can allow a variety of tax designations for corporations, only two general designations are discussed in this chapter: for-profit corporations and not-for-profit corporations.

RATIONALE FOR TAX-EXEMPT STATUS

tax-exempt
The status that allows an organization to pay no taxes, including sales tax, income tax, and property tax. Tax-exempt organizations may also raise capital by selling tax-exempt bonds, for which they can pay lower interest than comparable taxable bonds.

As a general rule, for-profit corporations pay taxes: federal and state income taxes on income; state and local sales taxes on purchased goods and, in some states, services; and local real estate and personal property taxes on land, buildings, and major equipment. Not-for-profit corporations pay no taxes; they are therefore **tax-exempt**. To be tax-exempt, corporations must meet certain criteria established by the federal government through the Internal Revenue Service (IRS) and state and local governments. Most state and local governments use either the same or similar criteria to those established by the IRS.

Why does the government grant tax-exempt status to corporations? The first reason is to relieve the government of the burden of providing the services itself. For instance, states grant healthcare organizations tax-exempt status, and in exchange the organizations provide healthcare services to state residents who cannot afford healthcare services. In the absence of this arrangement, the government presumably would provide these healthcare services itself. The second reason the government grants tax-exempt status to corporations is to reward the corporation for performing services that enhance community values and goals. For instance, governments reward healthcare organizations with tax-exempt status because the organizations provide uncompensated health-promotion programs to the community, which benefit the overall well-being of the community.

VALUE OF TAX-EXEMPT STATUS

Although the potential exposure of a corporation to taxes and fees depends on a variety of variables, including accounting practices, Witek, Milligan, and Ryan (1993) made the following general comments regarding valuing tax-exempt status. Federal income tax payments (approximately 34 percent, applied to net income) are generally the largest tax liability. State income tax payments average 6 percent, though not all states have a state income tax. Real estate and personal property taxes are significant tax liabilities; they are based on fair market value for land and appraised value for buildings and major equipment. In addition to eliminating tax liabilities, tax-exempt status also exempts the organization from paying most business fees and licenses. One of the most valuable benefits of tax-exempt status is the ability to issue tax-exempt bonds, whose yields are 4 to 5 percent below taxable bond yields.

Therefore, the value of tax-exempt status is the total value of taxes and business licenses and fees exempted and the value of access to tax-exempt bond markets. In 2013, these exemptions amounted to $12 billion for the nation's 5,000 community, tax-exempt hospitals (Rosenthal 2013).

QUALIFYING FOR TAX-EXEMPT STATUS

As previously mentioned, the IRS has developed the primary criteria for a corporation with tax-exempt status, designated under Section 501(c)(3) of the tax code. To qualify for tax-exempt status, corporations must

1. operate exclusively for charitable, scientific, or educational reasons;

2. serve public rather than private interests, in that the organization's income does not benefit individuals; and

3. not engage in prohibited transactions, including but not limited to

   - participating in political campaigns,

   - attempting to influence legislation,

   - lending any part of the organization's income without receiving adequate security and interest,

   - paying compensation in excess of reasonable salary levels,

   - making investments for more than adequate consideration,

   - selling an asset for less than adequate consideration,

   - subverting in any other manner substantial portions of its income or assets, or

   - making any part of its services available on a preferential basis.

In 1956, the IRS established that not-for-profit healthcare organizations qualified for tax-exempt status as charitable organizations under Revenue Ruling 56-185. In effect, this ruling established that healthcare organizations, in order to retain their tax-exempt status, are required to provide care to those unable to pay. This ruling was difficult to administer, and the term **charitable organization** was redefined in 1959 to include a concept of community benefit or public interest that was broader than just the provision of care to those unable to pay (Kuchler 1992). The standard has changed several times in the decades since, and today tax-exempt status in general and the community benefit standard specifically are under scrutiny from research, judicial, congressional, executive, and

charitable organization
An organization that provides community benefit or serves the public interest. In the case of healthcare, a hospital is a charitable organization if it provides care to people who cannot pay for their care or provides community health benefits.

public sectors. As the next section explains, the community benefit standard remains the primary IRS test for designating tax-exempt status.

COMMUNITY BENEFITS AND TAX-EXEMPT STATUS

Hospitals obviously benefit the community. However, do not-for-profit hospitals benefit their communities more than for-profit hospitals do? This question was raised in public in an exchange in the *New England Journal of Medicine* between Arnold Relman, the journal's editor, and Michael Bromberg, president of the American Federation of Hospitals, an association of for-profit hospitals.[1] In 1980, Relman wrote an article warning his readers of the medical-industrial complex—"a large and growing network of private corporations engaged in the business of supplying health-care services [exclusive of supplies and pharmaceuticals] to patients for a profit—services heretofore provided by nonprofit institutions or individual practitioners" (Relman 1980, 963). Relman worried that the medical-industrial complex would put the interests of stockholders before the interests of the community.

Answering Relman's claims, Bromberg wrote that for-profit hospitals provided capital that funded a technology boom; that for-profit hospitals paid significant taxes that supported social programs at the local, state, and federal levels; and that for-profit hospitals competed with not-for-profit hospitals, which would be good for the community by reducing costs and improving quality. Bromberg also criticized some of the early research that seemed to support Relman's claim. This research found that for-profit hospitals charge more per patient day; perform more ancillary tests per patient day; and "skim the cream," meaning that for-profit hospitals serve only paying patients and provide only profitable services (Bromberg 1983).

This issue has been studied many times since the Relman/Bromberg discussion. In 1987, an article in the *Harvard Business Review* found that little difference existed in community benefits provided by hospitals in for-profit systems and hospitals in not-for-profit systems.

> You are a tax attorney and consultant to Doctor's Hospital, a for-profit, physician-owned hospital. You are scheduled to give a presentation to the board regarding the advantages related to converting the hospital to not-for-profit tax status. What are your arguments? What are the board's likely arguments to remain for-profit?

For-profits do not deny access to care. In fact, we found the for-profits gave slightly more access to patients who carry little or no health insurance than did the nonprofits. The reasons are straightforward: hospital costs are mostly fixed, and the marginal costs of an additional patient generally are low. Even an indigent patient contributes somewhat to covering the hospital's fixed costs.

For-profits do not "cream" the affluent patients who have insurance coverage. There is no difference in accessibility between for-profits and nonprofits to the affluent patient.

While nonprofit hospitals receive more social subsidies than for-profits (exemptions from taxes, business fees and licenses, as well as access to tax-exempt bonds), they do not achieve better social results. They are not more accessible to the uninsured and medically indigent, nor do they price less aggressively. (Herzlinger and Krasker 1987, 103)

In 1993, Witek, Milligan, and Ryan reported that by including taxes as a community benefit, for-profit hospitals in Georgia actually provide substantially more community benefit than not-for-profit hospitals or county hospitals that receive direct tax support (see Exhibit 3.1).

In mid-2004, Richard Scruggs, an attorney who had successfully won billions of dollars in class-action lawsuits against asbestos manufacturers and the tobacco industry, began seeking class-action status in 49 lawsuits accusing 370 not-for-profit hospitals of overcharging the uninsured and using aggressive collection methods against poor patients. The lawsuit against the Providence Health System, which operates several hospitals in Washington and Oregon, is representative. Citing the Providence mission to provide "universal access to health care, social justice and compassion for all members of our society" with "special concern for the poor and vulnerable," Scruggs (2004) argued the following:

In fact, contrary to these representations, Providence discriminates against the very patients who are supposed to benefit most from its charity care by engaging in a pattern and practice of charging inordinately inflated rates to its uninsured patients,

Hospital Ownership	Indigent Care	Total Taxes	Total Benefit
County	6.0	(4.0)	2.0
Not-for-profit	4.1	0.0	4.1
For-profit	2.5	3.9	6.4

EXHIBIT 3.1
Community Benefit Comparison in Georgia Hospitals

Note: Amounts shown as percent of adjusted gross revenue.

Source: Data from Witek, J. E., D. L. Milligan, and J. B. Ryan. 1993. "Managing Charitable Purpose: Issues and Answers." Presented at the American College of Healthcare Executives Congress on Healthcare Management, Chicago, March 4.

including Plaintiffs and the Class they seek to represent, that are far higher than the rates it charges its insured patients for the same services.

Providence publicly represents itself as a 'not-for-profit medical care provider,' and it receives millions of dollars each year in tax exemptions under Section 501(c)(3) of the federal tax code, 26 U.S.C. §501(c)(3), as a charitable, 'nonprofit' organization that is required by law to engage in exclusively charitable purposes. Providence Oregon is similarly exempt from Oregon property taxes based on its charitable, 'nonprofit' status.

In fact, again contrary to its representations, Providence is extremely profitable. For example, in 2002, which is the most recent year for which data is available, Providence Oregon obtained over $1.2 billion in revenue, it held over $250 million in cash and investment securities, and the cost of its physical plant (land, buildings and equipment) was over $1.1 billion.

The same year, Providence Oregon's President and CEO, Henry G. Walker, received over $1.4 million in compensation and benefits, its four Vice Presidents received an average of over $565,000 in compensation and benefits, and the average compensation and benefits of its five highest paid employees other than officers and directors was $460,000.

In 2006, Providence Health System, along with Legacy Health System and Sutter Health, settled the uninsured billing cases while denying wrongdoing. As part of Providence's settlement, the system agreed to refund or adjust $1 million in past bills (Becker 2006).

In response to the increasing public pressure caused in part by the Scruggs lawsuits, the healthcare industry initiated a flurry of activity related to increasing community benefits. However, industry efforts to establish a voluntary standard for both the amount and what counts as community benefits have stalled as the American Hospital Association (AHA) and the Catholic Health Association (CHA) offered competing proposals. The AHA proposal counts the cost of bad debt and Medicare losses in addition to the cost of charity care and Medicaid losses as community benefit. But CHA argues that the costs associated with bad debts and Medicare losses should not be counted (*Modern Healthcare* 2006).

In December 2006, the Congressional Budget Office (CBO) released a report on the provision of community benefits by not-for-profit hospitals. Both for-profit and not-for-profit hospitals in five states—California, Florida, Georgia, Indiana, and Texas—were examined (n = 1,057). Acknowledging the lack of industry consensus on what constitutes community benefits and how such benefits should be measured, the CBO report defined community benefits as the provision of uncompensated care, the provision of services to Medicaid patients, and the provision of certain specialized services that have been traditionally identified as unprofitable. In general, comparing for-profit and not-for-profit hospitals produced mixed results. The CBO found, on average, that not-for-profit hospitals provided higher levels of uncompensated care and were more likely to provide unprofitable specialized services. For-profit hospitals provided care to more Medicaid patients as a percent of their total patient population and were found to operate in areas with lower average incomes, higher poverty rates, and higher rates of uninsurance (CBO 2006).

A study published in the *New England Journal of Medicine* (Young et al. 2013) found that community benefits averaged 7.5 percent of operating expenses in community, not-for-profit hospitals, and that 85 percent of the community benefits reported were charity care. The study also found great variation among hospitals in the amount of community benefits provided, ranging from 1 percent to 20 percent of operating expenses.

The CBO report also provided the results of the Joint Committee on Taxation, which valued the total 2002 tax exemptions for the nation's not-for-profit hospitals at $12.6 billion, with exemptions from federal taxes accounting for about half of the total (CBO 2006).[2]

JUDICIAL CHALLENGES TO TAX-EXEMPT STATUS

The previously mentioned research findings question the community benefits standard; courts have also reviewed the appropriateness of tax-exempt status. Since the 1980s, state attorneys general have challenged the tax status of many healthcare organizations. Here are some examples:

◆   A case in Utah (Utah State Tax Commission 1990) argued that not-for-profit
    hospitals had evolved to a position in the marketplace from which it was
    virtually impossible to distinguish them from their for-profit counterparts.
    The court ruled

> Tax exemptions confer an indirect subsidy and are usually justified as
> the quid pro quo [consideration] for charitable entities undertaking
> functions and services that the state would otherwise be required to
> perform. A concurrent rationale used by some courts is the assertion
> that the exemptions are granted not only because charitable enti-
> ties relieve government of a burden, but also because their activities
> enhance beneficial community values and goals. Under this theory, the
> benefits received by the community are *believed to offset the revenue
> lost by reason of the exemption* [emphasis added by author].

Under this court's rationale, the amount of community benefits provided
by the not-for-profit hospital should equal or exceed the amount of the
tax exemption. In this case, community benefits did not equal the tax
exemption, and the court required the not-for-profit hospitals to pay the
difference in taxes. Critics of this decision have argued that the community

benefit standard is too lenient. The standard defined community benefits as indigent care, community education and service, medical discounts, and donations of time, money, or services made by hospital employees acting as private individuals (Utah State Tax Commission 1990). In 2001, in Salt Lake County, the Board of Equalization voted to maintain tax exemption for four Intermountain Health Care facilities, but not before it required the system to once again present its case for exemption (Bellandi 2001).

◆ A case in Boise, Idaho, stated that a not-for-profit hospital was not sufficiently supported by donations; donations accounted for less than 2 percent of the hospital's total revenues. (Dutton 2013, Thompson Powers 1999).

◆ A hospital in Pennsylvania lost its tax-exempt status because the courts felt it had a profit motive, as evidenced by the CEO's $400,000 salary (in 1994), the fact that surpluses were sent to the corporate parent, and the fact that the hospital forced physicians to sign non-compete agreements (Thompson Powers 1999).

◆ A hospital in New Hampshire had its tax-exempt status revoked because its collection policy stipulated that it receive full payment for all services whenever possible; it provided only 2.9 percent of total revenue in charity care; and it used its surpluses to fund a for-profit subsidiary (Taylor 2001).

◆ The attorney general of Connecticut sued a hospital for hoarding $37 million in charitable funds in order to generate interest income instead of spending the funds to provide indigent care (Piotrowski 2003b).

◆ A clinic in Wisconsin lost its property tax exemption when the court ruled its property was not used exclusively for benevolent purposes as defined by state law (Taylor 2003).

◆ A medical center in Illinois lost its tax-exempt status because of aggressive patient-collection tactics and because the organization had contracted with several for-profit entities to fulfill key hospital functions (Pressey 2010).

IRS Challenges to Tax-Exempt Status

In 1987, in response to public pressure to reduce federal budget deficits, the IRS began auditing tax-exempt organizations, including healthcare

You are the president and CEO of St. Michael's Hospital for Children. You arrive at work to find TV cameras and news reporters in your office. A national news story had aired the previous evening calling into question the tax-exempt status of nonprofit hospitals related to the Illinois case referenced on this page. You feel compelled to address the issues raised in the Illinois case in particular and the general principles of tax-exempt hospitals from the local perspective. What does your press release say?

organizations. By the end of 1992, the IRS had audited 233 tax-exempt healthcare organizations. Most frequently reported irregularities included inappropriate physician recruiting arrangements and taxable unrelated business income. For instance, in 1994, a hospital in Houston agreed to pay nearly $1 million in federal income taxes and penalties in response to IRS allegations that the hospital had offered lucrative physician recruitment and retention incentives, including signing bonuses, income guarantees, free office space, malpractice insurance, equipment loans, and loan guarantees (Wang and Wambsganns 1997).

In 1991, the IRS initiated an audit program for tax-exempt healthcare systems called the coordinated examination program (CEP) (now known as the Coordinated Industry Case program). Using an interdisciplinary audit team of specialists in corporate restructuring, pensions, payroll taxes, income taxes, and tax-exempt bond financing, CEP audits examine the following (HFMA 1992):

◆ *Community benefit standard:* Auditors check composition of the governing board, amount of charity care provided, and complaints of patient dumping (i.e., denying or transferring patients based on inability to pay).

◆ *Unreasonable compensation and private **inurement**:* Auditors check physician relationships to identify prohibited instances of private benefit, unreasonable compensation, improper disclosure, and inappropriate physician recruiting practices.

inurement
Providing an employee benefit, such as salary, that is greater than the value of the employee's work.

◆ *Financial analysis:* Auditors check all affiliated entities to detect presence of prohibited proprietary purposes, inurement, serving of private interests, unrelated business income (i.e., income from business activities that is unrelated to the organization's tax-exempt purposes and therefore must be reported as taxable income), or lobbying activities.

◆ *Joint ventures:* Auditors check **joint ventures** (a relationship established between two business entities—for example, a hospital and radiologist purchasing and operating a computed tomography scanner together) to determine if the ventures violate prohibitions on private benefit, inurement, or kickbacks.

joint venture
A relationship between two business entities entered into for a specific purpose and period of time.

◆ *Independent contractors:* Auditors check hospital contracts to determine whether contractors should be treated as contractors or employees for tax purposes.

In 2009, the IRS released its final report on a study of nonprofit hospitals that began in 2006 (IRS 2009). The report was based on a survey sent to 500 nonprofit hospitals in four community settings: high-population urban, other urban and suburban, critical access hospitals, and other rural hospitals. The community benefit findings included substantial variation in the amount of community benefits provided by nonprofit hospitals. For instance, the report found that 20 percent of the survey hospitals accounted for 78 percent of the aggregate community benefits:

◆ There is considerable diversity in the demographics, community benefit activities, and financial resources among the hospitals in the sample.

◆ The average and median percentages of total revenues reported spent on community benefit activities were 9 percent and 6 percent, respectively, with the lowest percentages reported among the rural hospitals.

◆ Uncompensated care was the largest reported community benefit expenditure, accounting for 56 percent, followed by medical education and training at 23 percent, research at 15 percent, and community programs at 6 percent.

◆ The average excess profit margin for the sample was 5 percent, though 21 percent of the sample reported losses.

◆ The average and median total compensation amounts paid to the top management official were $490,000 and $377,000, respectively. Nearly all of the amounts were determined to be reasonable compensation by the IRS.

LEGISLATIVE CHALLENGES TO TAX-EXEMPT STATUS

At the federal level, significant activity related to the tax privileges of tax-exempt organizations has occurred with some success in recent years. Representative Charles B. Rangel (D-NY), who chaired the House Ways and Means Committee's panel on select revenue measures, held hearings in 2005 on tax-exempt status and has voiced concerns that existing law regarding tax-exempt status is too lenient and too difficult to enforce. Representative Brian Donnelly (D-MA) led legislative efforts to require tax-exempt hospitals to provide specific levels of charity care. In President Bill Clinton's health reform bill, tax-exempt healthcare organizations would have been required to assess the health needs of the community on an annual basis and develop plans to meet those needs (Blankenau 1994). The Taxpayer Bill of Rights II, which indirectly addresses tax-exempt issues, was signed into law in 1996. The act provides the IRS with intermediate sanctions prior to revoking an organization's tax-exempt status. According to Wang and Wambsganns (1997), the act also

◆ requires tax-exempt organizations to disclose excess benefit transactions (i.e., unreasonable compensation or any other transaction in which payment or benefit exceeds the value of the transaction) and excise taxes paid for such transactions on Form 990, which requires all not-for-profit organizations to substantiate their tax-exempt status;

◆ expands public access to Form 990; and

◆ subjects executives responsible for an excess benefit transaction, rather than the organization, to a 10 percent tax on the amount of excess benefit if corrected and reported, and a 200 percent tax on the amount of excess benefit if executives fail to correct a transaction in which they personally benefited.

In 2005, Senator Chuck Grassley (R-IA), ranking member of the Senate Finance Committee, sent letters to the nation's largest tax-exempt hospitals asking them for clarification of community benefits reported. In 2006, Senator Grassley convened hearings to release hospital responses to the 2005 letters and to investigate hospital executive compensation. In 2007, he released a draft of legislative reforms for tax-exempt hospitals and held roundtables to discuss the reforms. In 2008, he followed up with more letters to hospitals, and he requested a report from the Government Accountability Office. In 2009, Senator Grassley convinced the Democratic majority to include many of the reforms in the Affordable Care Act (ACA) (Grassley 2010):

Tax-exempt hospitals don't have many measures of accountability for their special status. The law hasn't given them much direction, and so they've defined standards for themselves. Sometimes that's resulted in providing very little charitable patient care or other community benefits, failing to publicize charitable care to patients, charging indigent, uninsured patients more than insured patients, and using very aggressive collection practices. The Government Accountability Office and others, including the former IRS commissioner, have said for a long time that there is often no discernible difference between the operations of taxable and tax-exempt hospitals. These new provisions are modeled after principles and policies that the Catholic Health Association has had in place for years.

The ACA imposes four new requirements for tax-exempt hospitals (AHA 2010):

1. Complete a community health needs assessment and implementation strategy every three years and make it available to the public. Needs that are identified and not addressed with resources must be explained.

2. Develop, implement, and publicize financial assistance policies that include criteria for financial assistance, methods of applying for assistance, the basis for determining the amount charged to patients, permissible debt collection actions for patients on financial assistance, and the availability of emergency care regardless of the patient's ability to qualify for assistance.

3. Limit charges to patients eligible for assistance to no more than the lowest amount billed to insured patients.

4. Avoid extraordinary billing and collection activities until eligibility for financial assistance is determined.

Related to the earlier case regarding St. Michael's Hospital for Children, do you as the CEO have additional arguments against taxing authorities attempting to revoke a hospital's tax-exempt status in lieu of the Affordable Care Act? Does the board have a different position based on the act?

Projecting the effects of the ACA on hospital charity care is difficult. Both the individual mandate and the expansion of Medicaid eligibility in many states will replace charity care patients with insured patients. However, undocumented workers who are not covered under the ACA and individuals and small businesses who opt for the federal fines in lieu of purchasing coverage will continue to seek charity care at hospitals (Chazin et al. 2010).

Representative Charles W. Boustany (R-LA), who chairs the Subcommittee on Oversight of the Committee on Ways and Means, held hearings in 2012 to review the IRS oversight of tax-exempt organizations including hospital compliance with ACA (House Ways and Means Committee 2012).

The state level has also shown significant activity related to the tax privileges of tax-exempt organizations, and 39 states have passed legislation that challenges, or at least defines more narrowly, tax-exempt status and requires either voluntary or mandated reporting of community benefits (Somerville, Nelson, and Mueller 2013). For example, the 1993 Texas Charity Care Law requires tax-exempt healthcare organizations to provide a certain amount for community benefits and develop a mission statement and community benefits plan for serving the community's healthcare needs. The plan must be based on a community-wide needs assessment and must contain mechanisms for measuring the plan's effectiveness, including measurable objectives and a budget. The budget must include an amount for community benefits at least equal to one of the following (Texas Tax Code 1993):

◆ 4 percent of the hospital's net revenue

◆ 100 percent of the hospital's state and local tax exemptions

◆ an amount that is reasonable in relation to community needs, available resources, and the hospital's state and local tax exemptions

As of 2013, 23 states require nonprofit hospitals to provide community benefits (definitions of community benefits vary greatly among the states); nine states have unconditional community benefit requirements; six states require the provision of community benefits as a condition of certificate-of-need approval; six states require the provision of community benefits as a condition of property tax exemption; three states require the provision of community benefits as a condition of hospital licensure; two states require the provision of community benefits as a condition of sales tax exemption; and two states require the provision of community benefits as a condition of partial state reimbursement for charity care expenses.

In addition to Texas, Illinois, Utah, Nevada, and Pennsylvania require nonprofit hospitals to provide a specific amount of charity care (Somerville, Nelson, and Mueller 2013).

CHAPTER KEY POINTS

➤ Tax-exempt status has several advantages for healthcare organizations.

➤ Tax-exempt organizations must meet several criteria, including the provision of community benefits.

➤ Legislatures, courts, and the IRS have challenged tax-exempt organizations, including hospitals.

➤ The Affordable Care Act of 2010 provides national criteria for nonprofit hospitals.

DISCUSSION QUESTIONS

1. Explain the rationale for granting organizations tax-exempt status.

2. Identify the benefits and the burdens of tax-exempt status for hospitals.

3. What are the steps necessary to qualify for tax-exempt status?

4. What are the bases of legislative, judicial, and IRS challenges to tax-exempt status?

5. Will the Affordable Care Act of 2010 be viewed as friend or foe to tax-exempt hospitals?

6. Under the ACA, if more people are covered by insurance and fewer people need charity care, how will nonprofit hospitals justify their tax-exempt status?

NOTES

1. For an informative history of the for-profit healthcare industry, see *Columbia/HCA: Healthcare on Overdrive*, by Lutz and Gee (1998).

2. The charity care issue is not limited to hospitals. While physicians are typically not required or obligated to provide charity care, charity care provided by physicians has shown a steady decline over the last eight years, according to a 2006 study by the Center for Studying Health System Change. According the study, 68 percent of physicians provided free care in 2004–2005, down from 72 percent in 2001–2002

and 76 percent in 1996–1997. The amount of hours of free care provided was also substantially down, according to the study (Romano 2006).

RECOMMENDED READINGS—PART I

Berger, S. 2005. *The Power of Clinical and Financial Metrics: Achieving Success in Your Hospital.* Chicago: Health Administration Press.

———. 2003. *Understanding Nonprofit Financial Statements,* 2nd ed. Washington, DC: BoardSource.

Betbeze, P. 2011. "Nonprofit Hospitals: Will Margin Change Mean Mission Change?" *HealthLeaders.* Published June 13. www.healthleadersmedia.com/content/MAG-266991/Nonprofit-Hospitals-Will-Margin-Change-Mean-Mission-Change.html.

Congressional Budget Office (CBO). 2006. *Nonprofit Hospitals and the Provision of Community Benefits.* Washington, DC: CBO.

Eastaugh, S. R. 2004. *Health Care Finance and Economics.* Sudbury, MA: Jones and Bartlett.

Finkler, S. A., and D. M. Ward. 2006. *Accounting Fundamentals for Health Care Management.* Sudbury, MA: Jones and Bartlett.

Finkler, S. A., D. M. Ward, and J. J. Baker. 2007. *Essentials of Cost Accounting for Health Care Organizations,* 3rd ed. Sudbury, MA: Jones and Bartlett.

Foundation of the American College of Healthcare Executives. 2009. "Patient Handoffs: Effectively Managing Care Transitions." *Frontiers of Health Services Management* 25 (3).

———. 2008. "Managing Chronic Disease: Technology and Community Offer New Hope." *Frontiers of Health Services Management* 25 (2).

Gapenski, L. C. 2011. *Healthcare Finance: An Introduction to Accounting and Financial Management,* 5th ed. Chicago: Health Administration Press.

———. 2010. *Understanding Healthcare Financial Management,* 6th ed. Chicago: Health Administration Press.

Gray, B. H. (ed.). 1983. *The New Health Care for Profit: Doctors and Hospitals in a Competitive Environment.* Washington, DC: National Academies Press.

Hankins, R. W., and J. J. Baker. 2004. *Management Accounting for Healthcare Organizations.* Sudbury, MA: Jones and Bartlett.

Herzlinger, R. E., and D. Nitterhouse. 1994. *Financial Accounting and Managerial Control for Nonprofit Organizations.* Cincinnati, OH: South-Western Publishing.

Lutz, S., and E. P. Gee. 1998. *Columbia/HCA: Healthcare on Overdrive.* New York: McGraw-Hill.

Maiuro, L. S., H. Schneider, and N. Bellows. 2004. "Endangered Species? Not-For-Profit Hospitals Face Tax-Exemption Challenge." *Healthcare Financial Management* 58 (9): 74–84.

Morrison, E. E. 2009. *Ethics in Health Administration: A Practical Approach for Decision Makers,* 2nd ed. Sudbury, MA: Jones and Bartlett.

Nowicki, M. 2006. *HFMA's Introduction to Hospital Accounting,* 5th ed. Chicago: Health Administration Press.

PricewaterhouseCoopers. 2006. "My Brother's Keeper: Growing Expectations Confront Hospitals on Community Benefits and Charity Care." *Modern Healthcare* 36 (27, special supplement).

Somerville, M. H., Nelson, G. D., and Mueller, C. H. 2013. "Hospital Community Benefits after the ACA: The State Law Landscape." *The Hilltop Institute.* www.hilltopinstitute.org/publications/HospitalCommunityBenefitsAfterTheACA-StateLawLandscapeIssueBrief6-March2013.pdf.

Starr, P. 1982. *The Social Transformation of American Medicine.* New York: Basic Books.

Stevens, R. 1989. *In Sickness and in Wealth: American Hospitals in the Twentieth Century.* New York: Basic Books.

Thompson Powers, LLC. 1999. *The Politics of Exemption: Tax Revenue vs. Community Benefit—Not-For-Profit Hospitals Under Pressure.* Irving, TX: VHA.

Zelman, W. A. 1996. *The Changing Health Care Marketplace: Private Ventures, Public Interests.* San Francisco: Jossey-Bass Publishers.

Zelman, W. N., M. J. McCue, and N. D. Glick, and M.S. Thomas. 2014. *Financial Management of Health Care Organizations,* 4th ed. San Francisco: Jossey-Bass Publishers.

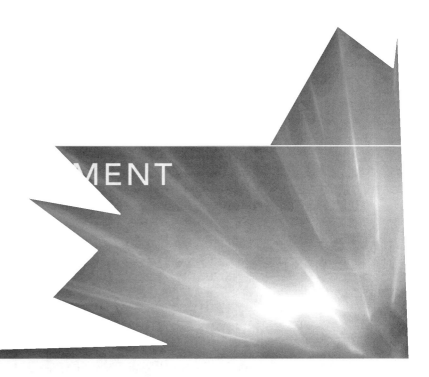

MENT

The most challenging situation that revenue cycle and finance departments are tackling right now is with their overall cost and charge structures relative to payer source agreements and reimbursements back to their organization. Healthcare organizations need to optimize their collection processes, to ensure they obtain every single dollar possible for services rendered, and they need a sound financial screening process for all patients entering their system.

Vince Schmitz, hospital senior vice president and chief
financial officer

LEARNING OBJECTIVES

After completing this chapter, you should be able to do the following:

➤ Review the history of third-party reimbursement

➤ Classify managed care organizations

➤ Examine new methods of financing and delivering healthcare

➤ Identify methods of payment, including bad debt and charity care

➤ Compute cost-shifting and cost-cutting problems

INTRODUCTION

Third-party payers are agents of patients who contract with providers (the second party) to pay all or a part of the bill to the patient (the first party). The most common third-party payers are insurance companies and the government (through Medicare and Medicaid). Third-party payers have had an important effect on healthcare organizations over the last 90 years. As mentioned in Chapter 1 and illustrated in Exhibit 4.1, third-party payment, including payments from the federal government, private insurance, and state and local government, will represent 79.8 percent of total personal healthcare expenditures in 2014 (CMS 2014).

HISTORY OF THIRD-PARTY PAYMENT

Third-party payment started in the 1920s, but not without significant opposition. Labor unions supported health insurance for their members as early as 1915, but their efforts failed as a result of opposition by the American Medical Association (AMA) and the anti-socialist mood of the country during and after World War I. Physicians were wary of approving a payment system that would change the **second-party payment** system—patients paying their own bills, rather than an insurance company paying the bills—already in place (see Exhibit 4.2).

The second-party payment system was economically efficient in that patients sought only the amount and quality of care they could afford. However, the second-party payment system created ethical concerns because some patients who needed care could not afford it, which prompted some employers to begin paying providers directly for the care received

second-party payment
Payment for healthcare that comes from the person receiving the service (i.e., patients paying their own bills).

EXHIBIT 4.1
Percentage of Total Healthcare Expenditures in the United States by Source of Funds, 2012, and Percentage of Total Health Insurance by Source of Funds, 2012

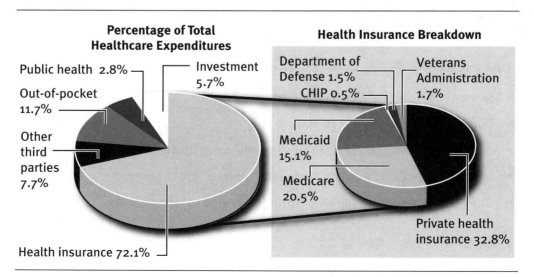

Source: CMS (2014).

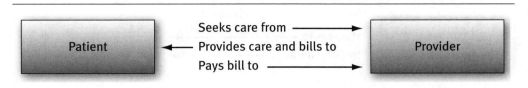

EXHIBIT 4.2
Second-Party
Payment

by their employees. The second-party system also created bad-debt concerns because some patients sought emergency care and could not afford to pay the bill after the care was provided. This concern prompted Baylor University Hospital in Dallas, Texas, to offer schoolteachers prepaid hospital care for $6 per year in 1929. In the next few years, several other hospitals offered similar arrangements to remain competitive with the Baylor plan, which later became the first Blue Cross plan. In 1933, Dr. Sidney Garfield began providing prepaid medical care to employees who worked on the California aqueduct system, and in 1938 he provided prepaid medical care to workers on the Grand Coulee Dam. Garfield's plan evolved into the Kaiser-Permanente health plan (Henry J. Kaiser was the employer who contracted with Dr. Garfield) (Starr 1982).

The Great Depression in the 1930s made it difficult for employers to pay providers directly for the care received by their employees and for hospitals like Baylor to accept the risk associated with offering prepaid plans. The AMA softened its position on voluntary health insurance during the mid-1930s, but the organization stipulated that hospital benefits (such as the charge for the hospital room) and medical benefits (such as the doctor's fee) be separate. For example, Blue Cross provided hospital benefits, and Blue Shield later provided medical benefits. The AMA remained adamantly opposed to **compulsory health insurance** and helped defeat proposals to include compulsory health insurance in President Roosevelt's Social Security Act in 1935.

DIRECT SERVICE PLANS

The defeat of compulsory health insurance in 1935 under President Roosevelt and again in the late 1940s under President Truman meant that health insurance in America would be largely voluntary and private. The early plans by Baylor University Hospital and Henry J. Kaiser were called **direct service plans** (employers prepaid specific hospitals and physicians to provide care to their employees) and were characteristic of most health insurance plans through the 1940s. Direct service plans were really an extension of second-party payment, in that the employer prepaid the provider on behalf of the employee (see Exhibit 4.3).

In the mid-1940s, plans called **commercial indemnity plans** allowed employers and/or employees to prepay an insurance company, which would reimburse a hospital or physician of the employee's choosing. These plans initiated the concept of the third party payer, because the insurance company was relatively independent from both the employer/employee and the provider (see Exhibit 4.4).

compulsory health insurance
A requirement that everyone have health insurance.

direct service plan
An arrangement whereby an employer prepays specific hospitals and physicians to take care of employees.

commercial indemnity plan
An arrangement whereby an employer pays an insurance company, which in turn reimburses hospitals and physicians chosen by the employees.

Exhibit 4.3
Direct Service
Plans

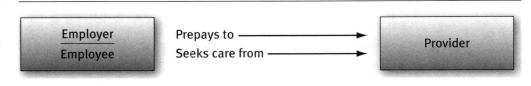

Exhibit 4.3
Direct Service
Plans

community rating
A premium-setting
method in which all
groups covered by an
insurance company pay
essentially the same
premiums, regardless
of their health risks.

Between 1945 and 1949, group commercial indemnity plans increased from 7.8 million subscribers to 17.7 million subscribers, and individual commercial indemnity plans increased to 14.7 million subscribers. By 1953, commercial insurance plans, which were for-profit, provided coverage to 29 percent of Americans. Blue Cross, which was a not-for-profit plan, provided coverage to 27 percent of Americans. Through the 1950s, use of commercial indemnity plans grew steadily, often at the expense of the less aggressive Blue Cross plans (Starr 1982).

Blue Cross typically set premiums using **community rating** (i.e., all groups paid essentially the same premium, resulting in low-risk groups subsidizing high-risk groups). Commercial insurance companies such as Prudential and Metropolitan, which had had significant histories in life insurance, set premiums using **experience rating** (i.e., groups paid different premiums based on their risk). Commercial insurance companies often solicited low-risk Blue Cross groups by offering lower premiums.

experience rating
A premium-setting
method in which
different groups
covered by an
insurance company
pay different premiums
based on their risk.

By the late 1950s, 66 percent of Americans had some form of health insurance; it was usually provided by the employer. Part of this increase is attributable to a 1954 Internal Revenue Service (IRS) tax ruling that confirmed that employers' contributions to health insurance plans were tax-exempt (Starr 1982). Medicare and Medicaid were introduced in 1966 (Medicare and Medicaid are discussed in more detail in Chapter 5); the percentage of covered Americans subsequently increased to 87 percent by 1968 (Harris 1975). Changes in federal Employee Retirement Income Security Act (ERISA) laws during the early 1980s allowed large employers to self-insure and gain the full benefit of any reductions in costs.

Exhibit 4.4
Commercial
Indemnity Plans

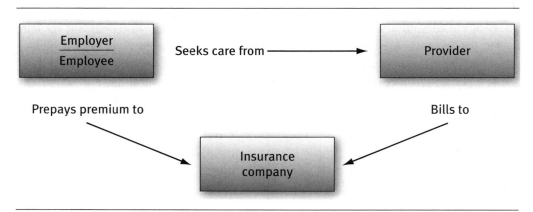

Some of these reductions were actually a transfer of costs to employees. With the Deficit Reduction Act of 1984, the federal government began limiting the amounts employers could deduct for health benefits. In 1987, the federal government began tracking healthcare spending by sponsor to determine the financial burdens placed on three sponsors: households, private businesses, and governments. In effect, most healthcare spending originates with these three sponsors. In the case of households, healthcare spending is composed of out-of-pocket spending (deductibles and co-pays), premiums (both private and public), and payroll taxes for public healthcare programs. In 2009, households paid for 29 percent of total healthcare spending and the trend has been decreasing. In 2009, private businesses paid for 21 percent of total healthcare spending and the trend has been decreasing. In 2009, governments paid for 44 percent of total healthcare spending and that trend has been increasing (CMS 2012).

While 18.5 percent of the total population was uninsured during the first half of 2009, there is wide variation by age, with 21 percent of those under 65 uninsured and 37 percent of those 19 to 24 uninsured (Roberts and Rhoades 2010).

managed care
organization
An organization that manages the cost and quality of and access to healthcare.

MANAGED CARE ORGANIZATIONS

Although the Baylor and Kaiser experiences with direct service plans were limited in the healthcare services they delivered, they were the first **managed care organizations** (MCOs). MCOs are organizations that manage the cost of healthcare, the quality of healthcare, and the access to healthcare. One way to classify MCOs is Kongstvedt's continuum (see Exhibit 4.5) (Kongstvedt 2013). At one end of the continuum is the commercial

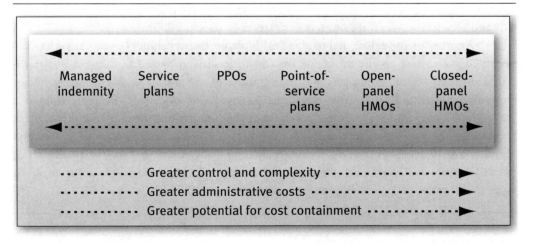

EXHIBIT 4.5
Managed Care
Continuum

Source: Adapted from Kongstvedt (2013).

indemnity plan, which requires precertification of elective admissions and case management of catastrophic illnesses.

Service plans, like the typical Blue Cross plans, add contractual relationships with providers that often include maximum fee schedules and prohibitions on balance billing (i.e., providers cannot bill the patient for amounts over the fee schedules agreed to with the service plan). **Preferred provider organizations** (PPOs) provide discounted provider services to insurance carriers and employers.

Providers usually agree to discount their prices in exchange for large volumes of patients. **Health maintenance organizations** (HMOs) integrate the financing and delivery of healthcare into one organization (see Exhibit 4.6). Financial risk, and opportunity, shifts from the employer/employee under the managed indemnity plans (i.e., the employer/employee pays for inappropriate use through increased premiums) to the HMOs (i.e., under prepayment, the HMO assumes the financial risk, and opportunity, for inappropriate use).

In response to a growing anti–managed care sentiment and in the face of possible legislation designed to hold managed care companies legally accountable for directly managing care through preadmission authorizations and utilization review, managed care companies like UnitedHealthcare are pursuing new methods to finance and deliver improved care while holding down costs. One method is evidence-based case management, where managed care companies partner with providers to determine the best, and thereby the most efficient, way to manage a case based on current evidence. For instance, in the late 1990s Anthem Blue Cross and Blue Shield collaborated with physicians and hospitals in Indiana, Ohio, and Kentucky and established a goal of administering ACE inhibitors to 60 percent of health plan members diagnosed with congestive heart failure. In Indiana hospitals from 1998 to 2001, the use of ACE inhibitors increased from 52 percent to 60 percent. Hospitals and physicians who met the targets were reimbursed more than hospitals and physicians who did not meet the targets (Nowicki 2003).

Another method designed to give health plan members choices in coverage that also seems to save money is the move toward consumer-driven plans. As the cost of healthcare continues to rise, employers are passing more of the cost to their employees or not providing healthcare at all. This economic phenomenon occurs at the same time as a demographic phenomenon—a large portion of the population, the baby boomers, are in their 60s and need more healthcare. Baby boomers are used to getting what they want and should have large amounts of discretionary income from inheritance to pay for what they want. Consumer-driven health plans allow consumers to select the coverage they need or want and pay the corresponding premiums (Millenson 2003).

preferred provider organization
An organization that provides discounted healthcare services to insurance carriers and employers.

health maintenance organization
An organization that integrates the financing and delivery of healthcare into one organization.

EXHIBIT 4.6
Health Maintenance Organizations

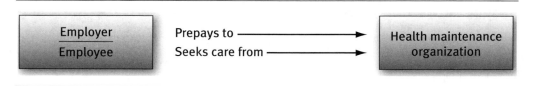

| Employer / Employee | Prepays to ⟶ Seeks care from ⟶ | Health maintenance organization |

Humana, one of the nation's largest health plans, may have been the first to try a consumer-driven plan with its own employees. Humana's chief executive officer, Michael McCallister, said "I'm a big believer that the most powerful player in understanding and managing costs is going to be the individual consumer. When people are spending their own money, given good and actionable information, they're going to do much better at controlling costs than the current model" (Rauber 2003a). From July 2001, when Humana replaced its traditional coverage with consumer-driven coverage for its Louisville-area employees and their dependents, through June 2002, Humana saved more than $2 million from its anticipated health benefits' costs.

To manage increased risk, MCOs contain costs with aggressive methods of controlling utilization that include carefully selecting subscribers and providers, providing physician incentives, and providing subscriber/employer incentives. Eastaugh (1992) reported that HMOs, the most aggressive form of MCOs, used 37 percent fewer hospital days (341 days per 1,000 enrolled) for their nonelderly enrolled populations than commercial indemnity plans, which used 542 days per 1,000 enrolled.

Historically, MCOs have been classified on the basis of the degree of control they have over their physician providers. Point-of-service (POS) plans are MCOs that exert minimum to no control over their physician providers because they allow enrollees to seek care from providers not on contract with the POS plans (i.e., out of network). Although POS plans reimburse the provider's fees, the POS plan usually requires the enrollee to pay out-of-network providers larger deductibles and coinsurance, as well as higher premiums to the POS plan, for the privilege of going out of network.

In 2013 Kaiser Family Foundation reported that POS plans represent about 9 percent of all covered workers while PPOs represent the majority of covered workers, 57 percent. About 14 percent of the employed population chose HMOs, 20 percent were covered by high-deductible health plans, and less than 1 percent chose conventional indemnity plans (Kaiser Family Foundation 2013a).

HMOs

Open-Panel HMOs

Open-panel HMOs exert moderate control over physician providers; they contract with physicians to provide care for enrollees in the physicians' offices. Open-panel HMOs include the direct-contract model and the independent practice association (IPA) model. Direct-contract HMOs contract with individual physicians to provide care, and IPAs contract with associations of physicians. Member physicians are not employees of the association. IPAs may be previously existing associations of physicians that contract with multiple HMOs, or the HMO may organize the association to provide physician services. In either model, as well as in the direct-contract model, physicians see their own patients and HMO patients. The open-panel HMO reimburses the physicians either on a fee-for-service basis, often with a discount, or by capitation (Kongstvedt 2013).

open-panel HMO
An HMO that exerts moderate control over physicians by contracting with them to provide care for enrollees. However, these physicians can see other patients.

Closed-Panel HMOs

Closed-panel HMOs exert maximum control over physician providers because the HMO contracts with or employs physicians to provide care for enrollees on an exclusive basis. Closed-panel HMOs include the group model and the staff model. Group-model HMOs contract with a multispecialty group of physicians to provide all physician care to enrollees, typically on capitation. In the group-model HMO, physicians are employed by the group, not the HMO. Staff-model HMOs employ individual physicians to provide all physician care to enrollees; primary care physicians are always employed, and some specialty and subspecialty physicians may actually be on contract. Closed-panel HMOs provide incentive payments to physician providers based on performance (Kongstvedt 2013).

Network HMOs

Network HMOs exert moderate to maximum control over physician providers because they contract with physician groups to provide care for enrollees. Network HMOs may be either open panel or closed panel. Typically, the network HMO relies on groups of primary care physicians and reimburses the groups on capitation. The primary care groups are often responsible for referring and reimbursing referrals to specialty physicians (Kongstvedt 2013).

Post–Managed Care

When the managed care industry had a tough few years in the late 1990s—with declining enrollments, poor public relations, and threatened anti–managed care legislation—many were predicting managed care's demise (Clarke 2000). The managed care industry adjusted with a "softer image" and more popular methods of controlling costs. Managed care continues to be a reliable method for payers, including employers and the government, to control healthcare costs. However, employers and the government continue to investigate new ways to control costs, such as defined-contribution plans, direct contracting, a more generous interpretation of consumer-driven plans than previously mentioned, and national health insurance. Depending on the configuration, these new ways of controlling healthcare costs might be considered under the managed care umbrella of products.

Defined-Contribution Plans

Employers—faced with the reality that employees who experience no personal economic consequences regarding healthcare spending will want, but not necessarily need, more healthcare and higher-quality healthcare—are turning from **defined-benefit plans** to **defined-contribution plans**. Under defined-benefit plans, the employee receives a defined-benefit package, and the employer/employee pays the premium, which is adjusted each year based on experience. Employers have absorbed large, unpredictable premium increases

closed-panel HMO
An HMO that contracts with or employs physicians to treat enrollees exclusively (i.e., the physicians do not treat other patients).

network HMO
An HMO that contracts with physician groups to provide care for enrollees. A network HMO may be either open or closed panel.

defined-benefit plan
A health plan in which the employer pays the premium, or an established part of the premium, regardless of the cost.

defined-contribution plan
A health plan in which the employer pays a set amount toward the cost of the premium and the employee pays the rest. Thus if an employee chooses an expensive plan, he pays more than if he chose a less expensive plan.

for several years under these plans. Under defined-contribution plans, employees typically choose from a variety of healthcare options, with a specified amount of the premium paid for by the employer. Any healthcare costs above this amount are paid for by the employee. Defined-contribution plans shift more of the financial responsibility to the employee, who becomes more aware of utilization and price as a result (Emery 2001).

DIRECT CONTRACTING

Direct contracting is when large employers contract directly with integrated delivery systems or systems of healthcare providers capable of accepting a financial risk and delivering a full range of healthcare services. Direct contracting reduces the administrative costs of insuring employees, since the third-party insurer is cut out of the deal. Direct contracting also stimulates competition between integrated delivery systems and encourages local control and innovation (Burrows and Moravec 1997).

CONSUMER-DRIVEN PLANS

Consumer-driven health is a movement that includes empowering healthcare consumers with control, choice, and information (Herzlinger 2004). **Consumer-driven plans** help individuals wisely choose their healthcare providers, and financial incentives encourage them to request only the appropriate amount of healthcare services. Consumer-driven plans come in two primary models: spending-account models and tiered models. Spending-account models include some type of health reimbursement account, such as a health savings account, which provides consumers a fund to spend on healthcare expenditures. Once a consumer has depleted the account, and for some expenses not eligible to be reimbursed from the account, a high-deductible PPO-style plan kicks in. Tiered models allow the consumer to customize cost-sharing parameters, such as the amounts of deductible and coinsurance, with commensurate adjustments to the amount of premiums paid by the consumer (Rosenthal, Hsuan, and Millstein 2005).

Many consumer-driven plans, whether they are spending-account or tiered models, are now categorized as high-deductible health plans. These are the fastest growing plans on the market,

direct contracting
The practice of contracting directly with an integrated health organization to service the health needs of a large employer.

consumer-driven plan
A health plan that provides information and incentives to encourage enrollees to make wise healthcare choices.

As the new benefits manager at Riley Industries, you have decided to implement a high-deductible health plan (HDHP) for the employees. You have heard that HDHPs have many benefits, such as substantial cost savings resulting from employees taking charge of their health. You have also heard there are disadvantages. For instance, employees are unaware of how to manage these plans. How should you educate the employees of Riley Industries on HDHPs? What if the employees want to keep their previous insurance plans instead? Discuss the other advantages of HDHPs to both the employer and the employees, including how employees are able to promote better health through these plans. Name some other disadvantages of the plans, including the inability to save for possible deductible costs. What is your opinion on companies moving toward HDHPs?

increasing from 4 percent of all managed care enrollees in 2006 to 20 percent of all managed care enrollees in 2013 (Kaiser Family Foundation 2013a).

STATE HEALTHCARE REFORM

As healthcare is increasingly viewed as a social good and right, businesses and states are looking to the federal government to provide for that right under some type of national health insurance. Some businesses see national health insurance funded by taxes as a more equitable way of financing and a more comprehensive way of delivering healthcare than the current method of voluntary coverage provided by employers. Businesses are hoping that spreading the tax burden for national health insurance would result in their tax increases being less than their healthcare costs now, which would make American business more competitive in an increasingly global economy (Salb 2008). However, other businesses see national health insurance as too expensive and lacking appropriate cost controls (US Chamber of Commerce 2010). While the US Chamber of Commerce admits that the ACA is here to stay, it continues to fight the employer mandate as too expensive for small businesses and the additional taxes mandated by ACA as unaffordable (Zigmond 2014).

At the same time, state governments are concerned about their increasing Medicaid costs and about providing healthcare to uninsured people who are not eligible for Medicaid. Massachusetts passed legislation in 2006 to address some of these concerns. The Massachusetts law includes the following:

◆ Individuals are required to carry health insurance, or face an annual fine of $1,069.

◆ Employers with 11 or more employees must provide health insurance coverage for their employees, or face fines of $295 per year per employee (in 2013 the fines were on a sliding scale based on income and age and range from $240 to $1,272 per year).

◆ Eligibility for Medicaid and the State Children's Health Insurance Program (SCHIP) was expanded to include families who earn 150 percent of the amount designated as the poverty level.

◆ Families earning between 150 percent and 300 percent of the poverty level can purchase subsidized insurance.

◆ Individuals earning above 300 percent of the poverty level and small businesses can purchase insurance at group rates.

By 2010, the percent uninsured in Massachusetts had dropped to 6.3 from 10.9 in 2006. However, the deliberate absence of cost controls imposed by the state has resulted in per capita health spending that is 15 percent higher than the national average (Kaiser Family Foundation 2012a).

NATIONAL HEALTHCARE REFORM

In March 2010, President Obama signed into law the Patient Protection and Affordable Care Act (ACA) and the Health Care and Education Reconciliation Act (HCERA), which made important modifications to the ACA (for a detailed analysis of the law by each of its nine titles, go to dpc.senate.gov/healthreformbill/healthbill04.pdf, and for a detailed analysis of the law by subject area, go to www.kff.org/health-reform/). The law followed a century of debate on universal healthcare coverage and months of legislative maneuvering by Democrats and Republicans.

The ACA is intended to provide insurance coverage to 32 million Americans who otherwise would be uninsured, leaving about 6 percent of the nation uninsured. The original cost estimate for the act is $940 billion over ten years; however, the Congressional Budget Office (CBO) estimates the laws will reduce the federal deficit by $143 billion over the same time period (CBO 2010) (2013 CBO estimates put the ten-year cost at $1.363 trillion). While a more detailed analysis of the reform laws is provided in Chapter 5 and Chapter 15, the Kaiser Family Foundation (2013b) has provided the following analysis of the reform law's impact on third-party reimbursement:

◆ *Insurance reform* (intended to provide insurance coverage to more citizens):

  ○ In 2010, seven provisions include providing programs to insure people with pre-existing conditions; requiring coverage for adult dependents on parent's policies to age 26; prohibiting insurance plans from lifetime limits on benefits; guaranteeing an appeals process in new insurance plans; creating a temporary reinsurance program for employers providing coverage for retirees over 55 who are not yet eligible for Medicare; requiring HHS to develop a website for consumers; and requiring insurance plans to provide certain preventive services without deductibles or co-pays.

  ○ In 2011, two provisions include requiring insurance plans to provide rebates to consumers if the proportion of premiums spent on clinical services is less than 85 percent in large group markets and 80 percent in individual and small group markets; and providing grants to states to establish insurance exchanges to be operational in 2013.

  ○ In 2012, one provision includes requiring insurance plans to provide to consumers a uniform benefit summary to help consumers compare health plans.

○ In 2013, three provisions include requiring states to notify the secretary of the Department of Health and Human Services of their intent to develop an insurance exchange or to rely on the federal insurance exchange; creating the Co-Op Health Insurance Plan to help develop nonprofit and member-run insurance plans; and authorizing and funding the Children's Health Insurance Program (CHIP) through 2015.

○ In 2014, 12 provisions were required, including: requiring US citizens and legal residents to obtain qualifying health insurance; creating state-based American Health Benefit Exchanges to provide affordable insurance coverage to individuals and small businesses with fewer than 100 employees; providing tax credits and cost-sharing subsidies to eligible individuals with incomes from 133 percent to 400 percent of the federal poverty level; guaranteeing the issue and renewal of health insurance regardless of health status with the following justifications for differences in insurance rates: age, geographic area, family composition, and tobacco use; creating an essential health benefits package that limits cost-sharing to $6,350 for individuals and $12,700 for families and identifying four types of plans offered through the exchanges: bronze, silver, gold, and platinum; fining employers with more than 50 employees who do not offer health insurance ($2,000 per employee, excluding the first 30 employees)(this provision was delayed until 2015); permitting employers to offer employees incentives up to 30 percent of the total cost of coverage for participating in wellness programs and meeting certain health-related standards; permitting employers to offer rewards for employees participating in wellness programs; and expanding Medicaid eligibility in many states (this provision was required in the original law, but was struck down by the Supreme Court in 2011—the federal government responded by agreeing to absorb all of the state's costs related to expanding Medicaid eligibility to 138 percent of the federal poverty level for seven years, and 75 to 90 percent of the of the state's costs with the expansion for three years more).

○ In 2015, there are no provisions.

○ In 2016, one provision includes allowing states to develop healthcare choice compacts that would allow insurers to sell policies in any state participating in the compact.

◆ *Payment and revenue reform* (intended to reduce the rate of increase in Medicare and Medicaid spending):

○ In 2010, three provisions include reducing Medicare annual updates for inpatient and outpatient hospital services, long-term care hospitals, inpatient rehab facilities, and psychiatric hospitals and adjusting payment for productivity; providing Medicare beneficiaries with rebates to cover the "donut hole" in Part D (outpatient prescription drug) coverage; and establishing the Federal Coordinated Health Care Office to improve coordination of care for dual eligibles (beneficiaries eligible for both Medicare and Medicaid).

○ In 2011, seven provisions include requiring pharmaceutical companies to provide a 50 percent discount on brand-name prescriptions filled under Medicare Part D and beginning federal subsidies for generic prescriptions under Part D; providing a 10 percent bonus in Medicare payment to providers for primary care services and general surgeons practicing in health professional shortage areas; eliminating cost sharing for Medicare-provided preventive services; creating the Center for Medicare and Medicaid Innovation to test new payment and delivery system models; freezing income threshold for Medicare Part B premiums resulting in higher Part B premiums for beneficiaries with higher incomes; restructuring payments to private Medicare Advantage plans and limiting cost-sharing opportunities for private plans; and authorizing a Medicare Independent Payment Advisory Board to submit legislative proposals to reduce per capita rate of growth in Medicare spending if spending exceeds targeting growth rates (note: Medicare spending has not exceeded the targeted growth rates through 2013).

○ In 2012, seven provisions include allowing providers to organize as accountable care organizations (ACOs) that meet quality standards and share Medicare savings that result; reducing rebates for Medicare Advantage Plans while providing bonus payments to high-quality plans; creating the Medicare Independence at Home demonstration program to provide high-need Medicare beneficiaries with primary care services provided in their home under the direction of physicians or nurse-practitioners; adding a productivity adjustment to the market basket update for certain providers; establishing a value-based purchasing program for hospital payment based on performance on quality measures with plans to extend value-based purchasing to skilled nursing facilities, home health care agencies, and ambulatory surgical centers; establishing procedures for screening, oversight, and reporting for providers in order to avoid Medicare fraud and abuse; and reducing Medicare payments to hospitals with excessive and preventable hospital readmissions.

○ In 2013, four provisions include establishing a national Medicare pilot program to develop and evaluate making bundled payments for acute, inpatient hospital services, physician services, outpatient hospital services, and post–acute care services for an episode of care; increasing the Medicare Part A tax rate on wages from 1.45 percent to 2.35 percent on earnings over $200,000 for individual taxpayers and $250,000 for married couples filing jointly, and imposing a 3.8 percent assessment on unearned income for higher-income taxpayers; eliminating the tax deduction for employers; and reducing Medicare Disproportionate Share Hospital payments by 75 percent and then increasing payments based on the percent of the population uninsured and the amount of uncompensated care provided.

❍ In 2014, two provisions include requiring Medicare Advantage Plans to have medical loss ratios no lower than 85 percent, and reducing Medicare payments by 1 percent to hospitals with hospital-acquired infections.

❍ In 2015, one provision includes an increase in the federal match for CHIP.

❍ In 2016, one provision includes the development of health insurance compacts allowing insurance companies to sell insurance in any state participating in the compact.

❍ No provisions in 2017.

❍ In 2018, one provision includes an excise tax on insurers of employer-sponsored plans with aggregate expenses that exceed $10,200 for individual coverage and $27,500 for family coverage.

METHODS OF PAYMENT

Third parties and patients use a variety of methods to pay providers for healthcare services. Methods of payment to healthcare organizations and other providers can be classified according to the amount of financial risk assumed by the healthcare organization.

CHARGES

charge
The amount patients are charged for services; also called *prices* or *rates*.

Every healthcare organization has a list of **charges** (also called prices or rates) for care provided to patients. The organization may set charges based on the care provided; several other methods of setting charges are discussed in Chapter 7. If the healthcare organization sets charges correctly, and if the third party or patient pays the charges, the organization assumes no financial risk—it provides the service, it gets paid. Using set charges as the method of payment provides no financial incentive for the healthcare organization to provide only what is medically appropriate.

CHARGES MINUS A DISCOUNT

Healthcare organizations sometimes offer discounted charges to third parties. For example, if an insurance company provides a large volume of patients to a healthcare provider, the provider may reward the insurer with a discount. If the healthcare organization does not discount its charges below its costs, it assumes little financial risk with this arrangement. As with charges, a healthcare organization that offers charges minus a discount has little financial incentive to provide only care that is medically appropriate.

COST

In the "cost" form of payment, healthcare organizations receive the cost for care provided to the patients of third-party payers, plus a small percentage that allows the organization to develop new services and products. Typically, the healthcare organization bills charges to the third party, which reimburses the organization for the projected cost, often expressed as a percentage of the charges. At the end of the year, the third party audits the healthcare organization to determine actual cost and adjusts accordingly what it has reimbursed to the organization. In this system, no incentive exists for the healthcare organization to contain costs. If the third party recognizes and approves the costs of the organization, the organization assumes little financial risk accepting this method of payment. However, in many cases, the third-party payers do not recognize the full costs incurred by healthcare organizations. As a result, organizations that accept the "cost" form of payment do assume some financial risk for the patient and must pass on losses to other third parties and patients who pay more than cost (usually those paying charges and discounts from charges).

PER DIEM

In this payment system, healthcare organizations receive a per-day reimbursement for care provided to the patients of third-party payers. Because the third-party payer sets the per diem rate prospectively, or prior to the provision of care, per diem provides financial risks and financial incentives to the healthcare organization. If the organization provides care for a cost greater than the per diem rate, the organization loses money. If it provides care for a cost less than the **per diem rate**, the organization makes money. However, if the healthcare organization unnecessarily extends lengths of stay, and the third-party payer does not protest, the provider can make more money than it is truly entitled to. Because per diem rates are generally the same for each day of a stay, this method of reimbursement assumes that costs are the same for each day. This assumption is true for many extended care organizations, but not for acute care organizations. In acute care organizations, the patient usually incurs a greater proportion of the costs during the early days of the admission.

per diem rate
A method of paying for healthcare in which the hospital is paid a flat fee per day, regardless of the service delivered on any given day.

PER DIAGNOSIS

per diagnosis rate
A method of paying for healthcare in which the hospital is paid a flat fee for each given diagnosis, regardless of the actual service provided.

Healthcare organizations using this system receive reimbursement from the third-party payer based on the diagnosis of the patient. The **per diagnosis rate** provides financial risks and financial incentives for the healthcare organization. The better the organization controls costs, the more profit it makes. However, there is no way an organization can "pad the bill" the way it can in a per diem system (by extending the length of stay), since the third-party payer is reimbursing per the diagnosis instead of per day.

CAPITATION

Under capitation, healthcare organizations receive a fixed amount of money each month for every person enrolled in the plan, regardless of whether or not a given person receives care. Capitation as a payment method provides the most financial risk and opportunity to the healthcare organization because the fixed amount is based on the cost of care projected to be used by the covered population, rather than the cost of care actually used. If the costs to care for the covered population fall below the capitated amount, the healthcare organization makes money. If the costs exceed the capitated amount, the organization does not profit. The other payment methods mentioned previously provide financial incentives to healthcare organizations to contain costs *after* the patient seeks care, primarily by controlling use, but capitation also provides financial incentives to healthcare organizations to contain costs *before* the patient seeks care, primarily by encouraging prevention. Third-party payers and healthcare organizations negotiate capitated payments, often called premiums, based on their perceptions of the actuarial experience of the covered population. Whether the healthcare organization realizes a profit or incurs a loss depends on its ability to project demand for care by the covered population and negotiate the appropriate capitation, and then to contain costs when a member of the enrolled population—a subscriber—seeks care.

BAD DEBT AND CHARITY CARE

Although they are not methods of third-party payment, bad debt and charity care are important concepts to discuss in this context because the amounts are substantial in healthcare organizations.

BAD DEBT

bad debt
A healthcare organization's unpaid patient bills.

Bad debt refers to unpaid healthcare bills. Healthcare organizations that use accrual accounting incur bad debt expense when they receive no payment or partial payment on an invoice and then write off all or part of the account. The *AICPA Audit and Accounting Guide for Health Care Entities* (2010) requires that healthcare organizations report bad debt expense as an operating expense based on charges, not costs. While reporting charges overstates the value of bad debt, hospitals can uniformly report charges for bad debt, whereas hospitals would have some difficulty reporting costs for bad debt because of the variety of ways to determine cost. The *AICPA Audit and Accounting Guide for Health Care Entities* (2012, p. 170) requires that a

> health care entity that recognizes significant amounts of patient services revenue at the time the services are rendered even though it does not assess the patient's ability to pay should present all of the following as separate line items on the face of the statement of operations:
>
> a. Patient services revenue (net of contractual allowances and discounts)
> b. The provision for bad debts (the amount related to patient services revenue and included as a deduction from patient services revenue)
> c. The resulting net patient services revenue less the provision for bad debts

Charity Care

Healthcare organizations incur **charity care** expense when they provide care to patients who they know are unable to pay. *The AICPA Audit and Accounting Guide for Health Care Organizations* (2010) requires that healthcare organizations not report charity care as revenue, a deduction from revenue, or an operating expense. Rather, it requires that healthcare organizations report the level of charity care (at full cost) in a note to the statement of operations in the annual report, along with the organization's policy for providing charity care and the method used to determine cost.

charity care
Care provided to patients who the organization knows cannot pay for the care.

Uncompensated Care

According to American Hospital Association (AHA) data for 2012 (see Exhibit 4.7), hospital spending for uncompensated care, which is the total of bad debt and charity care,

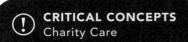

CRITICAL CONCEPTS
Charity Care

You are the CEO of Kind Heart Hospital, which is located in a low-income area and has spent millions of dollars over the years on charity care patients. Unfortunately, this has placed your hospital in a tough financial position, because Medicare and Medicaid continue to reduce reimbursements for their patients and your percentage of commercial insurance patients (or patients who pay more than your cost) continues to decline. Discuss what you can do to continue to provide care to the needy but reduce the amount of the loss. Will national health reform laws help your reimbursement or hurt it?

EXHIBIT 4.7
Uncompensated
Hospital Care and
Medicare and
Medicaid Losses

Year	Uncompensated Care (in billions)	Percentage of Total Expenses	Medicare Loss (in billions)	Medicaid Loss (in billions)
1997	$18.5	6.0		
1998	$19.0	6.0		
1999	$20.7	6.2		
2000	$21.6	6.0		
2001	$21.5	5.6		
2002	$22.3	5.4		
2003	$24.9	5.5		
2004	$26.9	5.6		
2005	$28.8	5.6	$15.5	$9.8
2006	$31.2	5.7	$18.6	$11.3
2007	$34.0	5.8	$21.5	$10.4
2008	$36.4	5.8	$22.0	$10.4
2009	$39.1	6.0	$25.2	$11.3
2010	$39.3	5.8	$20.1	$7.8
2011	$41.1	5.9	$23.8	$6.0
2012	$45.9	6.1	$42.3	$13.7

Source: American Hospital Association (AHA). 2013. *TrendWatch Chartbook 2012: Trends Affecting Hospitals and Health Systems, March 2013.* Chapter 4. www.aha.org/aha/research/reports/tw/chartbook/ch4.shtml.

continued to climb from its low point in 2002. Uncompensated hospital care was $39.1 billion in 2009 and represented 6.0 percent of hospital total expenses (AHA 2011). A relatively strong economy before the 9/11 attacks and the relative success of public programs such as SCHIP were likely reasons for the decrease beginning in 2001. Hospitals often attempt to shift these costs to paying patients through increased charges. To the extent they cannot shift these costs, hospitals cut costs in other areas.

cost shifting
The practice of shifting costs to some payers to offset losses from other payers.

COST SHIFTING

Cost shifting is the practice of shifting costs to some payers to offset losses from other payers. It occurs in every industry, usually to offset losses from bad debt. Evidence of cost shifting in healthcare is based on the fact that different payers pay different prices (charges minus a negotiated discount) for similar services. For instance, in 2012 Medicaid paid an average of 89 percent of the hospital's costs for caring for Medicaid patients, Medicare paid an average of 86 percent of the hospital's costs for caring for Medicare patients, while private payers paid an average of 135 percent of the hospital's costs for caring for private-pay patients. Employers believe that cost shifting is unfair, and the elimination of cost shifting is the primary reason that large employers favor an "all payer" system where each payer pays the same price for similar services (American Hospital Association 2014).

Recent evidence provided in Exhibit 4.8 shows that cost shifting was on the decline in the late 1990s as healthcare organizations lowered their costs in response to the Balanced Budget Act of 1997 and as competition lowered prices to private payers, thus making it more difficult for healthcare organizations to shift large losses to private payers. However, in the early 2000s, as Medicare margins declined for hospitals, cost shifting increased again, as shown in the most recent years in Exhibit 4.8.

Exhibit 4.9 demonstrates the impact of the cost shift in what is described as the cost-shift payment hydraulic for the average hospital. As payments for Medicare, Medicaid, other government programs, and uncompensated care decrease below cost, the charges to private payers (including patients not covered by insurance) must increase to avoid a loss to the hospital. The amount of the increase to private payers is a function of not only the below-cost reimbursement the hospital receives from certain payers, but also the amount of payers available and the amount of operating margin desired by the hospital.

In the event that hospitals cannot shift the costs of uncompensated care and government program losses to private payers because the private payers either refuse to pay increased charges (by using competitors instead) or because the private payers refuse to pay for costs unrelated to their patients, the hospital must cut costs. Problem 4.1 demonstrates cost shifting first and then cost cutting. The following problems project how much cost

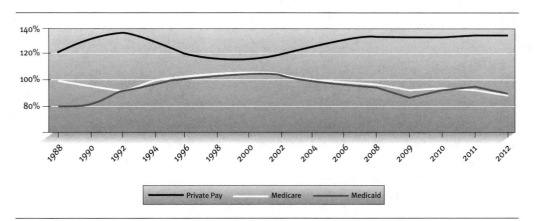

Exhibit 4.8

Aggregate Hospital Payment-to-Cost Ratios for Private Payers, Medicare, and Medicaid, 1988–2012

Source: American Hospital Association (AHA). 2013. *TrendWatch Chartbook 2013: Trends Affecting Hospitals and Health Systems, March 2013.* Chapter 4. www.aha.org/research/reports/tw/chartbook/ch4.shtml.

EXHIBIT **4.9**
Cost-Shift Payment
Hydraulic, 2012

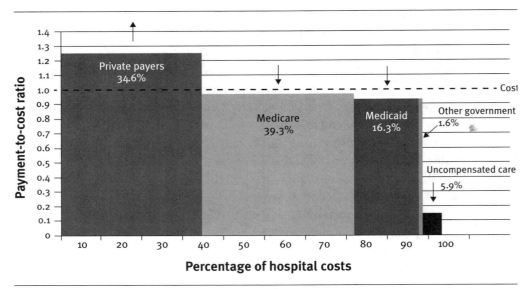

Source: Adapted from Dobson, A., J. DaVanzo, and S. Namrata. 2006. "The Cost-Shift Payment 'Hydraulic':
Foundation, History, and Implications." *Health Affairs* 25 (1): 22–23.

must be shifted or cut. The actual shifting takes place in the pricing of the products and services that make up a patient day and will be discussed in Chapter 7 on setting charges (see Appendix 7.1, Cost-Shift Pricing).

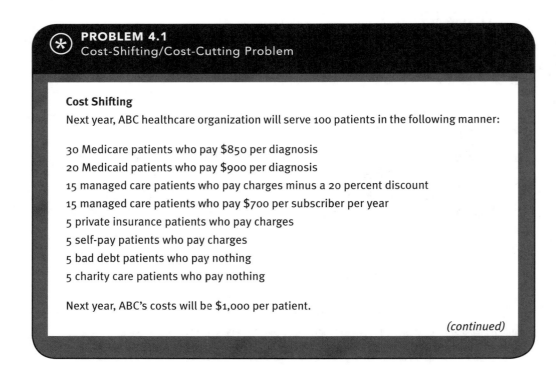

PROBLEM 4.1
Cost-Shifting/Cost-Cutting Problem

Cost Shifting

Next year, ABC healthcare organization will serve 100 patients in the following manner:

30 Medicare patients who pay $850 per diagnosis
20 Medicaid patients who pay $900 per diagnosis
15 managed care patients who pay charges minus a 20 percent discount
15 managed care patients who pay $700 per subscriber per year
5 private insurance patients who pay charges
5 self-pay patients who pay charges
5 bad debt patients who pay nothing
5 charity care patients who pay nothing

Next year, ABC's costs will be $1,000 per patient.

(continued)

PROBLEM 4.1
Cost-Shifting/Cost-Cutting Problem

Calculate the charge necessary to recover ABC's cost (called cost-led pricing).

Step 1:
Calculate the total projected loss by assuming the charge per patient equals the cost per patient.

Financial Class	No.	Costs	Charges	Collections	Profit
Medicare	30	30,000	30,000	25,500	−4,500
Medicaid	20	20,000	20,000	18,000	−2,000
Managed care #1	15	15,000	15,000	12,000	−3,000
Managed care #2	15	15,000	15,000	10,500	−4,500
Private	5	5,000	5,000	5,000	0
Self-pay	5	5,000	5,000	5,000	0
Bad debt	5	5,000	5,000	0	−5,000
Charity	5	5,000	5,000	0	−5,000
Total	100	100,000	100,000	76,000	−24,000

Step 2:
Calculate the charge necessary to recover ABC's cost by dividing the loss by the number of patients who will pay an increased charge, or portion thereof, and then add the cost per patient to the answer.

$$\frac{24,000}{15(.80) + 5 + 5 + 1,000} = \$2,091$$

Step 3:
Check the answer by calculating the loss using the new charge.

Financial Class	No.	Costs	Charges	Collections	Profit
Medicare	30	30,000	62,730	25,500	−4,500
Medicaid	20	20,000	41,820	18,000	−2,000
MC #1	15	15,000	31,365	25,092	10,092

(continued)

PROBLEM 4.1
Cost-Shifting/Cost-Cutting Problem

MC #2	15	15,000	31,365	10,500	−4,500
Private	5	5,000	10,455	10,455	5,455
Self-pay	5	5,000	10,455	10,455	5,455
Bad debt	5	5,000	10,455	0	−5,000
Charity	5	5,000	10,455	0	−5,000
Total	100	100,000	209,100	100,002	2

Note: The table produced in Step 3 can also be used to calculate contractual allowances (charges minus collections) for Medicare, Medicaid, and managed care. The total profit should be zero; "2" is due to a rounding error.

Cost Cutting

For the previously referenced cost-shifting problem, assume that those payers that pay charges, or charges minus a discount, limit ABC's charges to $1,070 per patient. Calculate the amount of costs that ABC will need to cut, or cover with additional revenues, to break even (i.e., realize no profit or loss).

Step 1:
Calculate the total costs to be cut by using the new charge per patient to determine profit/loss.

Financial Class	No.	Costs	Charges	Collections	Profit
Medicare	30	30,000	32,100	25,500	−4,500
Medicaid	20	20,000	21,400	18,000	−2,000
MC #1	15	15,000	16,050	12,840	−2,160
MC #2	15	15,000	16,050	10,500	−4,500
Private	5	5,000	5,350	5,350	350
Self-pay	5	5,000	5,350	5,350	350
Bad debt	5	5,000	5,350	0	−5,000
Charity	5	5,000	5,350	0	−5,000
Total	100	100,000	107,000	77,540	−22,460

(continued)

PROBLEM 4.1
Cost-Shifting/Cost-Cutting Problem

Step 2:

Step 1 showed that the hospital needs to cut $22,460 in order to break even. This can be accomplished by reducing the total patient costs to the total amount collected, $77,540. Calculate a new cost per patient day by dividing the total amount collected by the number of patients, 100. That calculation results in $775.40. Check the answer by calculating the profit/loss using the new cost per patient.

Financial Class	No.	Costs	Charges	Collections	Profit
Medicare	30	23,262	32,100	25,500	2,238
Medicaid	20	15,508	21,400	18,000	2,492
MC #1	15	11,631	16,050	12,840	1,209
MC #2	15	11,631	16,050	10,500	−1,131
Private	5	3,877	5,350	5,350	1,473
Self-pay	5	3,877	5,350	5,350	1,473
Bad debt	5	3,877	5,350	0	−3,877
Charity	5	3,877	5,350	0	−3,877
Total	100	77,540	107,000	77,540	0

CHAPTER KEY POINTS

➤ Third-party payments come from federal, state, and local government programs and private insurance.

➤ Blue Cross was the first pre-paid health insurance plan.

➤ Managed care organizations control costs and monitor quality and access to healthcare.

➤ HMOs allow for integration of the finance and delivery of healthcare.

➤ Other developments that help control healthcare costs are defined-contribution plans, direct contracting, consumer-driven plans, and state and national health insurance plans.

➤ Third parties and patients pay (or do not pay) providers in a variety of ways, including charges, cost, per diem, bad debt, and charity care.

➤ Cost shifting allows providers to offset losses from certain payers by charging other payers more.

DISCUSSION QUESTIONS

1. Discuss the differences between second-party payment and third-party payment. What led to the creation of the third-party payment system?

2. Which groups were considered the first managed care organizations? Distinguish between a managed care organization, preferred provider organization, and health maintenance organization.

3. Why did employers prefer managed care organizations? How have MCOs changed over the years?

4. Name some of the differences between open-panel HMOs and closed-panel HMOs.

5. What are the benefits to the employer of a defined-contribution plan?

6. Explain the two models of consumer-driven plans: spending account models and tiered models.

7. What are the different forms of payment to providers?

8. Why do organizations choose to shift costs to other payers?

Cost Shifting/Cost Cutting

Cost-Shifting Practice Problem

Next year, XYZ Healthcare Organization will serve 100 patients analyzed in the following manner:

20 Medicare patients, who pay $950 per diagnosis
30 Medicaid patients, who pay $900 per diagnosis
25 managed care patients, who pay charges minus a 15% discount
10 managed care patients, who pay charges minus a 25% discount
5 private insurance patients, who pay charges
5 charity care patients, who pay nothing
5 bad debt patients, who pay nothing

Next year, XYZ's costs will be $1,000 per patient. Calculate the charge necessary to recover XYZ's cost.

Cost-Shifting Practice Problem Solution

Step 1: Calculate the total projected loss by assuming the charge per patient equals the cost per patient.

Payer	No.	Costs ($)	Charges ($)	Collections ($)	Profit ($)
Medicare	20	20,000	20,000	19,000	–1,000
Medicaid	30	30,000	30,000	27,000	–3,000
MC #1	25	25,000	25,000	21,250	–3,750
MC #2	10	10,000	10,000	7,500	–2,500
Private insurance	5	5,000	5,000	5,000	0
Charity	5	5,000	5,000	0	–5,000
Bad debt	5	5,000	5,000	0	–5,000
Total	100	100,000	100,000	79,750	–20,250

Step 2: Calculate the charge necessary to recover XYZ's cost by dividing the loss by the number of patients who will pay an increased charge, or portion thereof, and then add the cost per patient to the answer.

$$\frac{\$20,250}{25(.85) + 10(.75) + 5} + \$1,000 = \$1,600$$

Step 3: Check the answer by calculating the profit/loss using the new charge.

Payer	No.	Costs ($)	Charges ($)	Collections ($)	Profit ($)
Medicare	20	20,000	32,000	19,000	–1,000
Medicaid	30	30,000	48,000	27,000	–3,000
MC #1	25	25,000	40,000	34,000	9,000
MC #2	10	10,000	16,000	12,000	2,000
Private insurance	5	5,000	8,000	8,000	3,000
Charity	5	5,000	8,000	0	–5,000
Bad debt	5	5,000	8,000	0	–5,000
Total	100	100,000	160,000	100,000	0

Cost-Cutting Practice Problem

Using the practice problem on cost shifting, assume that those payers that pay charges, or charges minus a discount, limit XYZ's charges to $1,050 per patient. Calculate the amount of costs that XYZ will need to cut, or cover with additional revenues, to break even (realize no profit or loss).

Cost-Cutting Practice Problem Solution

Step 1: Calculate the total costs to be cut by using the new charge per patient to determine the profit/loss.

Payer	No.	Costs ($)	Charges ($)	Collections ($)	Profit ($)
Medicare	20	20,000	21,000	19,000	−1,000
Medicaid	30	30,000	31,500	27,000	−3,000
MC #1	25	25,000	26,250	22,313	−2,687
MC #2	10	10,000	10,500	7,875	−2,125
Private insurance	5	5,000	5,250	5,250	250
Charity	5	5,000	5,250	0	−5,000
Bad debt	5	5,000	5,250	0	−5,000
Total	**100**	**100,000**	**105,000**	**81,438**	**−18,562**

Step 2: Check the answer by calculating the profit/loss using the new cost per patient:

$$\frac{\$100,000 - \$18,562}{100} = \$814.38$$

Payer	No.	Costs ($)	Charges ($)	Collections ($)	Profit ($)
Medicare	20	16,288	21,000	19,000	2,712
Medicaid	30	24,431	31,500	27,000	2,569
MC #1	25	20,360	26,250	22,313	1,953
MC #2	10	8,144	10,500	7,875	−269
Private insurance	5	4,072	5,250	5,250	1,178
Charity	5	4,072	5,250	0	−4,072
Bad debt	5	4,072	5,250	0	−4,072
Total	**100**	**81,439**	**105,000**	**81,438**	**−1**

Cost-Shifting Self-Quiz Problem

Assume your organization has 100 patients analyzed in the following manner:

15 Medicare patients, who pay $2,000 per diagnosis *Collect*

25 Medicaid patients, who pay $1,800 per diagnosis *"*

20 managed care patients, who pay charges minus a 20% discount ◦ $80\% \times 2,000 \times 20$

10 managed care patients, who pay charges minus a 25% discount ◦ $75\% \times 2,000 \times 10$

10 private insurance patients, who pay charges $2,000 \times 10$

10 charity care patients, who pay nothing $\emptyset$

10 bad debt patients, who pay nothing $\emptyset$

Your organization's average cost per patient is $2,000. Calculate the charge necessary to recover your cost.

Cost-Cutting Self-Quiz Problem

Using the data from the self-quiz problem on cost shifting, assume those who pay charges will allow a maximum charge of $2,100. Calculate the amount of costs you will need to cut to break even.

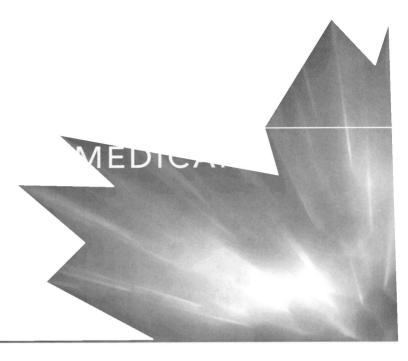

When President Lyndon B. Johnson signed Medicare and Medicaid into law on July 30, 1965, millions of Americans and about half our nation's seniors lacked health care coverage, unable to afford basic health care services or weather a medical emergency. The signing of Medicare forged a promise with older Americans—that those who have contributed a lifetime to our national life and economy can enjoy their golden years with peace of mind and the security of reliable medical insurance. Medicaid created an essential partnership between the federal government and the states to provide a basic health care safety net for some of the most vulnerable Americans: low-income children, parents, seniors, and people with disabilities. Forty-five years later, we must ensure this inviolable trust between America and its citizens remains stronger than ever.

President Barack Obama, 45th Anniversary of Medicare
and Medicaid, July 30, 2010

LEARNING OBJECTIVES

After completing this chapter, you should be able to do the following:

➤ Understand the history of Medicare and Medicaid

➤ Identify the current benefits of and financing for Medicare and Medicaid

➤ Analyze legislative attempts to control Medicare and Medicaid costs

➤ Understand the important provisions of the fraud and abuse laws and regulations

INTRODUCTION

President Lyndon B. Johnson and the 89th Congress changed the philosophy of healthcare in the United States from an individual responsibility to a social responsibility and changed access to healthcare from a privilege to a right for some Americans. The country's empathy after the assassination of President John F. Kennedy in 1963 and President Johnson's adroit legislative skills facilitated the passing of 12 major pieces of health legislation by Congress as part of President Johnson's Great Society[1] (Hepner and Hepner 1973). President Johnson signed Medicare and Medicaid into law as part of the Social Security Amendments of 1965 (P.L. 89-97).

Many believe that President Johnson's Great Society was built on the backs of future generations. When President Johnson assumed office in 1963, the economy was projected to soar to extraordinary levels by the end of the century. This projected growth in the economy would pay later for the "guns and butter" agenda of the president. This agenda included escalating the conflict in Vietnam while initiating significant social programs in the United States—a costly agenda funded without significant tax increases. President Johnson thought that proposing tax increases would have forced Congress to choose between fighting the Communists in Southeast Asia and fighting poverty in the United States (Peterson 1996).

Medicare was initially passed as two parts, Part A for hospital care and Part B for outpatient care, including physician care. The Balanced Budget Act of 1997 introduced Medicare Part C, which folded Parts A and B into a voluntary managed care program called Medicare+Choice (later changed to Medicare Advantage). The Medicare Modernization Act of 2003 introduced Part D, which included outpatient prescription coverage. The federal healthcare reform legislation that was signed into law by President Obama in March 2010 was made up of two specific laws: the Patient Protection and Affordable Care Act (ACA)(signed into law on March 23) and the Health Care Education Reconciliation Act of 2010 (signed into law on March 30), collectively referred to as the healthcare reform laws.

MEDICARE

MEDICARE ELIGIBILITY

Medicare, Title XVIII of the Social Security Amendments of 1965, is a federally funded program that provides health insurance to Americans at age 65. Medicare was expanded in 1972 to include coverage for people younger than 65 with disabilities who qualify for Social Security disability benefits and those with end-stage renal disease. Within the context of balancing the federal budget, considerable discussion has taken place regarding increasing the eligibility age of Medicare in a fashion similar to Social Security (people born in 1960 or later cannot collect full Social Security benefits until they reach age 67).[2]

Medicare
A federally funded program that provides health insurance to Americans at age 65.

MEDICARE BENEFITS

In 1966, Medicare covered seven basic services, including inpatient hospital services, out-patient diagnostic services, physician and other medical services, and outpatient thera-peutic services. Since 1966, a large number of services have been added, including some preventive services, hospice coverage, and skilled nursing facility coverage. (See Exhibit 5.1 for details.)

EXHIBIT 5.1
What Does
Medicare Cover?

Part A (Hospital Insurance, or HI)
Helps cover inpatient care in hospitals, including critical access hospitals, rehabilitation hospitals, and long-term care hospitals, and helps cover hospices, home health care ser-vices, and skilled nursing facilities not for custodial care or long-term care.

Part B (Supplemental Medical Insurance, or SMI)
Helps cover physician services and outpatient care, and helps cover some preventive services to maintain health and to keep certain illnesses from getting worse.

Part C (Medicare Advantage)
An expanded set of options for the delivery of healthcare under Medicare. While all Medi-care beneficiaries can receive benefits through the original fee-for-service program, most beneficiaries enrolled in HI and SMI can now choose to participate in a Medicare Advan-tage plan instead. Medicare Advantage plans include health maintenance organizations, preferred provider organizations, private fee-for-service plans, special needs plans, and Medicare medical savings account plans. Organizations that contract as Medicare Advan-tage plans must meet specific organizational, financial, and other requirements. Primary types of Advantage plans include

- coordinated care plans, including health maintenance organizations (HMOs), provider-sponsored organizations (PSOs), and preferred provider organizations, as well as other coordinated care plans certified by Medicare;
- private, unrestricted fee-for-service plans that allow beneficiaries to select certain private providers; and
- medical savings account (MSA) plans that provide benefits after a single, high deductible is met.

Most Medicare Advantage plans offer prescription drug coverage negating the beneficiary from enrolling in Medicare Part D.

Part D
Provides outpatient prescription coverage. Part D is voluntary, and the premium for Part D is paid for by the beneficiary.

MEDICARE FINANCING

Medicare was initially (1966) financed by assessments on employers for Part A (0.35 percent of payroll up to $6,500), by a coinsurance of $3 per month paid by beneficiaries for Part B, and by general revenue allocations to Part B (Harris 1975). Initial Medicare expenditures had been grossly underprojected, however. President Johnson reportedly believed that Medicare spending would run about $500 million a year (Peterson 1996). Medicare expenditures were $4.2 billion in 1967, the first full year of the program (Helbing 1993). The growth of Medicare expenditures was also grossly underprojected. Even critics of the program underestimated—they guessed that Medicare would cost $1 billion by the end of the twentieth century; in fact, it cost $205 billion per year by 2000. In 2011, Medicare spending was $554.3 billion, and it is expected to surpass $1 trillion by 2022. The ACA includes $716 billion in net Medicare spending reductions by 2022 through reducing annual payment updates to hospitals and other providers and payments to Medicare Advantage plans (CMS 2012a).

In 2010, Medicare was financed from three primary sources: general revenues (40 percent), payroll tax contributions (38 percent), and beneficiary premiums (13 percent). The different parts are funded as follows (Kaiser Family Foundation 2012a):

◆ Part A is financed through a 2.9 percent tax on earnings. This tax is split evenly between the employer and the employee; it accounts for 85 percent of all Part A revenue. ACA increases the payroll tax contributions to 3.8 percent starting in 2013 for individuals earning more than $200,000 and couples earning more than $250,000.

◆ Part B is financed through general revenues (72 percent), beneficiary premiums (25 percent), and interest (3 percent). Beneficiaries earning more than $85,000 per individual and $170,000 per couple pay a higher premium related to their income. The ACA freezes the income limits at 2010 levels through 2019.

◆ Part D is financed through general revenues (74 percent), beneficiary premiums (13 percent), and state payments for Medicare beneficiaries also eligible for Medicaid (13 percent). As with Part B, beneficiaries with higher incomes pay a larger share of the cost of Part D coverage.

Regarding cost sharing by Medicare beneficiaries, see Exhibit 5.2 for a listing of Medicare premium, deductible, and coinsurance rates that were in effect in 2014 (CMS 2013).

Note that Medicare pays only about half of a beneficiary's healthcare expenditures. For instance, in 2009 (the most current year for which data have been analyzed), the average Medicare beneficiary spent $17,231 on healthcare, of which Medicare paid 48 percent

EXHIBIT 5.2
Medicare Premium,
Deductible, and
Coinsurance Rates,
2014

Part A

Monthly premium: Most beneficiaries pay no monthly premium because they (or their spouses) have 40 or more quarters of Medicare-covered employment.

Annual deductible: $1,216

Coinsurance: $304 per day for days 61–90; $608 lifetime reserve day after day 90 of each benefit period (up to a maximum of 60 days over the beneficiary's lifetime)

Skilled nursing coinsurance: $152 per day for days 21–100 of each benefit period

Part B

Monthly premium:
    single income up to $85,000 and couple income up to $170,000 is $104.90
    single income up to $107,000 and couple income up to $214,000 is $146.90
    single income up to $160,000 and couple income up to $320,000 is $209.80
    single income up to $214,000 and couple income up to $428,000 is $272.70
    single income over $214,000 and couple income over $428,000 is $335.70

Annual deductible: $147

Part D

Premiums: Set by private plans (range from $17.60 to $105.50 per month)

(see Exhibit 5.3). The average beneficiary paid $4,308 of her own funds on healthcare in 2006, of which 60 percent was attributable to Medicare cost sharing.

Total Medicare payments for 2010 were $509 billion. Twenty-seven percent of that money paid for hospital inpatient services and 14 percent paid physicians (see Exhibit 5.4).

Slowing the growth of Medicare spending is particularly important in relation to the "graying of America"—the increasing proportion of the population that is aged 65 years or older. This demographic phenomenon is caused by the baby boom population (those born between 1946 and 1964) that makes up approximately 26 percent of the existing US population. In 2011 this age segment began turning 65 and began drawing Medicare benefits.

The healthcare reform laws of 2010 have substantially improved the financial outlook for Medicare; it is now projected to remain solvent through 2024, seven years longer than projections made prior to the laws. The improvement in future Medicare financing is based on increased tax contributions by the wealthy as well as reduced payment updates for most Medicare goods and services. To accommodate the reduced payment updates, the federal government is assuming productivity growth in healthcare can match the productivity growth in the overall economy. To facilitate this growth in productivity, the healthcare reform laws provide for demonstration projects in delivery and payment systems to improve efficiency (Social Security and Medicare Trustees 2011).

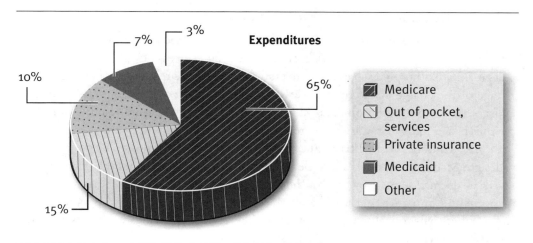

Exhibit 5.3
Personal Healthcare Expenditures for Medicare Beneficiaries, by Source of Payment, 2009

Source: Centers for Medicare & Medicaid Services (CMS). 2013. "Medicare Current Beneficiary Survey." Table 4.1. www.cms.gov/Research-Statistics-Data-and-Systems/Research/MCBS/Data-Tables.html.

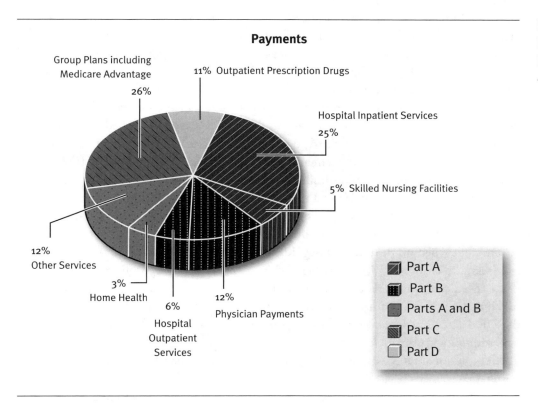

Exhibit 5.4
Medicare Benefit Payments by Type of Service, 2013

Source: CBO (2014).

MEDICARE REIMBURSEMENT TO PROVIDERS

Funded by the federal government, Medicare Part A reimbursed hospital services based on retroactive, reasonable cost—that is, cost-based reimbursement—from 1966 until 1983. Recognizing that hospitals charged more than cost, Medicare reimbursed hospitals a percentage of the charge at the time of service and then made adjustments based on cost reports that it required hospitals to file. To ensure quality, Medicare required hospitals to either pass a Joint Commission accreditation visit, called deemed status, or undergo a Medicare certification visit. This certification visit was thought by most to be more difficult by design; Medicare did not want to be in the inspection business and preferred that hospitals seek deemed status provided by The Joint Commission. Medicare Part B reimbursed physician and outpatient services based on "reasonable and customary charges," which allowed physicians to realize a profit by providing services to Medicare patients since the charge for a service is always more than its cost.

President Ronald Reagan introduced the first significant reimbursement reform in his Tax Equity and Fiscal Responsibility Act (TEFRA) of 1982. While the act reduced taxes in response to President Reagan's campaign promise, it also contained significant reimbursement reform for Medicare. Specifically, the act introduced cost limits per case and cost limits per year (known as TEFRA limits). The act directed the Department of Health and Human Services (HHS) to develop a prospective payment system (PPS) for hospitals (for a definition of *prospective payment*, see Chapter 1). It also introduced the option of managed care plans to beneficiaries and made Medicare the secondary payer when beneficiaries had additional insurance.

President Reagan signed into law the Social Security Amendments of 1983, which included provisions for prospective payment. Prospective payment applied to Part A reimbursement only, and it was intended to replace cost-based reimbursement. The amendments established prospective payment rates for **diagnosis-related groups** (DRGs), or similar cases that should require similar resource consumption.[3] Hospitals that provided care for less cost than the established rate for a DRG realized a profit. Hospitals that provided care for more cost than the established rate realized a loss. Because the DRG system gave hospitals a financial incentive to provide less service to Medicare patients, the federal government relied on **peer review organizations** (PROs), established under the TEFRA legislation, to ensure that Medicare beneficiaries were receiving appropriate care.[4]

Medicare implemented the PPS over a three-year period to give hospitals time to adjust their costs. During that time, Medicare used hospital-specific data to establish the DRG rates. At the end of the three-year period, hospitals were subject to a national rate with an adjustment for labor costs, which varied between regions. Currently, three different national rates exist: a teaching hospital rate, an urban hospital rate, and a rural hospital rate.[5]

Medicare used the DRG rate schedule to provide incentives and penalties for certain physician ordering patterns. For instance, hospitals that performed open-heart surgery before trying angioplasty were punished with a low rate of reimbursement, whereas

diagnosis-related group
A grouping of similar healthcare cases that should require similar resource consumption. DRGs are used by Medicare to calculate prospective payments.

peer review organization
An organization that ensures that providers give appropriate care to Medicare recipients.

hospitals that performed successful angioplasty without open-heart surgery were rewarded with high reimbursement.

Capital costs were not initially affected by the DRG system. Prior to 1990, Medicare had reimbursed capital costs based on reasonable cost, meaning that Medicare reimbursed its share of capital costs regardless of use. For instance, if Medicare patients were responsible for 35 percent of the hospital's operating costs based on the cost report, Medicare would reimburse 35 percent of the hospital's capital costs.

The Omnibus Budget Reconciliation Act (OBRA) of 1990 folded capital costs into the DRG rate over a ten-year period. This meant hospitals risked losing substantial reimbursement if their buildings and equipment were not sufficiently used by Medicare patients. For instance, Medicare now reimburses hospitals their CT scanner capital costs based only on those DRGs where a CT scan is medically necessary. If hospitals provide CT scans that are unnecessary for a certain DRG, the hospital's costs for that DRG would exceed the reimbursement and the hospital would lose money, Hospitals that had overextended (acquired more capital costs than would be reimbursed based on their DRGs) their capital were forced to consolidate their assets through a sale or a joint venture (joint ventures with for-profit organizations were popular because the for-profits had access to additional sources of capital).

The Health Care Financing Administration (HCFA) **resource-based relative value system** (RBRVS) of 1992 changed the way Medicare reimbursed physicians under Part B. Prior to 1992, Medicare had reimbursed physicians on the basis of reasonable and customary charges. By reimbursing physicians on an RBRVS, Medicare established a prospective, flat fee per visit, similar to DRGs for hospitals. Physicians who provided care for less cost than the established rate realized a profit; those who provided care for more cost than the established rate realized a loss. Furthermore, Medicare used the RBRVS rate schedule to provide incentives and penalties for certain medical specialties. Visits to primary care physicians resulted in favorable reimbursement, but visits to specialists resulted in unfavorable reimbursement.

The Balanced Budget Act (BBA) of 1997 reduced Medicare reimbursements to providers by $115 billion over five years (Ernst & Young 1997) (see Exhibit 5.7 for details), established the Children's Health Insurance Program (CHIP), and introduced the sustainable growth rate (SGR), a method used by Medicare to determine annual updates (increases) in payment for physician services. The Balanced Budget Refinement Act (BBRA) of 1999 provided approximately $16 billion in Medicare relief over five years after the government discovered that the BBA of 1997 had cut two to three times more than the $115 billion originally intended. The Medicare, Medicaid, and State Children's Health Insurance Program (SCHIP) Benefits Improvement and Protection Act (BIPA) of 2000 provided $35 billion in reimbursement relief over five years by increasing certain Medicare and Medicaid provider payments; adding preventive benefits and reducing beneficiary cost sharing under Medicare; and improving insurance options for low-income children, families, and seniors (HFMA 2000a).

resource-based relative value system
A Medicare reimbursement system that provides a flat, per-visit fee to physicians rather than reimbursing them according to their customary charges.

The Deficit Reduction Act (DEFRA) of 2005 achieved $8.3 billion in savings from Medicare and $4.7 billion in savings from Medicaid, including the SCHIP, over five years. Related to reimbursement, the act did the following (HFMA 2006):

◆ Starting in 2008, reduced Medicare payments for services provided as a result of certain hospital-acquired infections

◆ Addressed the calculation of a hospital's Medicare **disproportionate share hospital** (DSH) adjustments

◆ Provided that Medicare-dependent hospitals (MDHs)—those with 100 or fewer beds and a high proportion of Medicare patients—can receive special payments

◆ Reduced the reimbursement to ambulatory surgery centers (ASCs) if the ASC payment exceeds the hospital outpatient department fee schedule

The Tax Relief and Health Care Act of 2006 included provisions to prevent a 2007 cut in Medicare physician payments mandated under DEFRA of 2005. Related to reimbursement, the act did the following (AHA 2006):

◆ Froze physician payments under Medicare at 2006 levels and provided for a 1.5 percent increase in payments for physicians who participate in a voluntary quality reporting system

◆ Established a maximum Medicaid provider tax at 5.5 percent

◆ Extended a requirement that Medicare pay labs directly for the technical component of physician pathology services furnished to hospital patients

◆ Extended cost reimbursement for outpatient lab payments to rural hospitals

◆ Extended Section 508 of the Medicare Prescription Drug, Improvement, and Modernization Act of 2003, which allows for geographical reclassification

◆ Starting in 2009, reduced by 2 percent the annual update factor for outpatient services provided by hospitals and ambulatory centers that fail to report certain quality measures

In 2007, President George W. Bush signed into law the Medicare, Medicaid, and SCHIP Extension Act of 2007, which extended funding for the State Children's Health Insurance Program (SCHIP) and provided a 0.5 percent Medicare payment increase for physicians.

In 2008, Congress overrode President Bush's veto of the Medicare Improvements for Providers and Patients Act of 2008, which replaced a planned 10.6 percent cut in

disproportionate share hospital

Hospitals that qualify for increased payments from Medicare because they treat a high percentage of low-income patients and patients on Medicare, early Medicare on disability, and Medicaid.

Medicare payments to physicians based on the SGR with a 1.6 percent increase in Medicare payment to physicians. This law also did the following:

◆ For physicians, in addition to the 1.6 percent increase in Medicare payments, the law provided a 2 percent increase in Medicare payments for quality reporting through 2010 and financial incentives to encourage physician use of electronic prescribing technologies.

◆ For hospitals, the law improved payments to sole community hospitals, critical access hospitals, and ambulance services; preserved payment equity to rural hospitals and rural physicians who operate clinical labs; increased access to telehealth and speech/language therapy; and retained rural access to Medicare Advantage.

◆ For beneficiaries whose annual income was below $14,040, the law extended and improved assistance programs. The law also added new preventive benefits and reduced the beneficiary out-of-pocket expense for mental healthcare.

◆ For pharmacies, the law required Medicare Advantage plans to pay promptly (within 14 days) and to update medication prices (reimbursements) weekly.

◆ For Medicare Advantage plans, the law took steps to reduce Medicare payments to private plans, which were being paid more than 100 percent of the amount paid under a fee-for-service environment, and phased out double payments for indirect medical education (IME).

The American Recovery and Reinvestment Act of 2009 was signed by President Barack Obama and was intended to provide federal spending to stimulate an economy in recession. The law provided $150 billion to healthcare, including $87 billion in Medicaid assistance to the states, $25 billion for extended COBRA benefits, and $19 billion for information technology (Lubell 2009).

The ACA, signed by President Obama in 2010, is projected to reduce growth in Medicare spending to 5.8 percent per year by reducing the growth in Medicare payments to providers and Medicare Advantage plans, establishing several new programs and policies designed to reduce costs and improve quality of patient care, and establishing the Independent Payment Advisory Board to recommend Medicare spending reductions if projected spending exceeds targets. Healthcare reform laws also increase payroll taxes for high-income taxpayers to help fund Part A and increase Part B and Part D premiums for high-income beneficiaries (Kaiser Family Foundation 2010).

The Budget Control Act of 2011 reduced discretionary spending by the federal government by $1.2 trillion over the next ten years by capping per-year discretionary spending.

If spending caps are exceeded, an automatic across-the-board cut, called sequestration, takes place. The act also maintained spending for fraud and abuse investigations and created a 12-member committee to recommend additional and specific ways to reduce the deficit.

The *fiscal cliff* was a term used to describe the fiscal conundrum faced at the end of 2012 due largely to the provisions of the Budget Control Act of 2011. In addition to the possibility of sequestration, many of the provisions of the Affordable Care Act of 2010 were due to begin. In response to the pending fiscal cliff, Congress passed and President Obama signed the American Taxpayer Relief Act of 2012 that delayed sequestration for two months; raised taxes for wealthy Americans, increasing federal revenue by $600 billion over ten years; and suspended for one year a 26.5 percent cut in Medicare Part B reimbursement to physicians mandated by the SGR formula (the 26.5 percent cut was the accumulated effect of physician reimbursement increasing more than the SGR mandated each year since 2000).

During the summer of 2013, the House Energy and Commerce Committee unanimously passed a bill to replace the SGR formula. The Medicare Patient Access and Quality Improvement Bill of 2013 would repeal the SGR formula; would provide physicians with a 0.5 percent increase each year for five years; and would provide a value-based approach to reimbursement in 2017 (i.e., a 1 percent increase in annual reimbursement if the physician achieves certain quality metrics and a 1 percent decrease in annual reimbursement if the physician does not achieve the quality metrics, or an alternative value-based method). At the end of 2013, the House Ways and Means Committee and the Senate Finance Committee were discussing the bill favorably. The bill would cost an estimated $175 billion over 10 years (CBO 2013b) and funding the bill would be political and contentious.

MEDICARE EXPENDITURES

The cost of the Medicare program has been a problem for Congress from the very beginning (see Exhibit 5.5). Use was underprojected and revenue sources, particularly those projected economic growth, were overly optimistic. Attempts have been made to control costs through federal legislation (which is discussed in the next section), increased assessments to employers and employees, increased cost sharing to beneficiaries, and increased program allocation from general revenues. Even with these attempts, HHS—which has the overall responsibility for administering the Medicare program—projects that the Medicare Trust Fund will go bankrupt in 2024 (Social Security and Medicare Board of Trustees 2011).

The low average growth rate in Medicare expenditures from 1996 to 2000 stands in stark contrast to previous years, which averaged more than 10 percent growth. The 1996 to 2000 rate can be attributed to the implementation of the BBA of 1997, the intense efforts to identify and correct fraud and abuse in the Medicare program, and the low rate of general and Medicare inflation (Foster 2000). The 9.6 percent rate of increase from 2006 to 2010 also needs some further explanation. The percent rate of increase for 2006 was 18.7 percent, reflecting the costs of a fully implemented MMA of 2003, which provided outpatient prescription medication coverage to Medicare recipients. However, the rate of increase for 2010 was a much more moderate 4.3 percent. The 5.5 percent projected rate

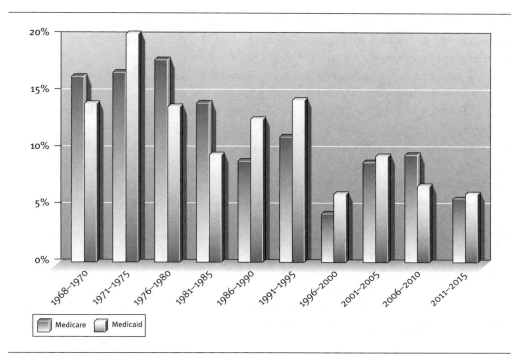

Sources: Data from CMS (2013) and Cuckler et al. (2013).

EXHIBIT 5.5
Average Annual
Percentage
Increase in
Total Medicare
and Medicaid
Expenditures

of increase from 2011 to 2015 includes a 2 percent reduction in payments in 2013 as a result of the Budget Control Act of 2011 and resulting sequestration (Cuckler et al. 2013).

The graying of America has special significance to healthcare organizations, because the population 65 years or older uses healthcare services at a much higher rate than the under-65 population, making their healthcare expenditures disproportionately high. Although 12.9 percent of the total population was 65 years or older in 2009 (US Census Bureau 2010b), they represented 34 percent of all personal health spending in 2004 (the latest year data are available) (Hartman et al. 2008). Baby boomers began turning 65 in 2011 (an estimated 7,918 baby boomers will turn 65 each day until 2029), and the US Census Bureau projects that 20.7 percent of the total population will be 65 years or older in 2029, when all of the baby boomers have reached age 65.

MEDICAID

MEDICAID ELIGIBILITY

Medicaid, Title XIX of the Social Security Amendments of 1965, provides health insurance to the medically indigent (i.e., individuals who may be able to pay for normal living expenses, but cannot afford healthcare expenses).[6] Historically, eligibility for Medicaid has been linked to eligibility for two federal cash assistance programs: Aid to Families

Medicaid
A program created
by the federal
government, funded
by the federal and
state government, and
administered by the
state government, to
provide free or low-cost
healthcare to low-
income recipients.

with Dependent Children (AFDC) and Supplemental Security Income. OBRA of 1986 expanded eligibility for low-income pregnant women, children, and infants, regardless of their eligibility for a state's AFDC program. The Medicare Catastrophic Coverage Act of 1988 required states to pay Medicare premiums, coinsurance, and deductibles for the elderly who earned less than the state's poverty limit.

The BBA of 1997 provided $23.4 billion over five years to the State Children's Health Insurance Program (now known as CHIP) a program to expand health coverage for children whose parents' income was too high to qualify for Medicaid, but too low to afford private insurance (Ernst & Young 1997). In 2009, President Obama signed the Children's Health Insurance Reauthorization Act, which expanded CHIP to an additional 4 million children and pregnant women, including coverage for the first time for legal child immigrants. In 2010, President Obama signed the healthcare reform laws, which will expand Medicaid eligibility for adults. The program had covered adults living at 100 percent of the poverty level; as of 2014, ACA encouraged states to increase the Medicaid eligibility from 100 percent of the poverty level to 138 percent of the poverty level. Until 2014, states were required to extend Medicaid benefits to children under 6 years old living in families with incomes up to 138 percent of the poverty level and to children 6 to 18 years old living in families with incomes up to 100 percent of the poverty level (Kaiser Commission on Medicaid and the Uninsured 2010).

MEDICAID BENEFITS

Although the federal government finances 50 to 83 percent of Medicaid costs in any given state, each state has significant authority in administering its Medicaid program. Each state is allowed considerable discretion in establishing its own income and resource criteria for program eligibility; determining the amount, duration, and scope of optional services beyond the mandatory services required by the federal government; and determining provider reimbursement methodologies. Optional services vary by state (HCFA 1996).

MEDICAID FINANCING

The Medicaid program has two categories of costs: costs for provider services, which are determined by formula (see Note 6); and costs for administrative services, which are shared equally by the federal and state government. The federal portion of costs is financed from general revenues. The state portion of costs for provider services may be financed from state and local revenues; however, the state's portion must be at least 40 percent. The state portion of costs for administrative services is financed by state revenues (HCFA 1996).

MEDICAID REIMBURSEMENT TO PROVIDERS

The Medicaid program operates as a vendor payment program—providers are reimbursed directly by the state. Reimbursement is subject to federal conditions that all states must satisfy. First, reimbursement must be such to recruit a sufficient number of providers. Second, participating providers must accept the Medicaid reimbursement as payment in full. Third, reimbursement to providers must be conditional on appropriate efficiency, economy, and quality standards. Each state has significant authority over reimbursement methods and rates with the following exceptions (HCFA 1996):

◆ Reimbursements to institutions cannot exceed amounts that would be paid for similar services under the Medicare program.

◆ DSHs are exempt from the Medicare limit.

◆ For hospice services, Medicaid reimbursements cannot be lower than Medicare reimbursements.

From the beginning, most states used reimbursement methodologies either identical to or similar to the reimbursement methodologies used by Medicare. For reimbursement to institutional providers, this meant that most Medicaid programs used cost-based reimbursement. As use and costs grew, most Medicaid programs implemented the same reimbursement controls as Medicare. During the late 1970s, many Medicaid programs were more aggressive than Medicare in recognizing reasonable costs. As Medicare moved into prospective reimbursement methodologies in the early 1980s, most Medicaid programs adopted methodologies based on case mix, or DRGs, similar to Medicare methodologies. However, some Medicaid programs set payment levels based on the historic costs of each institution. This practice had the effect of rewarding providers whose costs had historically been high and penalizing providers who had been cost-conscious in the past (Berman, Kukla, and Weeks 1994). Some Medicaid programs also deviated from Medicare's case-mix methodology, using other prospective methodologies, like rate-of-increase and negotiated budget methodologies. For reimbursement to physician providers, Medicaid programs used either fee schedules or reasonable charges methodologies. Medicaid programs using fee schedules set a flat maximum reimbursement for each service. Medicaid programs using reasonable charges limit reimbursement to the lowest of the physician's actual charge, the physician's customary charge for similar services, or the prevailing physicians' charges in the area.

A few Medicaid programs have requested permission, via Section 1115 research and demonstration waivers, to develop managed care programs for their Medicaid beneficiaries (HCFA 1996). The BBA of 1997 effectively eliminated this waiver requirement by giving states the option to require Medicaid beneficiaries to enroll in managed care plans. The act permitted managed care plans to bid on Medicaid business, which presumably could be capitated (Ernst & Young 1997).

The ACA, via the 2012 Supreme Court decision, encourages states to expand eligibility from 100 to 138 percent of the federal poverty level. The federal government will reimburse all of the costs associated with the expansion for the first seven years and 75 to 90 percent of the costs during the following three years.

MEDICAID COSTS

In the early 2000s, the Medicaid program experienced average annual expenditure increases of 9 percent (see Exhibit 5.5). State governments were concerned with the rate of Medicaid cost growth and the impact on state budgets.

Reflecting this concern, total federal and state Medicaid spending increased only 4.7 percent in 2008—the slowest rate of increase in ten years. Medicaid spending for hospitals, which represents 36 percent of all Medicaid spending, increased only 2.7 percent, as payments to hospitals and other providers were reduced (Hartman 2008). The 5.9 percent projected annual rate of increase from 2011 to 2015 continues at a moderate pace as states shift beneficiaries to managed care. However, in 2014, with the expansion of eligibility in some states, Medicaid expenditures are projected to increase 12.2 percent (Cuckler et al. 2013).

An analysis of the Medicaid beneficiary cost by eligibility grouping indicates that a relatively small proportion of Medicaid beneficiaries are responsible for the majority of Medicaid costs (see Exhibit 5.6). For instance, while the elderly and disabled represent 24 percent of all Medicaid beneficiaries, they account for 64 percent of all Medicaid payments (Kaiser Family Foundation 2013b).

EXHIBIT 5.6
Medicaid Beneficiaries and Payments by Medicaid Eligibility Category, 2010

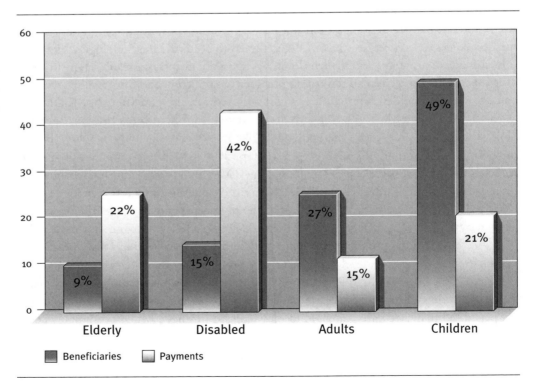

Source: Data from Kaiser Family Foundation (2013c).

LEGISLATIVE ATTEMPTS TO CONTROL COSTS OF MEDICARE AND MEDICAID

The federal government discovered early that Medicare and Medicaid use and resulting costs had been underprojected, and that retroactive, cost-based reimbursement to hospitals and charge-based reimbursement to physicians was inflationary. As early as 1971, the federal government attempted to control healthcare costs while maintaining benefits, and in some cases, improving benefits, through legislation and regulation. Exhibit 5.7 lists these attempts.

HEALTH INSURANCE PORTABILITY AND ACCOUNTABILITY ACT OF 1996

The Health Insurance Portability and Accountability Act (HIPAA) of 1996 was designed to improve the availability of health insurance to working families and their children. HIPAA includes important protections for an estimated 25 million Americans who move from one job to another, who are self-employed, or who have preexisting medical conditions. The law also provided administrative simplification standards intended to identify and secure protected health information (PHI).

Wage and Price Controls of 1971	Imposed wage and price controls in an attempt to deal with inflation throughout the economy. In the healthcare industry, price increases were limited according to federal price guidelines through 1974.	**EXHIBIT 5.7** Legislation and Regulation to Control Healthcare Costs
Social Security Amendments of 1972	Authorized price controls in the healthcare industry and directed the Department of Health, Education, and Welfare to develop a prospective payment method of reimbursement.	
Professional Standards Review Organizations (PSROs) of 1972	Established a peer-review program to determine appropriateness and quality of care delivered in hospitals to beneficiaries of federal programs. Inappropriate admissions, lengths of stay, or surgeries resulted in reductions in reimbursements.	
National Health Planning and Resource Development Act of 1974	Established certificate-of-need regulations, which required hospitals to obtain approval for capital expenditures and improvements that cost more than $100,000.	

EXHIBIT 5.7
Legislation and
Regulation to
Control Healthcare
Costs
(continued)

Omnibus Budget Reconciliation Act (OBRA) of 1980

Eliminated the "prior hospitalization" requirement for home health services reimbursement, and eliminated the limitation on the total number of home health services visits.

Tax Equity and Fiscal Responsibility Act (TEFRA) of 1982

Placed rate-of-increase limits on inpatient hospital services; replaced PSROs with peer review organizations; extended Medicare coverage to hospice care for those certified as terminally ill; made Medicare the secondary payer for working beneficiaries covered by their employers.

Social Security Amendments of 1983

Introduced hospital prospective payment based on DRGs to replace retroactive, cost-based payment; required federal workers to pay Medicare hospital insurance payroll tax (federal workers had been exempt from the tax prior to 1983).

Deficit Reduction Act (DEFRA) of 1984

Froze physician fees and established the Participating Physician and Supplies (PPS) program, which allowed physicians to accept assignment (i.e., physicians would accept the Medicare-approved charge as full payment and would not balance bill the Medicare beneficiaries). In return, Medicare would list physicians in a directory available to beneficiaries and expedite billing.

Consolidated Omnibus Budget Reconciliation Act (COBRA) of 1985

Made Medicare coverage mandatory for state and local government employees hired after 1985; directed HHS to develop a prospective payment system for physicians. As part of COBRA, Section 9121, or the Emergency Medical Treatment and Active Labor Act (EMTALA), also known as the antidumping law, requires that hospitals with emergency departments (1) provide a medical screening examination to anyone requesting such examination in order to determine whether the individual is in an emergency medical condition;

Consolidated Omnibus Budget Reconciliation Act (COBRA) of 1985 *(continued)*

(2) provide medical treatment to stabilize the condition if the hospital determines that the individual is in an emergency condition; and (3) must not transfer individuals in emergency medical conditions unless (a) the patient requests the transfer after knowing the hospital is obligated to continue treatment or (b) the transfer is medically appropriate. Hospitals and emergency room physicians that violate EMTALA can be fined up to $50,000 each per violation. Placed maximum allowable actual charge limits on the amounts physicians could bill Medicare beneficiaries above the Medicare-approved charge.

Medicare Catastrophic Coverage Act of 1988

Expanded Medicare benefits to include outpatient prescriptions, placed a cap on patient costs for catastrophic expenses, and expanded skilled nursing facility coverage. Funded by increases in the Part B premium and a new supplemental income premium.

Medicare Catastrophic Coverage Act Repeal of 1989

Restored benefits to previous levels and canceled new premium; directed HHS to develop a PPS for physicians.

Omnibus Budget Reconciliation Act (OBRA) of 1989

Introduced new fee schedule for physician services and limited the amount above the fee schedule that physicians could bill beneficiaries; tied increases in fee schedule to volume performance standards. Prohibited physician referrals under Medicare for clinical lab services when the referring physician has a financial relationship (known as self-referrals) with the lab unless the terms of certain statutory or regulatory exceptions are met (known as Stark I regulations, named after the bill's sponsor, Congressman Pete Stark [D-CA]).

EXHIBIT 5.7
Legislation and
Regulation to
Control Healthcare
Costs
(continued)

Omnibus Budget Reconciliation Act (OBRA) of 1990

Increased Part B deductible to $100; moved the reimbursement for inpatient hospital capital costs from cost-based reimbursement to prospective reimbursement based on DRGs.

HCFA Resource-Based Relative Value System (RBRVS) of 1992

Introduced a prospective payment system for physicians over a three-year implementation period.

Omnibus Budget Reconciliation Act (OBRA) of 1993

Removed cap on wages subject to Medicare Part A payroll tax; introduced new tax on Social Security benefits above certain incomes. Expanded Stark I prohibitions on physician self-referrals to include additional designated health services: physical therapy; occupational therapy; radiology, including MRI, CT, and ultrasound; radiation therapy; durable medical equipment and supplies; parenteral and enteral nutrients; orthotics and prosthetic devices; home health services; outpatient prescription drugs; and inpatient and outpatient hospital services (known as Stark II). Final rules, published in January 2001, "generally permit" self-referrals as long as compensation paid to the physician with an ownership interest is not more than would be paid to a physician who did not have an ownership interest.

Personal Responsibility and Work Opportunity Reconciliation Act of 1996

Made restrictive changes to welfare eligibility that in turn restricted eligibility to Medicaid.

Health Insurance Portability and Accountability Act (HIPAA) of 1996

Protected currently insured people from losing coverage because of job change or family illness; required insurers who offer small-group coverage to make policies available to all small groups; allowed for a pilot study of medical savings accounts or insurance accounts for the self-employed and small employers that would allow the beneficiaries substantial rebates if use is low; mandated standardized, electronic

EXHIBIT 5.7
Legislation and
Regulation to
Control Healthcare
Costs
(continued)

Health Insurance Portability and Accountability Act (HIPAA) of 1996
(continued)

billing by 2000; allowed the self-employed to increase their tax deduction for health insurance costs from 30 percent to 80 percent of the cost by 2006; and tightened fraud and abuse rules.

Balanced Budget Act (BBA) of 1997

Cut Medicare program expenditures by $115 billion over five years; froze DSH payments in 32 states and cut payments in 18 states; gave states the option to require Medicaid beneficiaries to enroll in managed care; allowed patient safety organizations to bid on Medicare and Medicaid business; and introduced SCHIP, which provided funding to expand health coverage for children.

Balanced Budget Refinement Act (BBRA) of 1999

Recognized as BBA relief, BBRA restored Medicare program expenditures by $16 billion over five years.

Medicare, Medicaid, and SCHIP Benefits Improvement and Protection Act (BIPA) of 2000

Recognized in part as BBA relief, BIPA restored Medicare program expenditures to hospitals by $35 billion over five years. The $109 billion appropriations bill included increased funding for the National Institutes of Health's medical research; increased funding for the Centers for Disease Control and Prevention; increased funding for Ryan White CARE Act; and increased funding for independent children's hospitals to train pediatricians.

Medicare Prescription Drug, Improvement, and Modernization Act (MMA) of 2003

Introduced prescription drug benefits; provided $25 billion in payment improvements for providers with incentives for hospitals to report quality data and bonuses to underserved areas; imposed an 18-month moratorium on new specialty hospitals; replaced Medicare+Choice with Medicare Advantage; allowed people with high-deductible policies to shelter some income from taxes in health savings accounts (HSAs); and allowed drug importation from Canada.

EXHIBIT 5.7
Legislation and
Regulation to
Control Healthcare
Costs
(continued)

Deficit Reduction Act (DEFRA) of 2005	Cut $8.3 billion from Medicare and $4.7 billion from Medicaid, including SCHIP, over five years. Also provided for reductions in Medicare payments for services provided as a result of certain hospital-acquired infections beginning in 2008; addressed the calculation of hospital Medicare DSH adjustments; and lowered the reimbursement to ASCs if the ASC payment exceeds the hospital outpatient department fee schedule.
Tax Relief and Health Care Act of 2006	Delayed a planned 5.1 percent cut in Medicare physician reimbursement for one year; provided a 1.5 percent incentive payment if physicians report on quality measures; and expanded the amount that individuals may contribute to HSAs.
Medicare, Medicaid, and SCHIP Extension Act of 2007	Extended funding for SCHIP and provided 0.5 percent Medicare payment increase for physicians.
Medicare Improvements for Providers and Patients Act of 2008	Overriding a presidential veto, the act replaced a pending 10.6 percent cut in Medicare reimbursement to physicians with a 2.0 percent increase for quality reporting; improved low-income assistance; reduced payments to Medicare Advantage plans that were paid in excess of fee-for-service counterparts; and improved payments to sole community hospitals, critical access hospitals, and ambulance services.
Patient Protection and Affordable Care Act of 2010	Provided comprehensive healthcare reform phased in over eight years and intended to provide insurance access to 32 million Americans, to make the healthcare delivery system more efficient, and to reduce the rate of increase in healthcare spending.
Health Care and Education Reconciliation Act of 2010	Amended the Patient Protection and Affordable Care Act to include provisions of the House bill on healthcare reform.

		Exhibit 5.7
Medicare and Medicaid Extenders Act of 2010	Delayed for one year a 25 percent reduction in Medicare physician payments due to take effect on January 1, 2011.	Legislation and Regulation to Control Healthcare Costs *(continued)*
Budget Control Act of 2011	Reduced and capped federal discretionary spending by $1.2 trillion over ten years. If caps are exceeded, across the board spending cuts, called sequestration, occur. (Sequestration did occur in March 2013, reducing Medicare payments to hospitals by 2 percent.)	
American Taxpayer Relief Act of 2012	Increased taxes for wealthy Americans, suspended a pending cut in Medicare reimbursement to physicians for one year, and delayed sequestration until March 2013 (the 2014 federal budget delayed the pending cut in Medicare reimbursement to physicians for three months and reduced some of the defense spending cuts ordered by sequestration).	

HIPAA Administrative Simplification Standards

As mandated by HIPAA, HHS has published final rules on five standards (transactions and code sets, national provider identifiers, national employer identifiers, privacy, and security) that make up the administrative simplification program, a program to streamline the processing of healthcare claims, reduce the volume of paperwork, and save the healthcare system billions of dollars while providing better service for providers, insurers, and patients. By promoting the greater use of electronic transactions and eliminating inefficient paper forms, HHS estimated that administrative simplification standards would provide a net savings of $29.9 billion to the healthcare industry over the next ten years. Although the 1996 act was passed with cost-saving rhetoric, no evidence exists that savings occurred through 2009. Implementing regulations set privacy compliance dates for 2003 and security compliance dates for 2005. In 2006, the American Health Information Management Association reported that only 39 percent of hospitals were fully compliant with privacy standards and only 25 percent of hospitals were compliant with security standards. The costs incurred implementing the standards are significant; it would follow that savings will not occur until after hospitals are fully compliant. Even after compliance is attained, healthcare organizations must report breaches of security to the Office for Civil Rights (OCR). Breaches of 500 or more records are reported on the HHS.gov website (see www.hhs.gov/ocr/privacy/hipaa/administrative/breachnotificationrule/breachtool.html), and hospitals are subject to significant civil monetary penalties.

HIPAA Civil Monetary Penalty Authority

HIPAA is nearly 20 years old, and compliance is now mandated, and fines and penalties are significant and deserve special attention. HIPAA provided the legislative power to the HHS Office of Inspector General (OIG) to implement changes to the agency's civil monetary penalty (CMP) authority, including

◆ expanding the OIG's authority to impose CMPs to all federal healthcare programs;

◆ increasing the maximum monetary penalty for violations occurring after January 1, 1997, from $100 per instance to a range of $100 per instance to $50,000 per instance; and

◆ creating additional CMPs for individuals retaining control or ownership interest in a facility to which they refer Medicare patients, upcoding and claims for medically unnecessary services, providing medically unnecessary services, inducing beneficiaries to choose a particular provider or supplier, and making false certification of patient eligibility to home health agencies.

Privacy Under HIPAA

The HIPAA privacy standard is a set of federal rules to protect the privacy of patients' medical records and other health information maintained by providers such as hospitals and physicians, health plans, and insurance companies. The privacy standard provides patients with access to their medical records while safeguarding the release of protected health information. Compliance with the privacy standard was required by 2003 for most entities. Complaints regarding the privacy standard are investigated by the OCR. Through August 2013, OCR had received 86,721 complaints. HHS has resolved more than 95 percent of complaints received through investigation and enforcement (25 percent); through investigation and finding no violation (11 percent); and through closure of cases that were not eligible for enforcement (59 percent). The most frequent compliance issue investigated is impermissible use and disclosure of PHI, and the most frequent covered entities required to take corrective action are private physician practices (HHS 2013a).

Most violations do not require a resolution agreement or CMP because the recipient of the complaint is willing to comply voluntarily. The first case requiring a resolution agreement and a fine of $100,000 was for Providence Health Services; the case was resolved in 2008. During 2005 and 2006, several subsidiaries of Providence Health Services left backup tapes, optical disks, and laptops unattended. The media and laptops were lost or stolen, and the health information of 386,000 patients was compromised. In 2009, CVS Caremark agreed to a $2.25 million settlement for failing to maintain protected health information in a secure manner. The OCR found that CVS failed to implement policies and procedures related to the disposal of protected patient information and failed to properly train employees in the disposal process (protected patient information was disposed in dumpsters accessible to the public) (HHS 2009). In 2013, the managed care company WellPoint agreed to pay HHS $1.7 million to settle potential violations of privacy and security standards. The OCR's investigation found that WellPoint did not adequately implement appropriate policies and procedures for authorizing online access. As a result, WellPoint could have potentially disclosed electronic PHI for 612,402 individuals by allowing unauthorized access to the application database (HHS 2013b).

SECURITY UNDER HIPAA

The HIPAA security standard is a set of federal rules to protect the security of electronic protected health information. Compliance with the security standard was required in 2003 for most entities; however, authority to administer and enforce the standard was not transferred to the OCR until 2009. Through August 2013, the OCR had received 750 complaints regarding the security standard, with 569 complaints closed after investigation and appropriate corrective action (HHS 2013a). Also in 2013, the Hospice of North Idaho agreed to pay HHS $50,000 to settle potential violations of the security standards. Although the settlement was relatively small, it was the first involving a breach of unsecured electronic PHI affecting fewer than 500 individuals (HHS 2013c).

RECOVERY AUDIT CONTRACTOR DEMONSTRATION PROJECTS

The Medicare Modernization Act of 2003 established a three-year demonstration project for **recovery audit contractors** (RACs). RACs detect and correct past improper payments from CMS to providers in order to prevent future improper payments by CMS (CMS 2011b). The demonstration project identified almost $1 billion in improper payments in the three states reviewed—the most common improper payment was for surgical procedures provided in the wrong setting (inpatient instead of outpatient). Because of this success, in 2007 the federal government authorized RAC audits in every state. In 2009, RAC audits recovered almost $1 billion in inappropriate payments (Forney and Phillips 2011).

recovery audit contractor
A private business that detects and recovers improper Medicare payments to providers.

PATIENT PROTECTION AND AFFORDABLE CARE ACT OF 2010

The Patient Protection and Affordable Care Act of 2010 will cost $940 billion over ten years and will provide insurance coverage to 32 million Americans, increasing health insurance coverage to 94 percent of the population (Lubell and DoBias 2010). Specifically, the law does the following (AHA 2010a):

◆ Expands coverage to 32 million people through a combination of public program and private-sector insurance expansions

◆   Reduces the rate of increase in Medicare and Medicaid spending through reduced payment updates, decreases in DSH payments, and financial penalties for unnecessary hospital readmissions and hospital-acquired infections

◆   Adopts several delivery system reforms to better align reimbursement with improved coordination of patient care and quality

◆   Provides grants and loans to improve workforce education and training on healthcare issues

◆   Includes provisions to reduce waste, fraud, and abuse in Medicare and Medicaid

◆   Imposes new reporting requirements for tax-exempt hospitals

◆   Places significant restrictions on the expansion of physician-owned hospitals and prohibits new physician-owned facilities

In 2012, the Supreme Court determined that the ACA was constitutional as a tax, but the requirement for states to expand eligibility for Medicaid or lose federal funding was unconstitutional. Reacting to this finding, the federal government offered significant incentives to states in return for eligibility expansion. At the end of 2013, 29 states were moving toward expansion.

MEDICARE/MEDICAID FRAUD AND ABUSE

fraud
An intentional misrepresentation of fact designed to induce reliance by another.

One of the most significant initiatives by the federal government to control healthcare costs has been the recent emphasis on enforcing fraud and abuse statutes (see Exhibit 5.8). **Fraud** is an intentional misrepresentation of fact designed to induce reliance by another. **Abuse** is an unintentional misrepresentation of fact. Typical examples of fraud include physician kickbacks for referral and intentional billings for services not rendered. Typical examples of abuse include unintentional billing and coding errors.

abuse
An unintentional misrepresentation of fact.

Fraudulent or abusive practices can result in criminal and civil liability and administrative sanctions. Criminal liability under the Fraud and False Statements Act can result in fines and imprisonment. Civil liability under the False Claims Act can result in fines of $10,000 for each false claim plus three times the total amount of the loss by the government. Civil liability under the False Claims Act extends to those who submit the fraudulent claim and to those who have knowledge that the claim is fraudulent. *Knowledge* is defined as either actual knowledge or reckless disregard for the claim's validity. Therefore, the government does not have to prove that false claims were submitted with the intent to defraud (i.e., the healthcare organization knew), but that the false claims were submitted in an environment that was likely to produce false claims (i.e., the healthcare organization should have known). Furthermore, the government must prove its case in civil cases by a preponderance of evidence, unlike in criminal cases, where the burden of proof is "beyond a reasonable doubt" (Russo 1997).

Violations of the Anti-Kickback Act, which is a criminal statute, can result in criminal fines up to $25,000 and civil fines up to $50,000 as well as five years in prison. Administrative sanctions can result in possible exclusion from federal programs. The Anti-Kickback Act was passed in 1972 and prohibits anyone from knowingly or willfully soliciting or accepting any type of remuneration to induce referrals for health services that are reimbursed by the federal government.

The Stark law is similar to the Anti-Kickback Act, and as a result is often confused with the Anti-Kickback Act. The Stark law is a federal civil statute passed in 1989 (Stark I) with amendments passed in 1993 (Stark II). It prohibits physicians from referring patients to an entity with which the ordering physician has an ownership interest or compensation arrangement if patient payments come from either Medicare or Medicaid (Watnik 2000). Final rules on Stark II were released in January 2001, after years of vigorous debate between the American Medical Association and the federal government. While prohibiting physician self-referral to most organizations that they own in whole or in part, the final rules "generally permit" self-referrals as long as compensation paid to the physician with an ownership interest is not more than would be paid to a physician who did not have an ownership interest (Romano 2001). The ACA made some changes to the Stark law, including a requirement that physician-owners of in-office ancillary services notify the patient in writing that the patient can obtain ancillary services elsewhere, and limitations on the scope of the whole-hospital exception to physician investments in whole hospitals that existed on or before December 31, 2010 (AHA 2010).

Violations of the fraud and abuse statutes appear to be both widespread and serious. Citing widespread violations in 1995, the OIG identified 4,660 hospitals (approximately 80 percent of all hospitals) that had violated the DRG payment window (OIG 1995). In 2007, Medtronic's spine subsidiary, formerly known as Kyphon, agreed to pay $75 million to settle a False Claims Act allegation that the company's marketing efforts caused hospitals and physicians to bill Medicare for inpatient kyphoplasty procedures that should have been completed and billed on an outpatient basis (Biesch 2009). In 2009, Pfizer and Pharmacia & Upjohn agreed to pay $2.3 billion (the largest fraud settlement in history) to settle both civil and criminal liability arising from the illegal promotion of certain pharmaceutical products (OIG 2009). In 2010, FORBA Holdings, which manages a nationwide chain of pediatric dental clinics, agreed to pay $24 million plus interest to settle allegations that it performed unnecessary and often painful dental services on children on Medicaid (OIG 2010a).

The OIG reported $3.8 billion in investigative receivables in the first half of 2013 and excluded 1,661 individuals and entities from participation in federal healthcare

EXHIBIT 5.8 Government Initiatives on Fraud and Abuse	**Health Insurance Portability and Accountability Act (HIPAA) of 1996**	Appropriates a new trust fund to pay for expanded investigations and broadens the authority of the FBI in investigations.
	Operation Restore Trust	A two-year pilot program initiated in 1995 to detect and punish fraud and abuse in the home health agencies, nursing homes, and durable medical equipment (DME) companies in five states (Texas, California, Florida, New York, and Illinois), which represent more than 50 percent of all Medicare business (HFMA 1997). This program was replaced by the recovery audit contractors (RAC) program in 2003.
	DRG Payment Window (72-Hour Rule)	Prohibits a hospital from billing for outpatient services provided by a controlling entity within 72 hours of an admission.
	Billings for Teaching Physicians	Prohibits a hospital from billing for teaching physician services when the teaching physician is not actually present at the time of service.
	Qui Tam Provisions	Protect and reward (15 to 25 percent of the total recovery) whistleblowers who identify instances of fraud and abuse to the federal government (HFMA 2000a). The Department of Justice takes court action on one of about 20 whistleblower complaints filed (HFMA 1999a).
	Voluntary Disclosure	Limits liability for healthcare organizations that discover, identify (to the federal government), and correct billing errors and other fraudulent or abusive practices.
	Federal Safe Harbors	Identifies payment practices to physicians that are safe from federal prosecution under the Anti-Kickback Act (see Appendix 5.1).
	Medicare Integrity Program	Permits HHS to contract with private organizations to decrease fraud and abuse.
	Hospital Outpatient Lab Project	Prohibits a hospital from improper unbundling and double-billing of laboratory tests.
	Prospective Payment System Patient-Transfer Project	Prohibits a hospital from billing for a discharge when the patient was in fact transferred and only eligible for a per diem of the DRG at discharge. Hospitals typically receive more reimbursement for a discharge than for a transfer. Medicare has specific conditions for both discharge billing and transfer billing. A discharge occurs when a patient is formally released from the hospital, dies in

		EXHIBIT 5.8
Prospective Payment System Patient-Transfer Project *(continued)*	a hospital, or is transferred to a non-PPS hospital or facility. A transfer occurs when a patient is moved from one PPS hospital or facility to another, moved to a non-PPS hospital that is under a statewide cost-control project or demonstration project, or moved to a PPS hospital whose first PPS cost-reporting period has not yet begun.	Government Initiatives on Fraud and Abuse *(continued)*
Pneumonia Upcoding Project	This initiative detects hospitals that upcode simple pneumonia to complex pneumonia in order to receive more reimbursement (see Gundling 1998).	
Corporate Integrity Agreements	Agreements between the Office of Inspector General and health-care organizations that are usually required as part of a settlement in a civil fraud investigation. The agreement identifies how the organization will ensure that compliance occurs after the settlement.	
Medicare Fraud Strike Force	Multiagency effort to analyze Medicare billings to determine fraudulent billing. Initiated in South Florida in 2007, the effort has been expanded to other states under the acronym HEAT, or Health Care Fraud Prevention Enforcement Action Team. The team is jointly directed by the secretary of HHS and the attorney general.	

programs. The OIG also reported 484 criminal actions and 240 civil actions during this period. Representative actions in the OIG report for the first half of 2013 included the following (OIG 2013):

◆ Abbott Labs agreed to pay $1.5 billion to resolve allegations that it violated the False Claims Act by improperly marketing and promoting the drug Depakote for uses not approved by the US Food and Drug Administration (FDA).

◆ Paul Boccone treated patients and prescribed narcotics by directing medical practitioners to endorse prescriptions that he wrote. According to the indictments, though Boccone was president of a pain management clinic, he lacked the proper medical education, qualifications, or licensing. Boccone was sentenced to 15 years imprisonment and ordered to pay $275,154 in restitution.

◆ Christopher Card, an optometrist, was sentenced to three years in prison and ordered to pay $1 million in restitution and a $100,000 fine after pleading guilty to charges of fraudulently billing Medicare, Medicaid, and other healthcare insurers for false diagnoses including glaucoma, color blindness, and macular degeneration.

The 2007 action against Medtronic and the 2009 action against Pfizer indicated an OIG willingness to investigate physicians. Lewis Morris, chief counsel to HHS, said, "Under the anti-kickback statute and Stark self-referral law, it takes two to tango. When we're doing our analysis of the fraud problem, we have come to recognize we're only going to get our arms around this if we address both parties to the scheme" (Biesch 2009, 1). That means the OIG is investigating physicians on the receiving end of kickbacks or referral relationships and CEOs and compliance officers who approved the relationships. In the Medtronic case, sales representatives promised physicians using their products that Medtronic would promote their practices and use of kyphoplasty to referring physicians. In the Pfizer case, the OIG alleged in the criminal complaint that Pfizer subsidiary Pharmacia held about 100 inappropriate "consultant" meetings for physicians from 2001 to 2003. Physicians at these meetings, which were held in the Bahamas, Virgin Islands, and elsewhere, received free airfare and resort accommodations, were entertained with golf outings and massages, and were paid honoraria of up to $2,000 per day (Biesch 2009).

Because fraud and abuse violations appear to be both widespread and serious, and because HHS Inspector General June Gibbs Brown declared in September 1997 a policy of "zero tolerance for fraud" (HFMA 1997), most healthcare executives are seeking ways to prevent and detect fraud in their organizations.

In 1991, the US Sentencing Commission issued guidelines for federal judges to use in sentencing corporations that had been found guilty of criminal misconduct, including fraud and abuse. The guidelines allow for lighter sentences for corporations that have corporate compliance programs in place (USSC 1991):

An effective program to prevent and detect violations means a program that has been reasonably designed, implemented, and enforced so that it generally will be effective in preventing and detecting criminal conduct. . . . The hallmark of an effective program to prevent and detect violations of the law is that the organization exercised due diligence in seeking to prevent and detect criminal conduct by its employees and other agents.

The guidelines provide seven requirements for an effective compliance program (Eiland 1996):

1. Establishes reasonable compliance standards and procedures that are organization-specific and that address the areas of greatest risk of liability, such as patient billing and medical record coding

2. Appoints a high-level employee, typically called a corporate compliance officer, who is charged with overseeing compliance with established standards and procedures

3. Exercises due care in delegating discretionary authority so that discretionary authority is not delegated to employees likely to engage in wrongdoing

4. Communicates compliance standards and procedures to employees through training programs on an initial and ongoing basis

5. Designs, implements, and monitors auditing systems to detect wrongdoing by employees, and has a system for employees to report suspected wrongdoing

6. Enforces compliance standards and procedures on a consistent basis through appropriate disciplinary mechanisms, including disciplining employees who fail to detect wrongdoing

7. Responds to wrongdoing in a consistent and timely manner, including disclosure of the wrongdoing to the appropriate government officials

HHS has published model corporate compliance plans for clinical laboratories, hospitals, home health agencies, third-party medical billing companies, durable medical equipment suppliers, hospices, Medicare Advantage plans, and nursing facilities. All model compliance plans are based on the following seven core elements (Federal Register 1998):

1. Implementation of written policies, procedures, and standards of conduct

2. Designation of a compliance officer[7]

3. Development of training and educational programs

4. Creation of a hotline or other measures for receiving complaints and procedures for protecting callers from retaliation[8]

5. Performance of internal audits to monitor compliance

6. Enforcement of standards through well-publicized disciplinary directives

7. Prompt corrective action in response to detected offenses

Corporate compliance with the core recommendations reduces the incidence of fraud and abuse and protects an organization from liability and administrative sanctions.

CHAPTER KEY POINTS

➤ Knowing the history of Medicare and Medicaid is important to understanding the current problems in both programs.

➤ Understanding the current benefits and financing of Medicare and Medicaid is relevant to any healthcare manager.

➤ Analyzing legislative attempts to control costs in Medicare and Medicaid helps place current legislative efforts in perspective.

➤ Understanding the important provisions of fraud and abuse laws is relevant to any healthcare manager.

DISCUSSION QUESTIONS

1. Discuss the history of Medicare and Medicaid, emphasizing the increasing cost of both programs.

2. What was the purpose of offering Medicare Advantage to Medicare beneficiaries?

3. Why was the year 2011 important in terms of Medicare viability?

4. In many states, Medicaid expenditures are the largest line item in the state budget. Why have Medicaid expenditures increased, and what can states do to contain Medicaid costs?

5. What are the major provisions of the Affordable Care Act?

6. Compare and contrast fraud and abuse.

7. What is the government's rationale for granting safe harbors?

NOTES

1. The purpose of President Johnson's legislative program was to eradicate poverty in the United States. While most health legislation in general—and Medicare in particular—was not aimed at those living in poverty, health legislation is often included in the Great Society. President Johnson benefited from a robust economy set in motion by President Kennedy's economic policies and by a liberal majority in Congress.

2. *Those born in   Can retire with full Social Security benefits at age*
    1937 and before 65
    1938–1942   Add 2 months to 65 for every year after 1937
    1943–1954   66
    1955–1959   Add 2 months to 66 for every year after 1954
    1960 and later   67

3. In *Who Will Tell the People,* Greider reports that the federal government used unaudited cost reports during the phase-in period, and as a result hospitals were grossly overpaid.

4. PROs replaced professional standards review organizations (PSROs) established by the Social Security Amendments of 1972. While PSROs were intended to protect the Medicare beneficiary from overuse rewarded under retroactive cost-based reimbursement, PROs were intended to protect the Medicare beneficiary from underuse rewarded under prospective DRG-based reimbursement.

5. Rural hospitals lost money under PPS for different reasons. First, the federal government set the rural hospital rate lower than the urban hospital rate, reflecting what it believed to be lower healthcare costs in the rural community. Second, rural hospitals were reimbursed a per diem rate of the final DRG rate if they transferred the patient. Because the majority of hospital costs occur in the first few days of hospitalization, a per diem rate seldom fully reimbursed a rural hospital for the costs incurred during the first few days.

6. Both the federal and state governments fund Medicaid. The state contribution ranges from 17 to 50 percent depending on the poverty status of the state (Gurny, Baugh, and Davis 1992) based on the following formula (Tudor 1995):

    $$\text{State share} = (\text{State per capita personal income}/\text{National per capita personal income}) \times 0.45$$

7. The OIG recommends that the chief compliance officer (CCO) not be the chief financial officer or anyone else who might have a conflict of interest pertaining to the billing process. When pressed on this point, the OIG has recommended the director of nursing or the director of medical records be the CCO.

8. Centralized billing operations present special problems for healthcare systems that must find a way to respond to patient complaints regarding billing problems at each institution.

Appendix 5.1
Federal Safe Harbors

The following 1989 safe harbors address the types of business and payment practices to physicians that are safe from federal prosecution when certain conditions are met:

- *Investment interests.* Protects payment to an investor that is a return on an investment interest if the investment is either (a) in an entity with assets greater than $50 million, of which payments are based solely on the amount of the investment interest, or (b) in a smaller entity where the activities of the investors are limited.
- *Space rental.* Protects payment by a lessee to a lessor for the use of space if the payment is set in advance and not based upon referrals or business between the parties.
- *Equipment rental.* Protects payment by a lessee of equipment to a lessor for the use of the equipment if the payment is set in advance and not based on referrals or business generated between the parties.
- *Personal services and management contracts.* Protects payment by a principal provided by the agent if the compensation is set in advance and not based on referrals or other business generated between the parties.
- *Sale of practice.* Protects payment to a practitioner by another practitioner for the sale of the former practitioner's practice.
- *Referral services.* Protects payment for the cost of operating the referral service made to an entity serving as a referral service.
- *Warranties.* Protects payment or exchange of anything of value under a warranty provided by a manufacturer or supplier to a buyer.
- *Discounts.* Protects a discount or other price reduction on a good or service received by a buyer if the discount is related to the purchase of a specific good or service and the discount is reported on a claim for payment.
- *Employment relationships.* Protects payments by an employer to an employee for employment in the furnishing of any item or service.
- *Group purchasing organizations.* Protects payments by a vendor of goods or services to a group purchasing organization as part of an agreement to furnish goods or services to an individual entity.
- *Waiver of beneficiary coinsurance and deductible amounts.* Protects the reduction or waiver of any coinsurance or deductible amount either by a hospital if the reduction is not related to the beneficiary's stay and is not made as part of a price reduction or to an individual if the patient qualifies for certain subsidized services.

The 1993 safe harbors address the types of business or payment practices to physicians that are safe from federal prosecution in managed care settings when certain conditions are present, such as

- increased coverage, reduced cost-sharing amounts, or reduced premium amounts offered by health plans to beneficiaries, and
- price reductions offered by health plans to beneficiaries.

The following 1999 safe harbors address the types of business and payment practices to physicians that are safe from federal prosecution when certain conditions are met (Glasser and Bloomquist 2000):

- *Investments* in ASCs. Protects certain investment interests in four categories of freestanding Medicare-certified ASCs: surgeon-owned ASCs, single-specialty ASCs, multispecialty ASCs, and hospital/surgeon-owned ASCs (hospital investors must not be in a position to influence referrals).
- *Joint ventures in underserved areas.* Relaxes several of the conditions of the 1991 Investment Interest safe harbor if the joint venture is in an underserved area as defined by OIG regulations.
- *Practitioner recruitment in underserved areas.* Protects recruitment payments made by entities to attract needed physicians and other healthcare professional to rural and urban health professional shortage areas (HPSAs). This safe harbor requires that at least 75 percent of the recruited practitioner's revenue be from patients who reside in the HPSA, and this safe harbor limits the duration of payments to three years.
- *Obstetrical malpractice insurance subsidies in underserved areas.* Protects a hospital or other entity that pays all or a portion of the malpractice insurance premiums for practitioners engaging in obstetrical practices in HPSAs. This safe harbor requires that at least 5 percent of the affected practitioner's patients be from the HPSA.
- *Sale of physician practices to hospitals in underserved areas.* Protects hospitals in HPSAs that buy and hold the practice of a retiring physician until a new physician can be recruited. This safe harbor requires that the sale be completed within three years and that the hospital engage in good-faith efforts to recruit a new practitioner.
- *Investments in group practices.* Protects investments by physicians in their own group practices, if the group practice meets the physician self-referral (Stark) law definition of a group practice.
- *Referral arrangements for specialty services.* Protects certain arrangements when an individual or entity agrees to refer a patient to another individual or entity for specialty services in return for the party receiving the referral to refer the patient back at a certain time and under certain conditions.
- *Cooperative hospital services organization.* Protects cooperative hospital service organizations (CHSOs) that qualify under section 501(e) of the IRS Code. CHSOs are organizations formed by two or more not-for-profit hospitals, known as patron hospitals, to provide specifically enumerated services, such as purchasing, billing, or clinical services solely for the benefit of patron hospitals.

The following 2006 safe harbor addresses the types of information technology that can be donated to physicians by healthcare organizations that are safe from federal prosecution when certain conditions are met (Conn 2006):

- *Information technology donations to physicians.* Protects certain arrangements when hospitals and other healthcare organizations donate e-prescribing, electronic health records technology, and related support services to physicians (This safe harbor was amended in 2013 to clarify exactly which information technology could be donated to physicians.)

The 2007 safe harbor addresses certain practices in federally qualified health center arrangements, including clarification of remuneration (OIG 2010b).

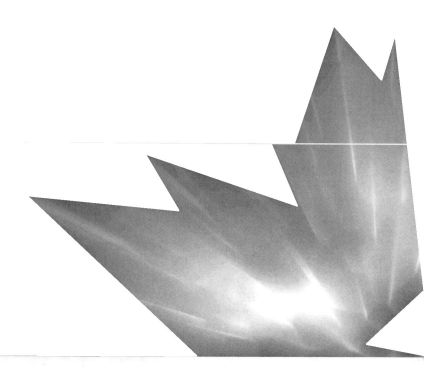

Value is defined as the relationship of quality to cost. High quality at inappropriately high cost does not produce value. Likewise, low quality at low cost also does not produce value. Relentlessly driving toward both high quality and low cost is what produces value.

Richard L. Clarke, president of the Healthcare Financial
Management Association, 1986–2012

LEARNING OBJECTIVES

After completing this chapter, you should be able to do the following:

➤ Explain the methods of classifying costs

➤ Explain the methods of allocating costs

➤ Explain the methods of assembling costs

➤ Understand the relationship of costs to volume and revenue

INTRODUCTION

Cost accounting is the analysis of costs, including methods for classifying costs, allocating costs, assembling costs, and determining product costs. The purpose of cost accounting is to provide management with cost information for a variety of reasons, including cost management, setting charges, and profitability analysis.

Cost accounting in healthcare increased in importance and degree of sophistication with the advent of prospective payment in 1983 and the rapid growth of managed care in the mid-1980s, both of which required cost information by product. With a fixed charge set by the government for diagnosis-related groups (DRGs) and by the managed care organizations for contracts, healthcare organizations need to know the cost of providing a service so they can determine profitability. Prior to 1983, the only cost accounting system available to hospitals was the Medicare cost report, which provided only aggregate data; most insurance companies paid the full amount hospitals charged for a service, regardless of how much a service cost the hospital.

METHODS OF CLASSIFYING COSTS

The first part of cost accounting involves understanding the various methods in which costs can be classified and defined. These costs are not mutually exclusive and the same examples can be used for different cost classifications.

ACCOUNTING FUNCTION

Costs can be classified by accounting function:

financial accounting costs
The amount of money used for a certain purpose.

- ◆ **Financial accounting costs** (also simply called accounting costs) are a measurement in monetary terms of the amount of resources used for a certain purpose. Technically, cost is a value placed on goods or services. When the value expires, the cost becomes an expense. Historical costs derived directly from the financial statements are an example of accounting costs.

managerial accounting costs
Costs that help management make better decisions.

- ◆ **Managerial accounting costs** (i.e., financial costs) are present and future costs that help management make better decisions. Costs derived from budget reports are an example of managerial costs.

MANAGEMENT FUNCTION

Costs can be classified by management function:

operating costs
Costs associated with producing a product or service.

- ◆ **Operating costs** are associated with producing the product or service. For example, supply costs associated with a patient visit to the emergency room would be considered operating costs.

◆ **Nonoperating costs** are associated with supporting the production of a product or service. For example, costs associated with borrowing money for the equipment in the emergency room would be considered nonoperating costs.

TRACEABILITY

Costs can be classified by traceability:

◆ **Direct costs** are costs that can be traced directly to a department, product, or service, such as labor and supplies.

◆ **Indirect costs** (i.e., overhead costs) cannot be traced directly to a department, product, or service. An example is costs associated with heating and cooling.

◆ Full costs include both direct and indirect costs.

◆ **Average costs** are full costs divided by the number of products or services.

BEHAVIOR

Costs can be classified by behavior in relation to volume of products or services:

◆ **Variable costs** vary directly and proportionately to changes in volume. For example, the cost of supplies is directly proportional to volume, so supply cost is a variable cost.

◆ **Fixed costs** remain constant in relation to changes in volume. The cost of heating and cooling a clinic is exactly the same whether there are many patients or just a few, so that cost is a fixed cost.

◆ **Semivariable costs** vary incrementally to changes in volume. For example, a hospital may not hire a new housekeeper if patient volume increases 1 percent, because the current housekeeping staff can probably handle the extra cleaning required because of that small increase. However, if patient volume jumps 5 percent, the hospital may decide to hire a new housekeeper. Thus, housekeeping staff costs are semivariable—they only go up when patient volume increases by a certain increment.

◆ **Marginal cost** is the cost of producing one more unit of something. In most cases, the marginal cost is simply the variable cost of each additional unit. For example, a medical lab may determine that if it performs 100 urinalysis tests per day, the cost per unit—which is the fixed cost plus the variable costs, divided by 100—is $10 per test. However, if it performed 101 tests on a given

nonoperating costs
Costs associated with supporting the production of a product or service.

direct costs
Costs that can be traced directly to a department, product, or service.

indirect costs
Costs that cannot be traced directly to a department, product, or service.

average costs
Full costs divided by the number of products or services.

variable costs
Costs that vary proportionately to volume.

fixed costs
Costs that remain constant in relation to changes in volume.

Semivariable costs
Costs that vary incrementally to changes in volume.

marginal cost
The cost of producing one more unit of something.

true costs
Hypothetical costs that are the most accurate representation of full costs that can be determined by management.

day, the marginal cost of that one additional test would be less than $10, since it would only be the variable cost associated with that one test (such as the supplies).

RELEVANCE TO DECISION MAKING

Costs can be classified by relevance to control and management decision making:

controllable costs
Costs that management can control.

◆   **True costs** are hypothetical costs that are the most accurate representation of full costs that can be determined by management.

◆   **Controllable costs** are costs under the manager's influence, such as labor.

uncontrollable costs
Costs that management cannot control.

◆   **Uncontrollable costs** cannot be influenced by the manager. Utility costs, for example, probably cannot be influenced by the manager, and thus they are uncontrollable.

◆   **Differential costs** (i.e., incremental costs) are the difference in costs between two or more alternatives.

differential costs
The difference in costs between two or more alternatives.

◆   **Sunk costs** are costs that have already been incurred and thus will not be affected by, and should not affect, future decisions. For example, if a CEO spends $1 million opening a new neighborhood clinic, that money is a sunk cost. If a year later it turns out the clinic is not profitable and should be closed, the CEO should not let the fact that he already invested $1 million affect his decision to close the clinic. The CEO might regret that he spent that $1 million, but there's no legitimate business reason to keep the clinic open just because he made that unwise decision in the beginning.

sunk costs
Costs that have already been incurred and thus will not play a role in future decisions.

◆   **Opportunity costs** are potential revenues forgone by rejecting an alternative. The opportunity cost of spending $1 million in opening a new clinic is the money that $1 million would have earned in another investment, such as by buying government bonds or buying a new X-ray machine.

opportunity costs
The cost of potential revenue forgone when an alternative is rejected.

◆   **Relevant costs** are costs that are important to a decision at hand. For example, if the CEO is deciding whether he should close his failing neighborhood clinic from the example above, the $1 million he spent when opening the clinic is not relevant to his decision, because that money is sunk. However, the cost of keeping the clinic open is a relevant cost, because that's how much he'll be spending if he doesn't choose to close the clinic.

relevant costs
Costs that are important to a decision at hand.

◆   **Actual costs** are the historic costs incurred. If the CEO budgeted $750,000 for bonuses to his nursing staff, but ended up paying only $650,000, his actual cost of the bonuses was $650,000.

◆ **Standard costs** are estimated or budgeted costs used for comparison purposes. For example, an ophthalmology practice manager may determine that the standard cost of performing a Lasik surgery is $400. If one of the practice's physicians routinely spends $450 for each Lasik operation (perhaps because she uses more supplies and technician time than the other physicians), the manager may ask this physician to watch her costs.

actual costs
Historic costs incurred.

standard costs
Estimated costs used for comparison.

METHODS OF ALLOCATING COSTS

As is the case with most organizations, healthcare organizations do not send a bill for every product or service they sell. For example, healthcare organizations do not send patients a bill for heating or cooling the hospital room. Instead, the costs of heating and cooling are **allocated** to a department that does generate patient bills, such as radiology and lab.

The process of allocating these indirect costs, and some direct costs, to departments that generate charges is called cost allocation (also called cost finding or cost analysis). The primary purpose of cost allocation is to assign the indirect costs and some direct costs in a way that ensures that patients are paying for only the costs of the services and products they received. Prior to choosing the best method of cost allocation, healthcare organizations must complete the following prerequisite steps (Berman, Kukla, and Weeks 1994).

allocate
Assign costs to a department.

ORGANIZATIONAL CHART

First, the healthcare organization must have an organizational chart and a commensurate chart of accounts. The organizational chart identifies who is responsible for each functional area, usually a department, in the organization. The chart of accounts identifies **cost centers** and **revenue centers** that correspond to the organizational chart. (Every department is a cost center, but only departments that make money are revenue centers.) This step is the basis for responsibility accounting, which means that the organization has identified and holds someone responsible for each revenue and cost center in the organization.

cost center
A department; from an accounting standpoint, a department that consumes money.

REVENUE CENTER IDENTIFICATION

Second, the healthcare organization must identify the cost centers that generate revenue and segregate them from the cost centers that do not generate revenue. The cost centers that do not generate revenue must allocate their costs to the cost centers that do generate revenue.

revenue center
A cost center (department) that generates revenue.

ACCOUNTING SYSTEM

Third, the healthcare organization must have an accounting system that accurately and promptly assigns costs and charges to the appropriate cost and revenue centers.

WORKLOAD STATISTIC

Fourth, the healthcare organization must have a comprehensive information system that generates accurate, nonfinancial statistics for every department. Each department should have a workload statistic that best reflects the work performed in the department. For instance, the workload statistic for the laundry department is usually pounds of laundry; for the personnel department, the statistic is usually number of employees in the organization; for the health information department, the statistic is usually discharges adjusted for outpatient visits; and for housekeeping, the statistic is usually square footage.

COST ALLOCATION METHODS

Fifth, the healthcare organization must have a predetermined cost allocation method. Several methods of cost allocation are used in healthcare organizations.

Direct Apportionment

Direct apportionment is the easiest method of allocation. It involves a one-time allocation of all costs from departments that have costs but do not generate revenue (NR), such as the housekeeping department, to cost centers of departments that do generate revenue (R), such as the laboratory (see Exhibit 6.1).

The main advantage of direct apportionment is its simplicity; the main disadvantage is that it does not take into account the costs of nonrevenue departments doing work for other nonrevenue departments. For instance, housekeeping does work for health information management. Because of this disadvantage, most third-party payers do not accept direct apportionment as a method of cost allocation.

Step-Down Apportionment

Step-down apportionment involves a two-time allocation and takes into account the disadvantage of direct apportionment. It involves a one-time allocation of all costs from cost

---

direct apportionment
A cost allocation method that moves costs from departments that do not generate revenue to departments that do generate revenue.

---

step-down apportionment
A cost allocation method that allocates costs from non-revenue-generating cost centers to other non-revenue-generating cost centers (as appropriate) and then to revenue-generating cost centers.

EXHIBIT 6.1
Direct
Apportionment

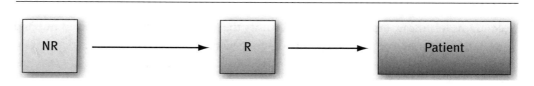

Note: NR = department that does not generate revenue

R = department that generates revenue

centers of departments that do not generate revenue to cost centers of other departments that do not generate revenue, and then a one-time allocation of all costs to cost centers of departments that do generate revenue (see Exhibit 6.2).

Step-down apportionment has two advantages: (1) it considers the costs of nonrevenue departments doing work for other nonrevenue departments before the final allocation to revenue departments, and (2) although burdensome, it can be performed by hand, without a computer. The disadvantage of step-down apportionment is that it does not consider revenue departments doing work for other revenue departments. For instance, the lab department may take cultures in radiology to determine the source of infections (in most healthcare organizations, this would result in an interdepartment charge, or a charge between departments).

Double Apportionment

Double apportionment also involves a two-time allocation and takes into account the disadvantage of step-down apportionment. Double apportionment involves a one-time allocation of all costs from cost centers of departments that do not generate revenue to cost centers of other departments that do not generate revenue. It also involves a simultaneous one-time allocation of costs between cost centers that do generate revenue to cost centers of other departments that do generate revenue before a one-time allocation of all costs to cost centers of departments that do generate revenue (see Exhibit 6.3).

Double apportionment has two advantages: (1) it takes into account the costs of revenue departments doing work for other revenue departments before the final allocation to revenue departments; and (2) considering value, or accuracy divided by cost,

double apportionment
A method that allocates costs from non–revenue-generating cost centers to other non–revenue-generating cost centers (as appropriate), then allocates costs from revenue-generating cost centers to other revenue-generating cost centers (as appropriate), and then allocates costs from non–revenue-generating cost centers to revenue-generating cost centers.

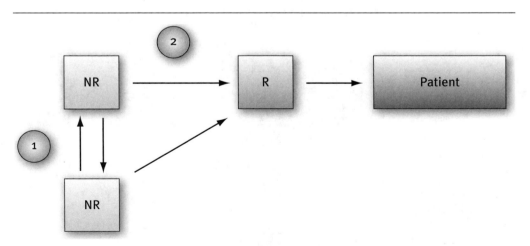

EXHIBIT 6.2
Step-Down Apportionment

EXHIBIT 6.3
Double
Apportionment

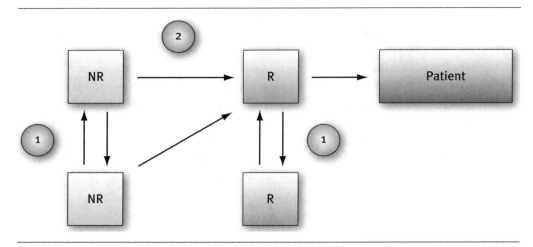

double apportionment is the most practical method of cost allocation because it maximizes accuracy in relation to cost. The disadvantage of double apportionment is that it requires significant computer time, which may make it cost-prohibitive for smaller healthcare organizations.

multiple apportionment
A two-step cost allocation method that makes multiple, simultaneous apportionments during the first step.

Multiple Apportionment

Multiple apportionment (sometimes called algebraic apportionment) also involves a two-step allocation, but it takes into account multiple, simultaneous apportionments during the first step (see Exhibit 6.4).

The more allocations the organization makes in the first step, the more accurate will be the costs reflected in the patient's bill. The advantage of multiple apportionment

EXHIBIT 6.4
Multiple
Apportionment

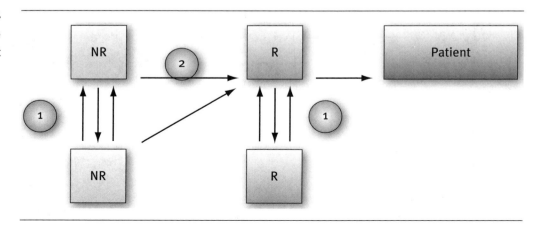

is that it is the most accurate method. The disadvantages are that multiple apportionment requires a computer with significant memory and significant computer time.

METHODS OF ASSEMBLING COSTS

After the healthcare organization has allocated the indirect costs and some direct costs by a method that ensures that patients are paying for only the costs of the services and products they received, the organization develops methods of assembling costs in ways that are meaningful for management. Three methods exist; most organizations use more than one method.

responsibility costing
A method of assembling costs by cost center or department.

RESPONSIBILITY COSTING

Responsibility costing is a method of assembling costs by responsibility center (cost center or department). In this way, the healthcare organizations can hold managers responsible for the controllable costs of the organization.

FULL COSTING

Full costing is a method of assembling direct costs and an allocated share of indirect costs to a product or service for the purpose of determining its profitability.

full costing
A method of assembling direct and indirect costs to a product or service to determine its profitability.

⚠ CRITICAL CONCEPTS

Mr. Shepard was a patient at Citizens Hospital, where he was admitted complaining of stomach pains. Tests revealed that Mr. Shepard had an inflamed appendix and surgery was indicated. Once the surgery was completed, Mr. Shepard spent one day recovering in the hospital. The surgery was routine and there were no complications; discharge was as planned. Using the following four departments as an example, explain how the different cost apportionment methods would work. Explain the advantages and disadvantages of each method as they relate to the case.

Human Resources	Surgery
Housekeeping	Laboratory

DIFFERENTIAL COSTING

Differential costing (sometimes called incremental costing or relevant costing) is a method of assembling costs and sometimes revenues to alternative decisions (Siegel and Shim 2006). In this method, sunk costs (i.e., costs that have already occurred) are not relevant; incremental or differential costs (i.e., costs that differ between the alternative decisions) are relevant. Generally, such an analysis involves the following steps, which are further explained in Problem 6.1:

differential costing
A method of
assembling costs and
sometimes revenues to
alternative decisions.

1. Gathering all costs and revenues associated with each alternative

2. Identifying and dropping all sunk costs

3. Identifying and dropping all costs and revenues that do not differ between the alternatives

4. Selecting the best alternative based on the remaining cost and revenue information

---

✳ PROBLEM 6.1
Differential Cost Analysis

Last week the ABC clinic bought a new piece of lab equipment for $100,000. The piece of equipment will perform 100,000 tests over its useful life. Total variable costs are $3 per test, and the clinic is planning to charge $5 per test. This week a competing lab equipment manufacturer introduced a similar piece of equipment for the same price. In effect, the introduction of this piece of equipment made the resale or trade-in value of the existing piece of equipment $0. Total variable costs for the new piece of equipment are $1 per test. Using differential cost analysis, should ABC clinic keep the existing piece of equipment or should the clinic buy the new piece of equipment?

Step 1:
Gather all costs and revenues associated with each alternative.

	Keep Old Equipment	Buy New Equipment
Revenue	$500,000	$500,000
Fixed cost		
Old	100,000	100,000
New		100,000
Variable costs	300,000	100,000
Full cost gain/(loss)	$100,000	$200,000

(continued)

PROBLEM 6.1
Differential Cost Analysis

Step 2:
Identify and drop all sunk costs (drop the $100,000 fixed cost for old equipment, since it has been spent already).

	Keep Old Equipment	Buy New Equipment
Revenue	$500,000	$500,000
Fixed cost		
Old	~~100,000~~	~~100,000~~
New		100,000
Variable costs	300,000	100,000

Step 3:
Identify and drop all costs and revenues that do not differ between the alternatives (since that figure is the same for both).

	Keep Old Equipment	Buy New Equipment
Revenue	~~$500,000~~	~~$500,000~~
Fixed cost		
Old		
New		100,000
Variable costs	300,000	100,000

Step 4:
Select the best alternative based on the remaining cost and revenue information.

Differential cost	($300,000)	($200,000)

Conclusion:
Using differential cost analysis, ABC should buy the new piece of lab equipment because it has a lower differential cost ($200,000) than the old piece of equipment ($300,000).

METHODS OF DETERMINING PRODUCT COSTS

After the healthcare organization has assembled costs in ways that are meaningful for management, the organization develops methods of determining product costs, or costs by products, such as DRGs, patient days, and outpatient visits. Product costs obviously cut across functional (department) lines of responsibility. Product costs are important in determining profitability in prospective payment arrangements, such as Medicare and managed care, where charges are published before the healthcare organization delivers products and services. Several methods of determining costs exist; organizations may use more than one. The following methods of determining costs are ordered from what are generally agreed to be the least accurate to most accurate methods.

RATIO OF COST TO CHARGES

ratio of cost to charges
A method of determining product cost by relating its cost to its charge. This ratio is usually calculated by dividing an organization's total operating expenses by the gross patient revenue. The resulting percentage is then applied to any product's charge in the organization to calculate the product's cost.

Ratio of cost to charges is a method of determining product cost by relating its cost to its charge. This is usually calculated by dividing an organization's total operating expenses by the gross patient revenue (obtained from the worksheet for the statement of operations).

The resulting percentage is then applied to any product's charge in the organization to calculate the product's cost. Ratio of cost to charges was the predominant method of calculating product cost during the cost-based reimbursement years prior to 1983. For instance, if an organization's total operating expenses are $50,000 and the total gross patient revenues are $100,000, the ratio of cost to charges would be 0.50. Applying that ratio to a CT scan with a charge of $1,000 would produce a product cost for each CT scan of $500.

This method has a serious flaw. It assumes a consistent relationship between cost and charge that simply does not exist because of the numerous ways healthcare organizations have set charges over the last 40 years (see Chapter 7). For example, to remain competitive, healthcare organizations may price a product or service below the actual cost of providing the product or service.

PROCESS COSTING

process costing
A method of determining product cost by dividing the full costs of the organization or department during a given accounting period by the number of products or services produced during the given accounting period.

Process costing is a method of determining product cost during a given accounting period. This number is usually calculated by dividing the full costs of the organization or department during a given accounting period by the number of products or services produced during the given accounting period. For instance, if the full costs of an imaging department are $10 million and the imaging department performs 10,000 procedures, the product cost of each procedure would be $1,000. This method of determining product cost might be appropriate in an organization or department that produces products similar in resource consumption. However, assuming similar resource consumption for most products in healthcare organizations is inappropriate. For instance, a CT scan in the radiology department consumes more resources than a hand X-ray does. Process costing would consider each procedure in the radiology department identical and therefore would assign both procedures the same cost.

JOB-ORDER COSTING

Job-order costing is a method of determining product cost by sampling the product's actual direct costs and developing a relative value unit (RVU)—a measure of resources consumed by each product—in varying amounts for each product. Total direct costs and indirect costs are then assigned to the product on the basis of the relationships established by the RVU. Problem 6.2 demonstrates the process of developing an RVU and determining product costing using the RVU.

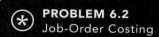

PROBLEM 6.2
Job-Order Costing

ABC Diagnostic Center is developing an RVU and product cost for the following CT procedures, given the projected volumes and sample direct costs. Projected total costs for the CT department are $10 million ($6 million in direct costs and $4 million in indirect costs). Calculate the cost per procedure using job-order costing.

Procedure	Projected Volumes	Labor Expense	Supply Expense
A: CT scan	1,000	$60	$30
B: Upper GI	2,000	50	20
C: Chest X-ray	4,000	25	10
D: Hand X-ray	5,200	20	5

Stage 1: Calculate the RVU for each procedure.

Divide total sample direct cost (labor expense + supply expense) by either the greatest common denominator (GCD) of the supply expenses, if there is one, or the average sample direct cost for each procedure.

Procedure	Total Sample Direct Expense	÷	GCD	=	RVU
A	90		5		18
B	70		5		14
C	35		5		7
D	25		5		5

(continued)

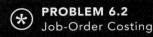

PROBLEM 6.2
Job-Order Costing

Stage 2: Calculate the total cost for each procedure.

Step 1:
Calculate the total projected RVUs by multiplying the RVUs per procedure by the projected volume of each procedure.

Procedure	RVU	×	Projected Volume	=	Total RVUs
A	18		1,000		18,000
B	14		2,000		28,000
C	7		4,000		28,000
D	5		5,200		26,000
Total					100,000

Step 2:
Calculate the cost per RVU by dividing total costs by total RVUs.
$10,000,000 ÷ 100,000 = $100

Step 3:
Calculate the cost per procedure by multiplying the cost per RVU by the RVUs of each procedure.

Procedure	Cost/RVU	×	RVU	=	Cost/ Procedure
A	$100		18		$1,800
B	100		14		1,400
C	100		7		700
D	100		5		500

activity-based costing
A method of determining product cost by using cost drivers to assign indirect costs to products.

ACTIVITY-BASED COSTING

Activity-based costing is a method of determining product cost by using cost drivers to assign indirect costs to products. While job-order costing assigns indirect costs to products proportionate to direct costs and volumes, activity-based costing uses cost drivers, or activity measures, that cause indirect costs to be incurred. Ideal cost drivers are activities that pertain to each procedure in varying amounts.

In Problem 6.2, labor expense and supply expense, which reflected activities and varied for each procedure, were used to determine both the direct and indirect costs for each procedure. Adding a cost driver that better represents the causal relationship of the indirect costs (such as equipment use, which represents a causal relationship to depreciation expense and repair expense) produces the most accurate cost-per-procedure information available, as demonstrated in Problem 6.3.

The difference in the costs per procedure for job-order costing and activity-based costing in Problem 6.3 are a result of the more accurate method of assigning indirect costs using activity-based accounting. Generally speaking, more cost drivers provide a more accurate cost; however, cost-driver information is often expensive to collect. Therefore, only cost drivers that have a high correlation to the consumption of overhead should be used (Siegel and Shim 2006).

(*) PROBLEM 6.3
Activity-Based Costing

ABC Diagnostic Center wants to develop a product cost for the following CT procedures using labor expense and supply expense to assign direct costs and machine minutes as a cost driver to assign indirect costs. Projected total costs for the CT department are $10 million ($6 million in direct costs and $4 million in indirect costs). Assign costs to each procedure using the following information.

Procedure	Projected Volumes	Labor Expense	Supply Expense	Equipment Use (min.)
A	1,000	$60	$30	30
B	2,000	50	20	30
C	4,000	25	10	20
D	5,200	20	5	10

Stage 1: Calculate the direct RVU and the cost driver for each procedure.

Step 1:
Divide total sample direct cost (labor expense + supply expense) by either the GCD, if there is one, or by the average sample direct cost for each procedure.

(continued)

(✳) **PROBLEM 6.3**
Activity-Based Costing

Procedure	Total Sample Direct Cost	÷	GCD	=	Direct RVU
A	$90		5		18
B	70		5		14
C	35		5		7
D	25		5		5

Step 2:

Divide total sample indirect cost by either the GCD or the average sample indirect cost for each procedure. Equipment use in minutes can be used as total sample indirect cost because it shows the same relationship as depreciation cost; however, if additional indirect cost drivers, such as the number of full-time equivalents, are used, then both would be converted to money, added together, and then divided by the GCD.

Procedure	Total Sample Indirect Cost	÷	GCD	=	RVU
A	$30		10		3
B	30		10		3
C	20		10		2
D	10		10		1

Stage 2: Calculate the total cost for each procedure.

Step 1:

Calculate the total projected direct RVUs by multiplying the direct RVUs per procedure by the projected volume per procedure.

Procedure	RVU	×	Projected Volume	=	Total RVUs
A	18		1,000		18,000
B	14		2,000		28,000
C	7		4,000		28,000
D	5		5,200		26,000
Total					100,000

(continued)

PROBLEM 6.3
Activity-Based Costing

Step 2:

Calculate the total projected cost drivers by multiplying the RVUs per procedure by the projected volume per procedure.

Procedure	RVU	×	Projected Volume	=	Total Indirect Cost Drivers
A	3		1,000		3,000
B	3		2,000		6,000
C	2		4,000		8,000
D	1		5,200		5,200
Total					22,200

Step 3:

Calculate the direct cost per RVU by dividing direct costs by total RVUs.

$6,000,000 ÷ 100,000 = $60

Step 4:

Calculate the indirect cost per cost driver by dividing indirect costs by total cost drivers.

$4,000,000 ÷ 22,200 = $180.18

Step 5:

Calculate the direct cost per procedure by multiplying the direct cost per RVU by the RVUs in each procedure.

Procedure	Direct Cost/RVU	×	RVU	=	Direct Cost/ Procedure
A	$60		18		$1,080
B	60		14		840
C	60		7		420
D	60		5		300

Step 6:

Calculate the indirect cost per procedure by multiplying the indirect cost per cost driver by the cost drivers in each procedure.

(continued)

> ### ✳ PROBLEM 6.3
> #### Activity-Based Costing
>
> | Procedure | Indirect Cost/
Cost Driver | × | Cost Driver | = | Indirect Cost/
Procedure |
> |:---:|:---:|:---:|:---:|:---:|:---:|
> | A | $180.18 | | 3 | | $540.54 |
> | B | 180.18 | | 3 | | 540.54 |
> | C | 180.18 | | 2 | | 360.36 |
> | D | 180.18 | | 1 | | 180.18 |
>
> Step 7:
> Calculate the total cost per procedure by adding the direct cost per procedure and in-direct cost per procedure.
>
> | Procedure | Direct Cost/
Procedure | + | Indirect Cost/
Procedure | = | Total Cost/
Procedure |
> |:---:|:---:|:---:|:---:|:---:|:---:|
> | A | $1,080 | | $540.54 | | $1,620.54 |
> | B | 840 | | 540.54 | | 1,380.54 |
> | C | 420 | | 360.36 | | 780.36 |
> | D | 300 | | 180.18 | | 480.18 |

STANDARD COSTING

Standard costing is not actually a method of determining costs; it is a method of establishing benchmark costs, or budgeted costs, for the purpose of comparing actual costs. This method of comparing standard costs to actual costs produces variances, or differences, that are useful to the manager in controlling costs.

IMPACT OF THE AFFORDABLE CARE ACT ON COSTING METHODS

The focus on costing methods in the past has been on costs per product and costs per payer, while the focus under the Affordable Care Act (ACA) will be on costs per patient population and costs per specific high-cost diagnoses and patients. The law moves providers toward assuming more risk for utilization through value-based purchasing, such as bundled payments and accountable care organizations. According to a study by the Agency for Healthcare Research and Quality (Bush 2012), 1 percent of the patients consumed 20 percent of all healthcare spending in 2009, or more than $90,000 per person that year. The same study found that 5 percent of the patients accounted for more than 50 percent of all healthcare spending. Data usage in the past has been on volume and profit, while data usage in the future will be on finding best practices and comparing costs between different treatment options (Selivanoff 2011). Also, costing methods in the past have included ratio of costs-to-charges and job-order costing, while costing methods in the future will be on activity-based costing in an attempt to identify and reduce both direct and indirect costs.

RELATIONSHIP OF COSTS TO VOLUME AND REVENUE

For purposes of determining profit or loss, managers must review costs in relation to associated volumes and revenues (sometimes referred to as cost-volume-profit analysis). The profit equation is

$$\text{Profit} = \text{Revenues} - \text{Expenses}$$

Therefore, the manager first must understand the relationship between costs and expenses. Within this context, cost is the amount spent to acquire an asset, and expense is the amount spent consuming the asset. Therefore, expense is an expired asset. As referenced earlier in this chapter, costs can be classified as fixed costs and variable costs. When classifying these costs in relation to an accounting period, fixed costs remain constant and variable costs change in relation to volume, as demonstrated in Exhibit 6.5.

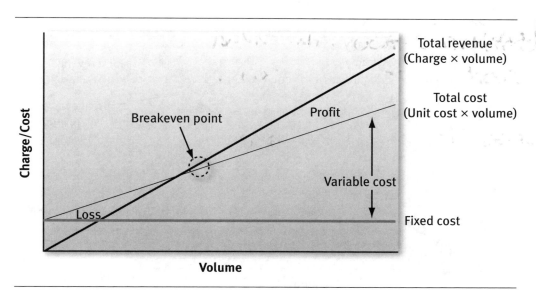

EXHIBIT 6.5
Costs per Period

Related to costs per period, the breakeven point is the volume in units at which the total revenue line intersects the total cost line, or where total costs equal total revenues, as expressed by the equation

$$\text{Breakeven quantity} = \frac{\text{Total fixed costs}}{\text{Charge} - \text{Variable costs per unit}}$$

When classifying these costs in relation to a unit of product or service, fixed costs change in relation to volume, and variable costs remain constant per unit, as shown in Exhibit 6.6.

Exhibit 6.6 is somewhat unorthodox, but it is important to understand the relationship in this way to understand breakeven analysis. At any point on the volume axis, total costs equal variable costs per unit, which remain constant, plus fixed costs per unit, which decline as volume increases. Using costs per unit, the breakeven point in units or revenues is the point at which fixed costs have been covered. Before that point, each unit sold has not only covered its variable costs, but has also contributed to fixed costs. This is called the contribution margin and can be expressed in dollars with the formula

You are the administrator of a physician's office practice, and the physician owners have asked you for a presentation on improving profitability without raising rates. Using both Exhibits 6.5 and 6.6, explain how profit can be increased.

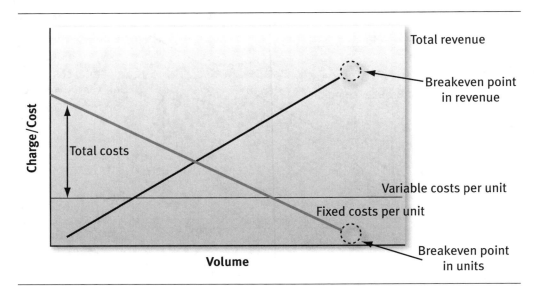

EXHIBIT 6.6
Costs per Unit

$$\text{Contribution margin \$} = \text{Charge} - \text{Variable costs per unit}$$

It also can be expressed as a percentage

$$\text{Contribution margin percent} = \frac{\text{Charge} - \text{Variable costs per unit}}{\text{Charge}}$$

and the breakeven point in dollars can be expressed with the formula

$$\text{Breakeven Point \$} = \frac{\text{Total fixed costs}}{\text{Contribution margin percentage}}$$

After the breakeven point has been reached and fixed costs have been covered, each subsequent unit produced contributes to profit, rather than to fixed costs.

To understand breakeven analysis in a capitated revenue environment, a more detailed profit equation is needed. (This equation is also useful in determining profit at different levels of volume and determining profit if variable costs per unit can be reduced.)

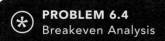 **PROBLEM 6.4**
Breakeven Analysis

ABC's home health care agency is considering a new product with a fixed cost of $1,000, a charge of $10 per unit, and a variable cost of $5.

What is the breakeven point in quantity and in dollars?

What is the contribution margin in dollars and in a percentage?

$$\text{Breakeven point quantity} = \frac{1,000}{10-5} = 200 \text{ units}$$

$$\text{Contribution margin \$} = 10 - 5 = \$5$$

$$\text{Contribution margin percent} = \frac{10-5}{10} = 50 \text{ percent}$$

$$\text{Breakeven point \$} = \frac{1,000}{0.5} = \$2,000$$

PROBLEM 6.5
Breakeven Analysis for Capitated Revenue

ABC Outpatient Clinic is considering a capitated agreement with an insurance company where the clinic would provide outpatient coverage to a 1,000-member plan at $100 per member per month. Variable costs are projected at $150 per clinic visit, and fixed costs allocated to the agreement are $600,000. What is the breakeven point in volume of clinic visits?

Profit = Revenue − (Fixed costs + [Variable cost per unit × Volume])

$0 = $1,200,000 − ($600,000 + [$150 × Volume])

Volume = 4,000 clinic visits (more than 4,000 clinic visits would result in a loss)

Profit = Revenues − Expenses
where Revenues = (Charge × Volume), and
where Expenses = (Fixed costs) + (Variable cost per unit × Volume)

In a capitated revenue environment, revenue is fixed, and what becomes important is controlling volume and variable costs. Exhibit 6.7 gives a graphic representation of the breakeven point in a capitated revenue environment.

EXHIBIT 6.7
Breakeven Point
for Capitated
Revenue

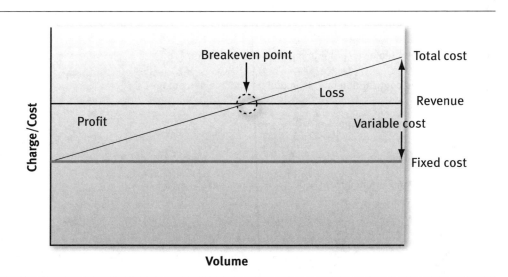

CHAPTER KEY POINTS

➤ Understanding the various methods of classifying costs is important in a cost containment environment.

➤ Knowing how indirect costs are allocated to direct costs and ultimately to the charge is necessary in order to understand the cost structure of a department.

➤ Understanding the relationship of costs to both volumes and revenues is important for the manager who wants to improve department efficiency and/or profit.

➤ Knowing how to isolate relevant costs in differential cost analysis improves decision making.

➤ Understanding how to allocate costs using activity-based costs better reflects costs for more accurate rate setting.

➤ Identifying new costing methods is necessary under the ACA.

DISCUSSION QUESTIONS

1. Why is it important for the healthcare manager to be able to classify costs a variety of different ways?

2. What is the point of allocating costs? After allocation, how is the resulting information used?

3. Cost information can be assembled in a variety of ways for a variety of reasons. List and explain three ways cost information is assembled and the reason for the assembly.

4. Explain how differential cost analysis might be used in the following nonroutine decisions: expanding an existing service, decreasing an existing service, starting a new service, and closing an existing service.

5. How will the ACA change how providers look at costs?

6. Compare and contrast breakeven points per period and breakeven points per unit of service.

DIFFERENTIAL COST ANALYSIS

Differential Cost Analysis Practice Problem

Beta Managed Care Corporation has approached XYZ Hospital for inpatient labor and delivery coverage for Beta's subscribers. Beta will pay $5,000 per delivery. XYZ's fixed costs per delivery are $3,000, and variable costs are $3,000. Using differential cost analysis, should XYZ Hospital accept Beta's offer?

Differential Cost Analysis Practice Problem Solution

Step 1: Gather all costs and revenues associated with each alternative.

	Accept	Reject
Revenue	$ 5,000	$ 0
Fixed Cost	3,000	3,000
Variable Costs	3,000	0
Full Cost Gain/(Loss)	($1,000)	($3,000)

Step 2: Identify and drop all sunk costs (drop $3,000 fixed cost for each alternative).

	Accept	Reject
Revenue	$5,000	$0
Fixed Cost	0	0
Variable Costs	3,000	0

Step 3: Identify and drop all costs and revenues that do not differ between the alternatives.

	Accept	Reject
Revenue	$5,000	$0
Fixed Cost	0	0
Variable Costs	3,000	0

Step 4: Select the best alternative based on the remaining cost and revenue information.

	Accept	Reject
Revenue	$5,000	$0
Fixed Cost	0	0
Variable Costs	3,000	0
Differential Cost Gain/(Loss)	$2,000	$0

Conclusion: Using differential cost analysis, XYZ should accept the offer because it has a higher differential gain ($2,000) than rejecting the offer ($0).

Differential Cost Analysis Self-Quiz Problem

The integrated delivery system you work for is thinking about dropping your sleep disorder program for financial reasons. The program serves 4,000 patients a year with annual revenues of $2 million. The variable cost per patient is $200 with allocated fixed costs to the program of $1.6 million. Should your program be dropped for financial reasons?

JOB-ORDER COSTING

Job-Order Costing Practice Problem

XYZ Reference Lab must calculate the relative value and cost per procedure given that the total lab expense is $851,455:

Procedure	Projected Volume	Labor Expense ($)
A	4,000	.10
B	3,500	.05
C	2,000	.05
D	4,000	.15
E	4,500	.10
F	6,000	.10
G	2,200	.15
H	1,800	.15
I	4,000	.05
J	3,000	.10

Job-Order Costing Practice Problem Solution

Stage 1: Calculate RVUs by dividing labor expense per procedure by the average labor expense.

Procedure	Labor Expense ($)	÷	Average Labor Expense ($)	=	RVU
A	.10		.10		1.0
B	.05		.10		.5
C	.05		.10		.5
D	.15		.10		1.5
E	.10		.10		1.0
F	.10		.10		1.0
G	.15		.10		1.5
H	.15		.10		1.5
I	.05		.10		.5
J	.10		.10		1.0

Stage 2, Step 1: Calculate total RVUs by multiplying RVUs per procedure by projected volume.

Procedure	RVU	×	Projected Volume	=	Total RVUs
A	1.0		4,000		4,000
B	.5		3,500		1,750
C	.5		2,000		1,000
D	1.5		4,000		6,000
E	1.0		4,500		4,500
F	1.0		6,000		6,000
G	1.5		2,200		3,300
H	1.5		1,800		2,700
I	.5		4,000		2,000
J	1.0		3,000		3,000
					34,250

Step 2: Calculate the cost per RVU by dividing total costs by total RVUs.

$851,455 ÷ 34,250 = $24.86

Step 3: Calculate the cost per procedure by multiplying the cost per RVU by RVUs per procedure.

Procedure	Cost/RVU	×	RVUs/Procedure	=	Cost/Procedure
A	24.86		1.0		24.86
B	24.86		.5		12.43
C	24.86		.5		12.43
D	24.86		1.5		37.29
E	24.86		1.0		24.86
F	24.86		1.0		24.86
G	24.86		1.5		37.29
H	24.86		1.5		37.29
I	24.86		.5		12.43
J	24.86		1.0		24.86

Job-Order Costing Self-Quiz Problem

Using the weighted procedure method of setting rates, calculate the relative value and cost per procedure for the following lab procedures given a total lab cost of $1.25 million and an average hourly lab tech rate of $15 (to calculate the RVU, divide the total sample expense by the common denominator of 5):

Procedure	Projected Volume	Labor in Minutes	Supply Expense ($)
Amylase	4,000	15	.75
Bleeding time	5,000	12	.50
Uric acid	3,000	10	.50
Platelet count	7,800	9	.25
Hematocrit	7,600	8	.25

ACTIVITY-BASED COSTING

Activity-Based Costing Practice Problem

XYZ Home Health Care Corporation wants to develop a product cost for the following home visits using labor expense and supply expense to assign direct costs and visit minutes as a cost driver to assign indirect costs. Projected total costs for the home health care corporation are $6 million ($5 million direct and $1 million indirect). Assign costs to each visit using the following information:

Visit	Projected Volumes	Labor Expense ($)	Supply Expense ($)	Visit Minutes
Physical therapy (PT)	2,000	60	30	60
Respiratory therapy (RT)	4,000	50	20	40
Nursing	9,000	25	10	30
Occupational therapy (OT)	7,000	20	5	40

Activity-Based Costing Practice Problem Solution

Stage 1: Calculate the direct RVU and the indirect RVU for each visit.

Step 1: Divide total sample direct cost (labor expense + supply expense) by either the greatest common denominator (GCD) (if there is one) or the average sample direct cost for each visit.

Visit	Total Sample Direct Cost ($)	÷	GCD	=	Direct RVUs
PT	90		5		18
RT	70		5		14
Nursing	35		5		7
OT	25		5		5

Step 2: Divide total sample indirect cost (visit minutes) by either the GCD or the average sample indirect cost for each visit.

Visit	Total Sample Indirect Cost ($)	÷	GCD	=	Indirect RVUs
PT	60		10		6
RT	40		10		4
Nursing	30		10		3
OT	40		10		4

Stage 2: Calculate the total cost for each visit.

Step 1: Calculate the total projected direct RVUs by multiplying the direct RVUs per visit by the projected volume per visit.

Visit	RVU	×	Projected Volume	=	Total Direct RVUs
PT	18		2,000		36,000
RT	14		4,000		56,000
Nursing	7		9,000		63,000
OT	5		7,000		35,000
					190,000

Step 2: Calculate the total projected indirect cost drivers by multiplying the indirect RVUs per visit by the projected volume per visit.

Visit	RVU	×	Projected Volume	=	Total Indirect Cost Drivers
PT	6		2,000		12,000
RT	4		4,000		16,000
Nursing	3		9,000		27,000
OT	4		7,000		28,000
					83,000

Step 3: Calculate the direct cost per RVU by dividing direct costs by total direct RVUs.

$5,000,000 ÷ 190,000 = $26.32

Step 4: Calculate the indirect cost per cost driver by dividing indirect costs by total indirect cost drivers.

$1,000,000 ÷ 83,000 = $12.05

Step 5: Calculate the direct cost per procedure by multiplying the direct cost per RVU by the direct RVUs in each procedure.

Visit	Direct Cost/RVU ($)	×	Direct RVU	=	Direct Cost/ Visit ($)
PT	26.32		18		473.76
RT	26.32		14		368.48
Nursing	26.32		7		184.24
OT	26.32		5		131.60

Step 6: Calculate the indirect cost per visit by multiplying the indirect cost per RVU by the indirect RVUs in each procedure.

Visit	Indirect Cost/RVU ($) ×	Indirect RVUs	Indirect = Cost/Visit ($)
PT	12.05	6	72.30
RT	12.05	4	48.20
Nursing	12.05	3	36.15
OT	12.05	4	48.20

Step 7: Calculate the total cost per procedure by adding the direct cost per procedure and the indirect cost per procedure.

Visit	Direct Cost/Visit ($) +	Indirect Cost/Visit ($) =	Total Cost/Visit ($)
PT	473.76	72.30	546.06
RT	368.48	48.20	416.68
Nursing	184.24	36.15	220.39
OT	131.60	48.20	179.80

Activity-Based Costing Self-Quiz Problem

Your wellness clinic wants to develop a product cost for the following activities using labor expense and supply expense to assign direct costs and visit minutes as a cost driver to assign indirect costs. Projected total costs for your wellness clinic are $600,000 ($300,000 direct and $300,000 indirect). Assign costs to each activity using the following information:

Activity	Projected Volumes	Labor Expense ($)	Supply Expense ($)	Visit Minutes
Evaluation	4,000	30	10	60
Education	3,000	50	20	40
Exercise	2,000	05	00	90

BREAKEVEN ANALYSIS

Breakeven Analysis Practice Problem

Assume the following for XYZ Medical Supply Vendor:

Fixed cost = $20,000
Selling price = $1,000
Variable cost = $600

What is the breakeven point in units? In dollars? What is the contribution margin in percent? In dollars?

Breakeven Analysis Practice Problem Solution

Breakeven point in units

$$\frac{\text{Total fixed costs}}{\text{Price} - \text{Variable costs}} = \frac{\$20,000}{\$1,000 - \$600} = 50 \text{ units}$$

Breakeven point in dollars

Breakeven units x Price = 50 x $1,000 = $50,000

Contribution margin in percent

$$\frac{\text{Price} - \text{Variable costs}}{\text{Price}} = \frac{\$1,000 - \$600}{\$1,000} = .40, \text{ or } 40\%$$

Contribution margin in dollars

Price − Variable cost = $1,000 − $600 = $400

Breakeven Analysis Self-Quiz Problem

Assume the following for your facility:

Fixed cost = $10,000
Selling price = $100
Variable cost = $20

What is the breakeven point in units? In dollars? What is the contribution margin in percent? In dollars?

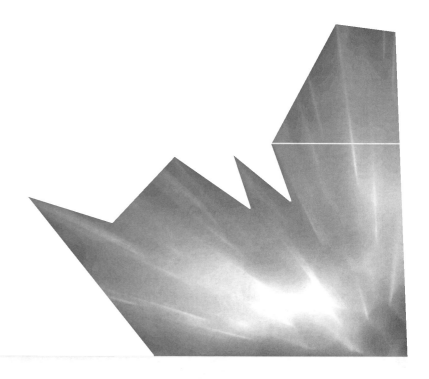

The economic "perfect storm" is coming to healthcare organizations: a rising tide of uninsured and underinsured patients, aging baby boomers that will present greater healthcare demands, a challenging economic climate, shifting eligibility requirements, and cultural obstacles regarding healthcare payments.

DeLuca and Smith (2010)

LEARNING OBJECTIVES

After completing this chapter, you should be able to do the following:

➤ Review the history of setting charges

➤ Understand the current concerns regarding charges

➤ Examine the various methods of setting charges

➤ Examine the future of setting charges

➤ Describe how cost shifting affects setting charges

➤ Review methods of reimbursement to providers

INTRODUCTION

In response to a report by ABC's *PrimeTime Live* on how charging practices affected rising healthcare costs, Humana, which at the time was a large for-profit chain of hospitals, responded (ABC News 1991):

> Hospital charges are inaccurate measurements of the cost of healthcare to patients, since the vast majority of patients and insurers no longer pay them in full.

Essentially, Humana was correct: Few patients or insurers pay what they are charged; most patients and insurers pay charges minus a negotiated discount.[1] Discounting charges and other charging practices have resulted in charges that have little, if any, relationship to costs. How did charges in the healthcare industry arrive at such a nonsensical point? The answer can be found in the history of healthcare charging practices.

HISTORIC CONTEXT

Healthcare charging practices have progressed through three distinct eras: consensus-driven charging, financial expediency–driven charging, and competition-driven charging. All of these have had a perverse effect on the relationship between charges and costs.

Prior to Medicare, charging was driven by consensus: Healthcare providers set charges consistent with other providers in the community. Providers sought consistent charges for fear that higher-than-average charges would signal inefficiencies to regulators or drive business to competing providers. Setting charges based on consensus resulted in cost shifting (i.e., the practice of shifting costs to some payers to offset losses from other payers). For instance, a new provider would set charges consistent with other providers in the community, even if the new provider had higher per-unit costs than its competitors. To make up the difference, the provider would charge more for procedures for which it had less competition from other providers (Finkler 1982).

With the advent of Medicare and Medicaid, charges became irrelevant for a substantial portion of the provider's business. Medicare—and usually Medicaid—paid hospitals on the basis of reasonable costs, not charges, and paid physicians on the basis of approved charge schedules. Realizing that only patients covered by commercial insurance and patients paying their own way (i.e., charge-based patients) would pay the provider based on charges, most providers set charges based on financial expediency—the financial needs of the provider. The financial needs of the provider obviously include the costs of providing services to charge-based patients, but they also include other factors, such as losses to both Medicare and Medicaid, the cost of bad debt, and the cost of charity care. Problem 4.1 (page 86) demonstrates how these costs are identified and shifted to charge-based patients during the budget process. The recovery of shifted costs occurs at the procedural level using **charge masters**, which are lists of items (e.g., medications, procedures,

charge masters
Lists of items providers charge for.

supplies, rooms) providers charge for. Providers developed software programs to show each item on the charge master and the item's use by the patient. If the item was frequently used by cost-based payers (i.e., those on Medicare or Medicaid), the charge was set close to allowable cost because allowable cost was the amount the provider would be reimbursed. If the item was not often used by cost-based payers, the charge was increased to maximize the collection from the charge-based patients (i.e., those who had commercial insurance or paid the bills themselves). Because providers, especially hospitals, set charges in this manner every year, it is easy to understand how some charges, over time, were increased thousands of percent over cost (see Appendix 7.1).

In the early 1980s, the consumer movement complicated charging based on financial expediency. Billing regulations mandated that Medicare patients receive a copy of their bill from the provider, even in cases where patients had no financial liability. In this way, patients could audit the bills to determine whether they had received the items listed on the bill. Patients often complained about high charges for items they could buy for less in their local drugstore (e.g., aspirin, facial tissues, toothbrushes), even when the charges were covered in part or entirely by Medicare. In response, many providers either reduced the charges for these consumer items or dropped the charges altogether. However, to recover the cost of these items, providers increased the charges for items that patients could not buy in their local drugstore.

Medicare's prospective payment based on diagnosis-related groups (DRGs) did not change the way providers set charges; however, it did provide the impetus for providers to implement sophisticated cost accounting systems so that they could determine their profits or losses per DRG. This proved to be an important precursor to the next era—competition-driven charging.

During the competition-driven charging era, which began in the mid-1980s and continues today, providers set charges based on what the market will bear, or what the charge-based patients and their insurers will pay. However, two factors have led to lower charges: (1) managed care, which demands that providers discount their charges significantly in exchange for business, and (2) the prospective payment system (PPS), which means providers are no longer guaranteed to cover their costs.[2, 3, 4]

The practice of charging payers different prices for the same products and services—which could be construed to be a violation of the 1890 Sherman Antitrust Act (15 USC 2), the 1914 Clayton Act (15 USC 13), and the 1932 Robinson-Patman Act (15 USC 13–13b, 21a)—may be thought to be essentially the same as discounting charges to different payers for the same products and services. However, third-party payers justified the demands for discounts on the basis of the high volumes of patients they brought to the providers. Because the third parties were a sure and predictable source of revenue, product costing became critical during the competition-driven era.[5] Providers needed sophisticated methods of determining product costs so they could negotiate discounts without discounting below cost, or at least below variable costs.[6]

During the early years of competition-driven charging, providers practiced price-driven costing, the practice of cutting costs to break even with charges, which were dictated by the insurer or determined by competition. However, price-driven costing, even when coupled with aggressive downsizing or reengineering strategies,[7] ultimately arrives at a point at which additional cost cutting may affect quality.[8] Furthermore, managing costs effectively is only half the strategy for economic survival. The other half is managing revenue effectively by making up for revenue lost as a result of discounting and competition.

> *charging analysis*
> An examination of charges to make sure maximum reimbursement is being received.

Most healthcare organizations have pursued relatively conservative revenue management strategies that have included charging analysis, charge master enrichment, and charge capture assessment (Murray et al. 1994). **Charging analysis** ensures that the charge set for a specific item results in maximum reimbursement related to the payer classification. For example, elective plastic surgery, which is normally paid for by private insurance, is marked up considerably in order to maximize profits. On the other hand, hip replacement surgery, which is usually Medicare reimbursed, is not marked up because Medicare pays a predetermined amount, thus limiting the reimbursement. **Charge master enrichment** ensures that healthcare organizations charge only for items that third-party payers recognize as legitimate charges. **Charge capture assessment** ensures that healthcare organizations do not lose charges within the organization. Charge capture assessment compares what patients receive, as documented by medical records, to what patients are billed, as documented in patient bills.

> *charge master enrichment*
> An analysis of charges to make sure every item is recognized by third-party payers as a legitimate charge.

Cross (1997) believed that the healthcare industry was ready for more aggressive revenue management strategies, including charging strategies that have been commonplace in other service industries for a long time, and to a certain extent that has happened. For instance, airlines offer significant discounts to travelers who are willing to travel during off-peak periods and make their reservations in advance. In this way, the airlines are better off using their fixed costs (i.e., airplanes) while ensuring that their variable costs are still met by the discounted charges. The discounted charges have created a new market without hurting the old market. In most cases, business travelers who fly during peak periods are willing to pay the higher charges because their company is reimbursing the cost; vacation travelers who fly during off-peak periods want the lower charges because they pay the cost themselves. Some healthcare organizations enhance their market share by discounting to fill excess capacity, especially during the weekends, or create new markets by discounting procedures that patients are likely to pay out of pocket.

> *charge capture assessment*
> A comparison of medical records to patient invoices to make sure the organization is not missing billable items.

HEALTHCARE PRICING COMES UNDER PUBLIC SCRUTINY

While most patients do not pay charges because their insurance company has negotiated a discount, patients without insurance have often been asked to pay the entire bill by healthcare organizations. Whether the organizations actually expect the uninsured patient to pay the entire bill is unclear (many of these bills ultimately become bad debt), but there is no doubt the healthcare industry has been widely criticized for these charges, especially because increasing numbers of uninsured are middle-class individuals and families with political and business clout. Why haven't hospitals offered the uninsured the same discounts offered to insurance companies? Historically, hospitals have not offered discounts to the uninsured because of concerns about Medicare payment and compliance. For example, if a hospital offered a big discount to everybody except Medicare, the hospital could run afoul of Medicare rules regarding charges that are "substantially in excess" of "usual charges" (Barry and Keough 2005). However, this situation may change. As noted in Chapter 3, the Affordable Care Act (ACA) requires nonprofit hospitals to limit charges to patients eligible for assistance to no more than the lowest amount billed to insured patients.

In addition to amending policies to allow additional write-offs to charity care, hospitals also revised their pricing policies and prices. Amending prices is difficult because of the number of managed care agreements that have negotiated discounts on the previous price. HFMA introduced the following strategy for rational pricing in 2005 (Clarke 2006):

1. Using a cost accounting system, identify and measure the costs associated with the product or service to be priced.

2. Gather data on prices for similar products and services offered by competitors.

3. Address contractual considerations to ensure the new price will result in the same or improved net revenue for the product or service.

4. Prepare for public scrutiny. Under consumer-driven healthcare, consumers are more financially responsible for their healthcare. As a result, they demand prices and information on how the prices were set. What most patients need is a detailed explanation of benefits that identifies what their out-of-pocket expense will be.

Many state legislatures have passed pricing transparency laws. New York passed such a law in 2007. The New York law, dubbed Manny's Law after a 24-year-old patient who died as a result of surgery postponed because he did not

You are the business office manager of a 26-bed rural hospital. The chairman of your governing body, who has been the chairman for more than 30 years, is discussing with you possible ways to improve the hospital's financial position. During the discussion, he asks you why you cannot increase the charges to Blue Cross to cover the losses to Medicare, Medicaid, and charity care. He goes on to say that this strategy was used in the 1970s and 1980s, and he does not understand why it will not work in 2014. What do you tell him?

have insurance, requires New York hospitals to establish financial-aid policies for low-income and uninsured patients. The law prohibits hospitals from charging patients earning less than 300 percent of the federal poverty level more than private or government insurers pay. California passed a similar law in late 2006. California's Hospital Fair Pricing Law prohibits hospitals from charging self-pay patients who earn less than 350 percent of the federal poverty level more than what Medicare and other government-sponsored programs pay for care (Benko 2006). The National Conference of State Legislatures disclosed a summary of signed laws and proposed state legislation relating to transparency and disclosure of health and hospital charges. Included are details concerning 31 state measures affecting disclosure, transparency, and reporting and/or publication of healthcare provider and hospital charges and fees (NCSL 2009).

The ACA includes requirements for hospitals to publicize an annual updated list of standard charges, including Medicare severity diagnosis-related groups (MS-DRGs) (AHA 2010a). The laws also require tax-exempt hospitals to limit their charges for emergency or other medically necessary care to patients eligible under the facility's financial assistance policy (charity care policy) to not more than the amounts billed to insured patients who receive the same care. According to the regulations, the financial assistance policy must include (IRS 2012, p. 5):

- eligibility criteria for financial assistance and whether such assistance includes free or discounted care;

- the basis for determining amounts charged to patients;

- the method for applying for financial assistance;

- in the case of an organization that does not have a separate billing and collections policy, the actions the hospital organization may take in the event of nonpayment; and

- measures to widely publicize the financial assistance policy within the community served by the hospital organization.

Subsequent to the 2012 Supreme Court decision on the ACA, states are encouraged to expand eligibility criteria for Medicaid from 100 percent of the federal poverty level to 138 percent of the poverty level. To encourage states to expand Medicaid, the federal government will pay all of the expansion costs for the first three years and 90 percent for the next seven years. States that are resisting the expansion are concerned about its effects on the federal debt and the federal government's ability to keep its funding promise for ten years. Hospital associations generally support the expansion, even though Medicaid seldom pays the full cost of providing care to its beneficiaries. These associations project increases in Medicaid volumes, even at a reimbursement less than cost, will be more than offset by the decline in charity care that will result from the expansion of Medicaid eligibility. This is especially true for safety-net hospitals that care for higher-than-average Medicaid loads (Betbeze 2013).

METHODS OF SETTING CHARGES

Given that many different influences affect the charge-setting decision, the initial charge, before comparisons to other facilities and before discounts, should reflect the healthcare organization's true cost of providing the product or service.[9] The following three methods of setting charges based on costs are well established in the literature (Suver, Neumann, and Boles 1992; Berman, Kukla, and Weeks 1994).

> You are the CEO of a nonprofit community hospital located in a small city. An influential patient is in your office with a hospital bill that he received recently for a one-day stay in your hospital (most of the time was spent in the emergency room). The bill, excluding physician charges, was $17,000. The patient thinks this is outrageous, and he wants to know what the care actually cost the hospital. What do you tell him?

RVU METHOD

The first method of setting charges is called the relative value unit (RVU) method (see Chapter 6 for an explanation of how RVUs are created). The RVU method is used in departments that have an established **RVU schedule**, such as laboratory and radiology. RVU schedules are recalculated every three to five years. Costs per RVU and corresponding charges per procedure are calculated more often, usually every year.[10] After full costs per procedure have been established (see problems 6.2 and 6.3 in Chapter 6), charges can be set to break even (i.e., charge the full cost only) or to realize a gain (i.e., charge the full cost plus a percentage) (see Problem 7.1).

RVU schedule
A list of charges, such as procedures performed by the radiology department, based on relative value units (RVUs).

⊛ PROBLEM 7.1
RVU Method of Setting Charges

Using job-order costing and activity-based costing from Problems 6.2 and 6.3, calculate the charge necessary to realize a 5 percent gain at the diagnostic center.

Using Job-Order Costing:

Step 3 (This example is a continuation of Problem 6.2 in Chapter 6):

Calculate the cost per procedure by multiplying the cost per RVU by the RVUs in each procedure.

Procedure	Cost/RVU	×	RVU	=	Cost/ Procedure
A	$100		18		$1,800
B	100		14		1,400
C	100		7		700
D	100		5		500

(continued)

PROBLEM 7.1
RVU Method of Setting Charges

Step 4:

Calculate the charge necessary to realize a 5 percent gain at the diagnostic center.

Procedure	Cost/ Procedure	+	5 Percent	=	New Charge
A	$1,800		90		$1,890
B	1,400		70		1,470
C	700		35		735
D	500		25		525

Using Activity-Based Costing

Step 7 (This example is a continuation of Problem 6.3 in Chapter 6):

Calculate the total cost per procedure by adding the direct cost per procedure and the indirect cost per procedure.

Procedure	Direct Cost/ Procedure	+	Indirect Cost/ Procedure	=	Total Cost/ Procedure
A	$1,080		$540.54		$1,620.54
B	840		540.54		1,380.54
C	420		360.36		780.36
D	300		180.18		480.18

Step 8:

Calculate the charge necessary to realize a 5 percent gain at the diagnostic center.

Procedure	Cost/ Procedure	+	5 Percent	=	New Charge
A	$1,620.54		81.03		$1,701.57
B	1,380.54		69.03		1,449.57
C	780.36		39.02		819.38
D	480.18		24.01		504.19

HOURLY RATE METHOD

The second method of setting charges is called the hourly rate method; it is used in departments that charge per hour (or per modality or segment of time) for their services. Respiratory therapy, physical therapy, and surgery are three examples of departments that use this method for setting charges. Problem 7.2 demonstrates the calculations involved in using the hourly rate method.

SURCHARGE METHOD

The third method of setting charges is the surcharge method. It is used in departments that know the cost of their products and add a surcharge to cover overhead. Pharmacy and central supply are two examples of departments that use the surcharge method for setting charges. This method is demonstrated in Problem 7.3.

STRATEGIC CHARGE SETTING

In 1987, Eastaugh predicted that increasing competitive pressures would drive healthcare organizations into the same strategic pricing options that other service industries use. Referring to Porter's 1980 book, *Competitive Strategy: Techniques for Analyzing Industries and Competitors*, Eastaugh identified the competitive pressures as they relate to the healthcare industry:

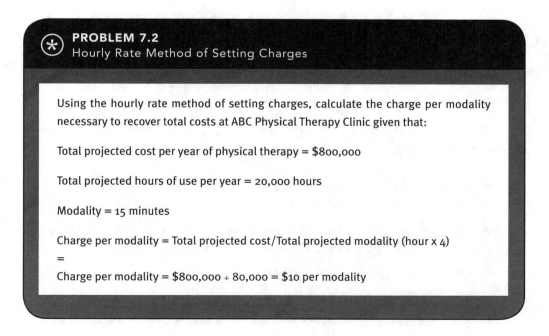

PROBLEM 7.2
Hourly Rate Method of Setting Charges

Using the hourly rate method of setting charges, calculate the charge per modality necessary to recover total costs at ABC Physical Therapy Clinic given that:

Total projected cost per year of physical therapy = $800,000

Total projected hours of use per year = 20,000 hours

Modality = 15 minutes

Charge per modality = Total projected cost/Total projected modality (hour x 4)
=

Charge per modality = $800,000 ÷ 80,000 = $10 per modality

✱ PROBLEM 7.3
Surcharge Method of Setting Charges

Using the surcharge method of setting charges, calculate the charge necessary to cover total costs for 100,000 admission kits at ABC Women's Hospital given that:

Overhead allocated to the admission kits project = $50,000

Total projected cost of admission kits = $100,000

Step 1: Overhead + Cost of kits = Total cost

$50,000 + $100,000 = $150,000

Step 2: Total cost ÷ Number of kits = Charge per kit to break even

$150,000 ÷ 100,000 = $1.50

- ◆ Rivalry among existing competitors

- ◆ Potential new entrants to the market

- ◆ Bargaining power of buyers (e.g., Medicare, Medicaid, managed care)

- ◆ Bargaining power of suppliers (e.g., physicians)

- ◆ Rivalry from substitute products (e.g., holistic medicine, natural cures, self-care)

These pressures ultimately forced healthcare organizations to review all of the following strategic pricing options:

- ◆ *Predatory pricing:* The practice of pricing products and services low in the short term to gain market share.

- ◆ *Slash pricing:* The practice of pricing products and services low in the long term by making fundamental changes in the product or service.

- ◆ *Follower pricing:* The practice of pricing products and services relative to the market leader.

- ◆ *Phaseout pricing:* The practice of pricing products or services high to eliminate poor quality or underused products and services.

◆ *Preemptive pricing:* The practice of pricing products and services low to discourage new entrants in the market.

◆ *Skim pricing:* The practice of pricing products and services high because of high quality or low availability in the market.

◆ *Segment pricing:* The practice of pricing products and services high relative to their "snob appeal," such as high charges for birthing centers.

◆ *Loss-leader pricing:* The practice of pricing products and services low to attract customers to complementary products or services that are priced high.

The changes occurring in the healthcare environment will require close attention to rate setting and pricing strategies. Sound pricing decisions remain critical to the successful operation of healthcare organizations.

METHODS OF REIMBURSEMENT TO PROVIDERS

Common methods of reimbursement to providers include the following:

◆ *Charges:* Retrospective reimbursement based on charges submitted by the provider to the patient or to the insurer on behalf of the patient.

◆ *Charges minus a discount:* Retrospective reimbursement based on charges minus a discount negotiated between the provider and the insurer (the usual method of reimbursement for preferred provider organizations).

◆ *Cost plus:* Retrospective reimbursement based on a cost report submitted by the provider to the insurer. The insurer reimburses the provider for reasonable cost plus a percentage for growth.

◆ *Cost:* Retrospective reimbursement based on a cost report submitted by the provider to the insurer (the predominant method of Medicare and Medicaid reimbursement from 1966 to 1983).

◆ *Per diem:* Prospective reimbursement based on a per-day rate established by the insurance company (the predominant method of reimbursement to nursing homes).

◆ *Per diagnosis:* Prospective reimbursement based on a per-diagnosis rate established by the insurer (the predominant method of Medicare and Medicaid reimbursement from 1983 to present).

◆ *Per head, or capitation:* Prospective reimbursement bases on a per-head rate negotiated between the provider and the insurer. The provider receives the capitation each month regardless of whether the patient is sick.

Most providers agree that reimbursement based on charges is the most favored method while reimbursement based on capitation is the least favored method of reimbursement. Under charges, charges minus a discount, cost plus, and cost, the strategy for successful providers is containing costs. Under per diem, per diagnosis, and capitation, the strategy for successful providers is not only containing cost, but controlling utilization. Capitation has a successful history of containing both costs and utilization in HMOs, and many believe that capitation can reduce healthcare costs in integrated delivery systems and accountable care organizations.

CHAPTER KEY POINTS

➤ The relationship between costs, studied in Chapter 6, and charges is important to understand.

➤ The history of setting charges in healthcare helps managers understand current practices.

➤ Healthcare pricing has come under public scrutiny. Knowing why this scrutiny has come about, and what can be done to restore the public's faith, is important for managers to articulate.

➤ Managers should know how healthcare prices are established both academically and in practice.

➤ Pricing in other industries may have relevance to healthcare in the future.

➤ Capitation supported by the Affordable Care Act may become a reality in coming years.

DISCUSSION QUESTIONS

1. Is there a relationship between cost and price for any given product or service in healthcare? Should there be?

2. Many would concede that healthcare prices are currently irrational. How did prices get that way?

3. The public and those that represent the public (legislatures, insurance companies, consumer groups) have concluded that healthcare prices are outrageous. What can the healthcare industry do to restore public confidence?

4. Healthcare prices are not, and perhaps should not be, set like prices in other industries. Compare how healthcare prices are set to how automobile prices are set.

5. From the provider's perspective, evaluate the common methods of reimbursement.

NOTES

1. *Charge*, *price*, and *rate* are often used synonymously.

2. Eastaugh (1987) compares the healthcare industry to the airline industry in explaining the competitive pressures brought about by the PPS. In the airline industry, routes were deregulated, resulting in airlines competing for the more favorable routes. The competition resulted in inefficient airlines going out of business and efficient airlines gaining market share and reducing prices. In the healthcare industry, the guarantee of reimbursed cost to hospitals ended in 1983 and to physicians in 1992; as a result, inefficient hospitals and group practices went out of business, and the remaining hospitals and group practices gained market share.

3. Some healthcare organizations and physicians have refused to discount their charges. Reid Hospital in Richmond, Indiana, refused to discount, citing the hospital's pricing policy, which states that "prices should be fair and reflective of the resources used to produce the services performed and uniformly applied" (Pallarito 1997a). Under this policy, which has since been changed, the hospital considered it unfair to discount to one payer and shift the costs to another payer.

4. The Center for Healthcare Industry Performance Studies reported that wage-adjusted and case mix–adjusted hospital prices increased only 0.6 percent during 1995, down from 2.4 percent the previous year (Pallarito 1997b).

5. Courts have consistently found that such practices did not lessen competition and therefore were not violations of antitrust law.

6. If fixed costs are covered, effective charges can be negotiated down to variable costs without realizing a relevant loss.

7. Downsizing (i.e., reducing resources to meet reduced demand) was an appropriate strategy for healthcare organizations that were losing business or had too many resources. Reengineering, that is, "the fundamental rethinking and radical redesign of business processes to achieve dramatic improvements in critical contemporary measures of performance, such as cost, quality, service, and speed," was an appropriate strategy for healthcare organizations that were experiencing the same or more demand, but at much reduced effective charges (Hammer and Champy 2001).

8. Anti–managed care laws (i.e., laws designed to control the growth and decision making of managed care organizations, length-of-stay laws, or those that mandate minimum lengths of stay for certain diagnoses such as obstetric delivery) and any-willing-provider laws (patient protection laws that allow patients to receive care from providers outside a network) are examples of patient reactions to cost-savings endeavors. Opponents of these laws are quick to point out that such laws would increase costs and, as a result, charges and premiums to patients.

9. *True cost* is a widely disputed term based largely on the Medicare interpretation of cost during the cost-based reimbursement days. Medicare "disallowed" portions of some costs because the costs were higher than the community standard and "unallowed" some costs in their entirety because the program did not recognize the nature of the cost (e.g., bad debt in the early days and shift differentials in the latter days of cost-based reimbursement). True cost is still important under prospective payment because the payment formulas for DRGs were determined on the basis of Medicare's interpretation of true cost. True costs could vary considerably between facilities on the basis of volume because high-volume healthcare organizations have less fixed cost per unit than low-volume healthcare organizations.

10. For the purpose of setting charges, the use of the same RVU schedule for several facilities or the adoption of a national RVU schedule could constitute price fixing.

Appendix 7.1
Cost-Shift Pricing

This problem demonstrates how cost-shift pricing, also referred to as financial expediency–driven pricing, works. For the sake of simplicity, this example uses only three procedures and only two types of reimbursement. The projected volume for each procedure is 10. Procedure A is reimbursed at allowable cost ($100) for all 10 procedures. Five of Procedure B's procedures are reimbursed at allowable cost, and five of Procedure B's procedures are reimbursed at the price charged. Procedure C is reimbursed at the price charged for all 10 procedures.

Procedure	Percentage Cost-Based	Projected Volume	Cost/ Procedure	Price/ Procedure	Total Collections
A	100	10	$100	$105	10 × $100 = $1,000
B	50	10	$100	$105	5 × $100 + 5 × $105 = $1,025
C	0	10	$100	$105	10 × $105 = $1,050
Average price					$105
Total true cost					$3,000
Total collections					$3,075

To generate collections that would cover costs without raising the average price, the healthcare organization could use cost-shift pricing. This would involve lowering the price of the cost-based Procedure A to $100 (without affecting the amount collected), lowering the price of Procedure B to $100 (with a minimal effect on collections), and raising the price of Procedure C to $115 (with a moderate effect on collections). In so doing, the average markup for all three procedures is 0 percent, while the effect on collections can be more—in this case, 2.4 percent.

Procedure	Percentage Cost-Based	Projected Volume	Cost/ Procedure	Price/ Procedure	Total Collections
A	100	10	$100	$100	10 × $100 = $1,000
B	50	10	$100	$100	5 × $100 + 5 × $100 = $1,000
C	0	10	$100	$115	10 × $115 = $1,150
Average price					$105
Total true cost					$3,000
Total collections					$3,150

RECOMMENDED READINGS—PART II

Andrianos, J., and M. Dykan. 1996. "Using Cost Accounting Data to Improve Clinical Value." *Healthcare Financial Management* 50 (5): 44–48.

Baker, J., and R. W. Baker. 2014. *Health Care Finance: Basic Tools for Nonfinancial Managers*, 4th ed. Boston: Jones & Bartlett Learning.

Berger, S. 2008. *Fundamentals of Healthcare Financial Management*, 3rd ed. San Francisco: Jossey-Bass Publishers.

Betbeze, P. 2004. "Aggressive Collections." *HealthLeaders* 7 (7): 38–44.

Cross, R. G. 1997. *Revenue Management: Hardcore Tactics for Market Domination*. New York: Broadway Books.

Cuckler, G. A., A. M. Sisko, S. P. Keehan, S. D. Smith, A. J. Madison, J. A. Poisal, C. J. Wolfe, J. M. Lizonitz, and D. A. Stone. 2013. "National Health Expenditure Projections, 2012–22: Slow Growth Until Coverage Expands and Economy Improves." *Health Affairs* 32: 1820–21.

Dobson, A., J. DaVanzo, and M. Sen. 2006. "The Cost-Shift Payment 'Hydraulic.' " *Health Affairs* 25 (1): 22–33.

Finkler, S. A. 2009. *Financial Management for Public Health and Non-Profit Organizations*. Upper Saddle River, NJ: Prentice Hall.

Finkler, S. A., D. M. Ward, and J. J. Baker, 2007. *Essentials of Cost Accounting for Healthcare Organizations*, 3rd ed. Boston: Jones & Bartlett Learning.

Gapenski, L. C. 2011. *Healthcare Finance: An Introduction to Accounting and Financial Management*, 5th ed. Chicago: Health Administration Press.

Gapenski, L. C., and G. H. Pink. 2010. *Understanding Healthcare Financial Management*, 6th ed. Chicago: Health Administration Press.

Healthcare Financial Management Association (HFMA). 2005. *What's Your Strategy for Developing Rational Pricing?* Chicago: HFMA.

Herzlinger, R. E. (ed.). 2004. *Consumer-Driven Health Care: Implications for Providers, Payers, and Policy Makers*. San Francisco: Jossey-Bass Publishers.

Porter, M. 1980. *Competitive Strategy: Techniques for Analyzing Industries and Competitors*. New York: Free Press.

Reinhardt, U. E. 2006. "Hospital Pricing: Chaos Beyond a Veil of Secrecy." *Health Affairs* 25 (1): 57–69.

Tompkins, C. P., S. H. Altman, and E. Eilat. 2006. "The Precarious Hospital Pricing System." *Health Affairs* 25 (1): 45–56.

Young, D. W. 2008. *Management Accounting in Health Care Organizations*, 2nd ed. San Francisco: Jossey-Bass Publishers.

Zelman, W. N., M. J. McCue, N. D. Glick, and M. S. Thomas. 2014. *Financial Management of Health Care Organizations, 4th ed*. San Francisco: Jossey-Bass Publishers.

RVU Rate-Setting Practice Problem

Referring to the job-order costing and activity-based costing practice problems from pages 157 and 161, respectively, calculate the charges necessary to realize a 10 percent gain at the XYZ Reference Lab using job-order costing and a 10 percent gain at the XYZ Home Health Care Corporation using activity-based costing.

RVU Rate-Setting Practice Problem Solution

Using Job Order Costing (continued from the job-order costing practice problem solution on page 157)

Step 3: Calculate the cost per procedure by multiplying the cost per RVU by the RVUs in each procedure.

Procedure	Cost/RVU ($)	× RVU	=	Cost/Procedure ($)
A	24.86	1.0		24.86
B	24.86	.5		12.43
C	24.86	.5		12.43
D	24.86	1.5		37.29
E	24.86	1.0		24.86
F	24.86	1.0		24.86
G	24.86	1.5		37.29
H	24.86	1.5		37.29
I	24.86	.5		12.43
J	24.86	1.0		24.86

Step 4: Calculate the charge necessary to realize a 10 percent gain at the XYZ Reference Lab.

Procedure	Cost/RVU ($) =	10%	=	Change/Procedure ($)
A	24.86	2.49		27.35
B	12.43	1.24		13.67
C	12.43	1.24		13.67
D	37.29	3.73		41.02
E	24.86	2.49		27.35
F	24.86	2.49		27.35
G	37.29	3.73		41.02
H	37.29	3.73		41.02
I	12.43	1.24		13.67
J	24.86	2.49		27.35

Using Activity-Based Costing (continued from the job-order costing practice problem solution on page 161)

Step 8: Calculate the charge necessary to realize a 10 percent gain.

Procedure	Cost/Procedure ($)	+	10%	=	Charge/Procedure ($)
PT	546.06		54.61		600.67
RT	416.68		41.67		458.35
Nursing	220.39		22.04		242.43
OT	179.80		17.98		197.78

RVU Rate-Setting Self-Quiz Problem

Referring to the job-order costing and activity-based costing self-quiz problems on page 160 and 165, respectively, calculate the charges necessary to realize a 10 percent gain at the lab using job-order costing and a 7 percent gain at the wellness center using activity-based costing.

HOURLY RATE-SETTING

Hourly Rate-Setting Practice Problem

Using the hourly rate method of setting rates, calculate the operating room rate to recover the costs at the XYZ Ambulatory Surgery Center:

Total projected cost of operating room = $130,000
Total projected hours of use = 2,000 hours

Hourly Rate-Setting Practice Problem Solution

Total projected cost ÷ Total projected hours of use = Hourly rate

$130,000 ÷ 2,000 = $65

Hourly Rate-Setting Self-Quiz Problem

Using the hourly rate method of setting rates, calculate the oxygen therapy rate per shift to break even at your nursing home:

Total projected cost of oxygen = $600,000
Total projected hours of use = 100,000 hours
Shift = 8 hours

Surcharge Rate-Setting

Surcharge Rate-Setting Practice Problem

Using the surcharge method of setting rates, calculate the average prescription rate for the XYZ Pharmacy to cover their costs given the following data:

Total projected cost of the pharmacy = $60,000
Projected cost of drugs billed to patient = $45,000
Number of prescriptions = 3,750

Surcharge Rate-Setting Practice Problem Solution

Step 1: Overhead + Cost of drugs = Total cost

$15,000 + $45,000 = $60,000

Step 2: Total Cost ÷ Number of prescriptions

$60,000 ÷ 3,750 = $16

Surcharge Rate-Setting Self-Quiz Problem

Using the surcharge method of setting rates, calculate the average rate to break even in your central supply given the following data:

Total projected cost of central supply = $900,000
Total projected cost of billable supplies = $750,000
Average cost per billable supply = $7

TAL

Evaluating-

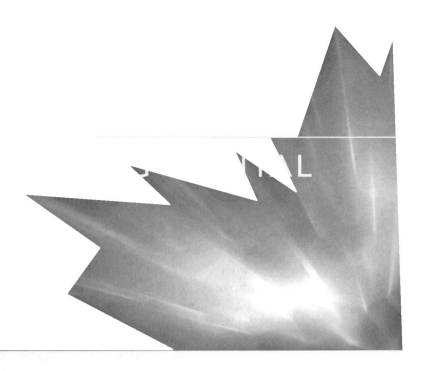

Our goal is to maintain financial viability and keep the hospital from any financial risk, even as our focus remains on expansion and growth.

Chrissy Yamada, hospital chief financial officer

After completing this chapter, you should be able to do the following:

➤ Define and understand the importance of working capital

➤ Identify the sources of working capital

➤ Explain the importance of managing cash flow

➤ Discuss the ratios used to evaluate capital and cash performance

INTRODUCTION

Every manager in the healthcare organization has either a direct or an indirect effect on working capital. Therefore, understanding working capital, the sources of working capital, and the financing of working capital is important.

DEFINITION OF WORKING CAPITAL

Working capital, properly defined, is the sum of a healthcare organization's investment in current assets; it can be simply defined as total current assets. Current assets are cash and other short-term assets that the organization expects to convert to cash within one year. Following is a list of typical current assets:

◆ *Cash:* Money on hand, and money that the organization has immediate access to that is deposited in a bank. Cash equivalents are reported as cash and include investments with a maturity of three months or less (e.g., treasury bills, money market funds).

◆ *Short-term securities:* Investments with a maturity date of less than one year.

◆ *Accounts receivable:* Money due to the organization from patients and insurers for services that the organization has already provided.[1]

◆ *Inventories:* The value of supplies on hand that are properly presented as a current asset on the balance sheet. When inventories are used, they are presented as a supply expense on the statement of operations.

◆ ***Prepaid expense:*** The money paid in one accounting period for value consumed in a later period. An example of prepaid expense is insurance premiums that are paid in one accounting period for protection in subsequent accounting periods. After the value is consumed, the value is reported as an expense.

prepaid expense
Money paid in one accounting period for something that will be consumed in a later period.

Current assets are often measured in terms of their liquidity, which is their ability to be consumed or converted to cash. Cash is considered the most liquid current asset, followed by cash equivalents, short-term investments, and accounts receivable. Prepaid expense is considered the least liquid current asset; inventories are only slightly more liquid than prepaid expense.

working capital
An organization's current assets; the assets available to run the organization in the short term.

The term **working capital** is often used synonymously with the term *net working capital,* so it is important to distinguish the difference.[2] Although working capital is the organization's total current assets, net working capital is the difference between current assets and current liabilities. Net working capital is an important measure of an organization's ability to meet its current liabilities, or its short-term debt-paying capacity.

Current liabilities include accrued wages payable and accounts payable. *Accrued wages payable* is money owed but not yet paid to employees for work already performed for the organization. *Accounts payable* is money owed but not yet paid to vendors for services and products already received by the organization.

IMPORTANCE OF WORKING CAPITAL

Working capital is important because it is the catalyst that makes fixed or long-term assets productive. For instance, although fixed and long-term assets consist of buildings and equipment, the buildings and equipment cannot be productive or produce revenue unless working capital in the form of employees and inventory is introduced. The costs of the employees and inventory, as well as the costs of the building and equipment in the form of depreciation, are reflected in the bill to the patient or the patient's insurance company. Until the bill is paid, the amount is carried as an account receivable. When the bill is paid, part of the money is used to start the process again.

Healthcare organizations that possess sufficient amounts of working capital also enjoy other benefits. Sufficient amounts of working capital enable organizations to pay their employees and vendors on time, and thus help ensure good employee and vendor relations. Sufficient amounts of working capital also demonstrate to lenders that organizations have sufficient resources to repay loans and are therefore creditworthy.

SOURCES OF WORKING CAPITAL

Sources of working capital include money invested in the organization (equity), net income, borrowed money (which is an increase in noncurrent liabilities), and the sale of a noncurrent asset, such as a building or piece of equipment. The sources and methods used to finance working capital, as well as the quantity of working capital to be maintained, are called the **working capital policy**.

Healthcare organizations obtain their permanent working capital (i.e., the minimum amount of working capital that is always on hand) from the owners to cover start-up costs. In the case of government organizations, the initial working capital comes from the government entity through taxes or bonds. In the case of not-for-profit organizations, the initial working capital comes from the community or religious order through tax-exempt bonds. In some cases, working capital may come from philanthropy. In the case of for-profit organizations, the initial working capital comes from the sale of stock.

For-profit organizations not only have greater access to working capital through stock markets, but also have greater flexibility in using the proceeds of stock transactions. For-profit organizations can choose the timing of the sale of stock and the volume of stock necessary to bring in the desired amount of working capital. And they have fewer restrictions on how they can use the proceeds of the sale of stock. The uses of capital in

working capital policy
Sources and methods used to finance working capital, as well as the quantity of working capital to be maintained.

governmental and not-for-profit organizations are often restricted by the philanthropists who provided it or by bond issuers. Because healthcare organizations do not generate sufficient working capital from patient revenues for months or even years, depending on the size of the organization and market conditions, the owners must be willing to support start-up working capital needs for an extended period.

At some point in a healthcare organization's life cycle, the organization's collected revenues will surpass its expenses. After this point, future working capital needs should be funded by net income. In addition to working capital, other demands on net income will arise. For-profit organizations, for instance, will use portions of net income to pay stockholders' dividends and retain part of the income for future expansion. Not-for-profit organizations will use portions of net income to fund reserves and expansion.

Sometimes healthcare organizations have an unexpected increase in business that depletes their working capital reserves. When that happens, they need temporary working capital, which comes from **equity, debt,** or **trade credit.** For instance, accrued wages payable is typically due every 14 days and accounts payable is typically due every 30 days, but accounts receivable may take as long as 60 days to collect. If the organization does not have enough cash to meet its obligations while waiting for the accounts receivable to be paid, it may need an infusion of cash from new investment (equity) or the bank or other lender (debt); or it may need to ask its creditors to extend its payment deadlines or enlarge its credit line (trade credit). Exhibit 8.1 reviews the working capital cycle.

Debt should not be used for permanent working capital needs, nor should it be used for temporary working capital needs unless there is reasonable assurance that the debt can be repaid. For instance, in situations where healthcare organizations lack the working capital necessary to pay employees and vendors because of a decline in business, increasing

equity
Money that comes into an organization from investors.

debt
Money that is borrowed by an organization.

trade credit
Credit extended to an organization by vendors.

EXHIBIT 8.1
Working Capital Cycle

	Day 1	Day 3	Day 14	Day 30	Day 63
Accounts Receivable	Patient seen	Patient billed			Patient pays
Accrued Wages	Employees work		Employees paid		
Accounts Payable	Supplies used			Vendors paid	

debt may be a mistake unless alternative sources of funds exist from which the debt can be repaid (see Exhibit 8.2).

FINANCING TEMPORARY WORKING CAPITAL NEEDS

Assuming that the organization does not have sufficient cash available to meet temporary working capital needs, two sources of short-term financing are available: debt and trade credit.

In the case of using short-term debt to finance temporary working capital needs, healthcare organizations with good credit histories have a line of credit with a commercial bank. At the beginning of the year, the commercial bank will notify the healthcare organization how much credit the organization has available for the coming year. During the year the organization can borrow against that line of credit. Because banks extend lines of credit to organizations with good credit histories, the interest rate charged to such organizations is generally the prime rate, or the lowest possible rate charged to creditworthy organizations. The interest on short-term loans can be expressed with the following equation (see Problem 8.1):

Interest = Amount borrowed × Annual interest rate × Percentage of the year

If the healthcare organization does not have a good credit history, the bank might lend the organization money at a prime rate plus a percentage to account for the risk that the organization might not pay on time, or might not pay at all. In such cases, the bank might also want to secure the loan with collateral. The organization can use marketable

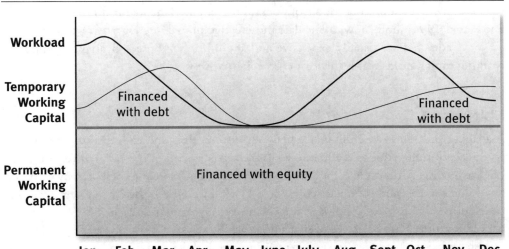

EXHIBIT 8.2

Sources of Working Capital

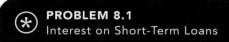

PROBLEM 8.1
Interest on Short-Term Loans

ABC Nursing Home borrows $100,000 for six months at a 3 percent annual interest rate. How much interest will ABC Nursing Home pay for the loan?

$$\text{Interest} = \$100{,}000 \times 0.03 \times \frac{6}{12}$$

$$\text{Interest} = \$1{,}500$$

securities, land, buildings, equipment, or inventory as collateral. For healthcare organizations, often accounts receivable are used as collateral. In such cases, the organization pledges the accounts receivable to the bank; the organization maintains control of the receivables unless the organization fails to repay the loan.

When an organization uses trade credit to finance temporary working capital needs, it is in effect borrowing money from a vendor by delaying payment to the vendor for goods or services already received by the organization. In using trade credit, the cost involved is either the cost of forgoing an incentive to pay on time or the cost of a late fee. Many vendors offer an incentive, or discount, if the organization pays on time. The term *2–10, net 30* means the organization receives a 2 percent discount if it pays within ten days. Applying 2–10, net 30 to a $100 purchase means that if the organization pays within ten days, the vendor will discount the purchase to $98. If the organization pays during days 11 to 30, the organization must pay $100. Thus, the organization is effectively paying $2 in interest to delay paying the bill for a couple of weeks. Problem 8.2 (adapted from Berman, Kukla, and Weeks 1994) shows how to calculate the effective annual interest rate for this situation.

Trade credit is usually expensive and should only be used to finance temporary working capital needs if it is the least costly alternative.

MANAGING CASH FLOW

Managing cash flow—the difference between cash receipts and cash disbursements for a given accounting period—is also known as the management of the cash conversion cycle. The **cash conversion cycle** is the process of converting resources represented by cash outflows into services and products represented by cash inflows. In healthcare organizations, cash outflows consist of employee wages and supply expenses; cash inflows consist of patient revenues. The objective of managing cash flow is to always have the right amount of cash on hand by maximizing and expediting cash inflows and minimizing and delaying cash outflows.[3] The organization must have cash on hand for the following reasons:

cash conversion cycle
The process of converting resources into products or services.

PROBLEM 8.2
Effective Annual Interest Rates on Trade Credit

ABC clinic makes a $100 purchase with a 2 percent in 10, net 30 provision. What is the effective annual interest rate if the clinic pays on day 11? On day 30? Think of the problem this way: How much *annual* interest is the clinic paying to keep its money *one extra day* (in the case of paying on day 11), or 20 extra days (in the case of paying on day 30)? In either case, the organization is paying a penalty of $2 (because it has to pay the full $100 instead of $98, which it would have paid had it paid within 10 days). If it pays on day 11, it is paying that penalty to keep its money just one extra day, so the equivalent *annual* interest would be $2 times 365, which, as you can imagine, equates to a giant interest rate. The story is similar if the organization pays on day 30; it is paying $2 for the privilege of holding onto its money for 20 extra days. There are 18.25 20-day periods in one year, so the equivalent annual interest is $2 times 18.25. That's much better than paying on day 11, but still much more than any other normal finance interest rate.

On day 11:

Step 1: Annual interest paid $= \dfrac{365}{1} = 365 \times \$2 = \$730$

Step 2: Amount borrowed = $98

Step 3: Annual interest rate $= \dfrac{\text{Annual interest paid}}{\text{Amount borrowed}}$

$$= \frac{\$730}{98} = 7.45 \text{ or } 745\%$$

On day 30:

Step 1: Annual interest paid $= \dfrac{365}{20} = 18.25 \times \$2 = \$36.50$

Step 2: Amount borrowed = $98

Step 3: Annual interest rate $= \dfrac{\text{Annual interest paid}}{\text{Amount borrowed}}$

$$= \frac{\$36.50}{98} = .372 \text{ or } 37.2\%$$

♦ *Transactions:* The expected demand for cash to pay employees and suppliers.

♦ *Precautions:* The unexpected demand for cash to pay for emergencies and other unplanned events.

♦ *Speculations:* The unexpected demand for cash when a vendor offers a price reduction or other good deal that the organization does not want to pass up. For example, sometimes a vendor offers a reduced price per unit if the organization buys a certain amount that exceeds its current needs.

You are the administrator of Lincoln Family Clinic, which has been hit hard by the current economic crisis and has been cutting expenses to survive. Your cash on hand is short, and it is the time of the month to pay your employees and vendors. The cash inflows from patient revenues supplied just enough to cover about half of your salaries and expenses. Explain the options for the clinic. What would you do?

Because cash inflows consist of patient revenues, maximizing and expediting inflows is the primary objective of managing accounts receivable (discussed in detail in Chapter 9). Cash outflows consist of employee wages and supply expenses, and to the extent possible, ethically and legally, they should be minimized and delayed.[4] Minimizing employee wages and supply expenses is a function of the budgeting process, during which managers should explore new ways to accomplish more work with fewer resources. In delaying cash outflows, the chief financial officer (CFO) or controller must determine when to pay employees and vendors. Typically, organizations pay employees every two weeks or every month, rather than at the end of each day. In this way, the organization holds and invests money that employees have already earned. Organizations pay vendors when the money is due, not when the organization receives the supplies or the bill. The organization determines the **float period,** which is the time difference between the day checks are written and the day checks are presented for payment. The organization uses the float period to transfer money from an interest-bearing account to the checking account as the money is drawn, a process called **book overdraft.**

float period
The time between when a check is written and when it is presented for payment.

book overdraft
Process of transferring money from an interest-bearing account to the checking account as the money is drawn.

cash budget
Predicts the timing and amount of cash flows and systematically examines the cost implications with each alternative.

CASH BUDGET

Larger healthcare organizations use a cash budget to help manage cash flows. A **cash budget** predicts the timing and amount of cash inflows and outflows, and systematically examines the cost implications of various cash management decisions. Basic steps in developing a cash budget for a specific period include the following:

♦ Prepare a list of all expected sources of cash inflows.

♦ Estimate the amounts to be received from each source.

♦ Prepare a list of all expected sources of cash outflows.

◆   Estimate the amounts to be expended to each source.

◆   Calculate the period-end cash balance.

◆   Determine how to finance deficit balances (see earlier section, Financing Temporary Working Capital Needs) or invest surplus balances.

The organization should have a board-approved **investment policy** that directs the CFO or controller in making short-term investment decisions. The investment policy should include objectives of investment, authority for investment, and types of investments to be made. Typically, the types of investments to be made include US Treasury bills, money market funds, and commercial certificates of deposit, all of which provide both **liquidity,** in the event the organization needs the money invested on short notice, and financial security. **Compounding** is used to determine the amount of income investments will generate. Compounding is a way of looking at a present amount of money, called **present value** (PV), and calculating the future amount of money, called **future value** (FV), using the following formulas:

$$FV = PV(1 + i)^n$$

where *i* is the annual interest rate at which the money is invested, and *n* is the number of years the money is invested; and

$$FV = PV(1 + i/m)^{mn}$$

where *m* is the number of times the money is compounded each year. Problem 8.3 shows how these formulas are used.

PROBLEM 8.3
Calculating the FV of an Investment

ABC Physical Therapy Clinic wants to invest $100,000. What is the FV compounded annually at 7 percent for five years? At 7 percent compounded semiannually for five years?

Compounded annually for five years:
FV = $100,000 (1 + .07)^5
FV = $140,255

(continued)

---

investment policy
Directs the chief financial officer or controller in making short-term investment decisions.

liquidity
A characteristic of an investment that pertains to how quickly it can be converted to cash.

compounding
The action of adding interest to interest on an investment.

present value
The current value of an investment.

future value
The future value of an investment, taking into account factors such as interest rate, time, and the frequency of compounding.

⊛ **PROBLEM 8.3**
Calculating the FV of an Investment

Compounded semiannually for five years:

FV = $100,000 (1 + [.07 / 2])$^{2 \times 5}$

FV = $141,060

NOTE: This answer is formula driven. Use of a calculator or spreadsheet may alter the answer slightly because of rounding or how interest is calculated (at the end of the period versus during the period).

HP 10BII Keys

Key	Store or Calculates
N	The number of payments or compounding periods
I/YR	The annual nominal interest rate
PV	The present value of future cash flows
PMT	The amount of periodic payments
FV	Future value
◐ P/YR	Store the number of periods per year. The default is 12.
◐	Shift key (orange on most models)

HP 10BII Solution to Problem 8.3 compounded annually

Keys	Display	Description
1 ◐ P/YR	1.00	Sets compounding periods per year to 1
5 N	5.00	Stores the number of compounding periods (1 x 5)
7 I/YR	7.00	Stores the interest rate
–100,000 PV	–100,000.00	Stores the PV as an annuity (–)
FV	140,255.17	Calculates the FV

(continued)

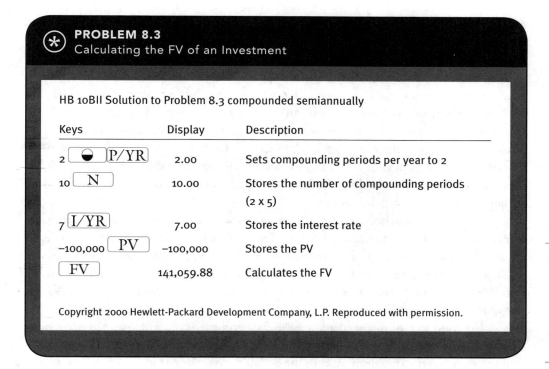

PROBLEM 8.3
Calculating the FV of an Investment

HB 10BII Solution to Problem 8.3 compounded semiannually

Keys	Display	Description
2 ⊖ P/YR	2.00	Sets compounding periods per year to 2
10 N	10.00	Stores the number of compounding periods (2 x 5)
7 I/YR	7.00	Stores the interest rate
−100,000 PV	−100,000	Stores the PV
FV	141,059.88	Calculates the FV

Copyright 2000 Hewlett-Packard Development Company, L.P. Reproduced with permission.

EVALUATING WORKING CAPITAL AND CASH PERFORMANCE

Financial analysis, covered in more depth in Chapter 14, is how investors, creditors, and management evaluate the past, present, and future financial performance of the organization. Financial analysis includes the following three steps (Berman, Kukla, and Weeks 1994):

1. Establishing the facts in the organization

2. Comparing the facts in the organization over time and also to facts in other similar organizations

3. Using perspective and judgment to make decisions regarding the comparisons

The first step, establishing the facts, usually relates to a review of the organization's financial statements, the accuracy of which has been confirmed by independent auditors. The second step, comparing the facts over time and comparing the facts to similar organizations, includes ratio analysis, **horizontal analysis,** and **vertical analysis.** Ratio analysis is the most common form of comparison and evaluates an organization's performance through computing and showing the relationships of important line items found in the financial statements. Typically, there are four kinds of ratios: liquidity, profitability, activity,

financial analysis
Methods used by investors, creditors, and management to evaluate past, present, and future financial performance.

horizontal analysis
An evaluation in the trend in a line item that examines the percentage change of that line item over time.

vertical analysis
Evaluation of the internal structure of an organization by focusing on a base number and showing percentages of important line items in relation to the base number.

and capital structure. Horizontal analysis evaluates the trend in the line items by focusing on the percentage change over time. Vertical analysis evaluates the internal structure of the organization by comparing important line items to a base number. For instance, vertical analysis could be used to show what percentage of gross revenue is net revenue, bad debt, charity care, or contractual allowance. After ratio analysis, horizontal analysis, and vertical analysis are complete, the organization can make trend and industry comparisons.

Trend comparisons assess the organization's present and past ratios, trends, and percentages to determine the organization's financial performance over time. However, trend comparisons only work with ratios, trends, and percentages that show **directionality**; this means that the numbers are always better as they move in one direction, and always worse as they proceed in the other direction.

Industry comparisons analyze the organization's ratios, trends, and percentages compared to the ratios, trends, and percentages of other similar organizations to determine the organization's financial performance relative to competitors. Several organizations publish key ratios, trends, and percentages: Moody's Investors Service publishes *Health Care Medians,* Dun & Bradstreet publishes *Key Business Ratios,* and CCH publishes the *Almanac of Business and Industrial Financial Ratios.*

The third step of financial analysis, using perspective and judgment to make decisions regarding the comparisons, uses the information obtained in the first two steps, coupled with information derived from the decision maker's unique perspective and judgment. Decisions that may at first be at odds with the information provided in the first two steps may make perfect sense based on pressures from internal and external constituents, including medical staffs, employers, regulators, donors, and others.

When evaluating working capital and cash performance, the following liquidity ratios are important. The first of these ratios does not show directionality: if the ratio is too low, the organization must borrow money to meet its obligations; if the ratio is too high, the organization loses the opportunity to invest in longer-term assets with a higher return. The remaining three do show directionality in that movement in the ratio in a specific direction is always better.

◆   Current Ratio

$$\frac{\text{Total current assets}}{\text{Total current liabilities}}$$

The basic indicator of financial liquidity, or an organization's ability to meet its financial obligations. Higher values indicate better debt-paying capacity. The current ratio does not take into account the relative liquidity of the different current asset accounts. The current ratio median for all hospitals reporting to Optum (2014) for 2012 audited financial statements was 2.15.

---

directionality
Statistical property for numbers that always improve in one direction and always worsen in the other direction.

◆ Days Cash on Hand, Short-Term Sources

$$\frac{\text{Cash} + \text{Marketable securities}}{(\text{Total expenses} - \text{Depreciation expense}) / 365}$$

◆ Days Cash on Hand, All Sources

$$\frac{\text{Cash} + \text{Marketable securities} + \text{Unrestricted long-term investments}}{(\text{Total expenses} - \text{Depreciation expense}) / 365}$$

An indicator of how long an organization could meet its obligations if cash receipts were discontinued. The days cash on hand, short-term sources median from all hospitals reporting to Optum (2014) for 2012 audited financial statements was 30.5. The days cash on hand, all sources median from all hospitals reporting to Optum for 2012 audited financial statements was 93.8.

◆ Average Payment Period

$$\frac{\text{Current liabilities}}{(\text{Total expenses} - \text{Depreciation expense}) / 365}$$

An indicator of the average time that passes before a current liability is paid. Higher values can indicate potential liquidity problems to creditors. The average payment period median from all hospitals reporting to Optum (2014) for 2012 audited financial statements was 51.8.

The analysis of working capital and cash performance is an important aspect of the financial management of healthcare organizations. Chapters 9 and 10 take a closer look at the management of two specific current assets: accounts receivable and materials.

CHAPTER KEY POINTS

➤ Working capital is an organization's total current assets.

➤ Working capital can be made up of equity, net income, an increase in noncurrent liabilities, and a decrease in noncurrent assets.

➤ Net assets, short-term debt, or trade credit finance temporary working capital needs.

➤ The management of cash flows is represented by cash outflows into services and cash inflows from patient revenues.

➤ Financial analysis is used to evaluate the past, present, and future financial performance of an organization using three steps.

DISCUSSION QUESTIONS

1. Define the terms *cash, short-term securities, accounts receivable, inventories,* and *prepaid expenses.*

2. What are some of the differences in sources of capital between not-for-profit organizations and for-profit organizations?

3. What is the formula for calculating interest on short-term loans?

4. What is the main objective of managing cash flows? What are the reasons an organization should have cash on hand?

5. Explain why healthcare organizations use present value of money and future value of money for their investments.

6. Why do organizations need to perform a financial analysis? Explain each of the steps involved.

NOTES

1. Healthcare organizations, like physicians' offices, that use cash accounting rather than accrual accounting will not have accounts receivable or bad-debt expense because cash accounting records revenue when paid, whereas accrual accounting records revenue when earned.

2. Net working capital is sometimes confused with cash flow, which is the difference between cash receipts and cash disbursements for a given accounting period.

3. The right amount of cash on hand is a function of both the timing and the amount of cash inflows and cash outflows. At a minimum, the right amount of cash on hand is the difference between cash inflows and cash outflows, as expressed in the following equation (Berman, Kukla, and Weeks 1994):

   Cash outflows – Cash inflows = Minimum cash balance on hand

4. Summers (1986) argues that the CFO's primary duty is to the organization; therefore, as long as the implied contract between the organization and its vendors is not violated, paying late is all right.

Effective Annual Interest Rate on Short-Term Loans

Effective Annual Interest Rate on Short-Term Loans Practice Problem

XYZ Assisted Living Center can borrow $150,000 for 1 year at 7.5 percent. Calculate the amount of interest they will pay.

Effective Annual Interest Rate on Short-Term Loans Practice Problem Solution

$$7.5\% = \frac{I}{\$150,000}$$

$$I = 7.5\% \times \$150,000$$

$$I = \$11,250$$

Effective Annual Interest Rate on Short-Term Loans Self-Quiz Problem

Your daycare center can borrow $50,000 for 1 year and pay $3,625 in interest. Calculate the interest rate you will pay.

EFFECTIVE ANNUAL INTEREST RATE ON

TRADE CREDIT

Effective Annual Interest Rate on Trade Credit Practice Problem

XYZ Hospital makes a $98 purchase on the first day of the month and must pay a $2 late fee if it does not pay within the first 10 days. What is the annual interest rate if the hospital pays on day 45? On day 30? On day 11?

Effective Annual Interest Rate on Trade Credit Practice Problem Solution

On day 45

Step 1: Annual interest paid $= \dfrac{365}{35} = 10.43 \times \$2 = \$20.86$

Step 2: Amount borrowed each time = $98

Step 3: Annual interest rate $= \dfrac{\text{Annual interest paid}}{\text{Amount borrowed each time}} = \dfrac{\$20.86}{\$98.00} = 21.3\%$

On day 30

Step 1: Annual interest paid $= \dfrac{365}{20} = 18.25 \times \$2 = \$36.50$

Step 2: Amount borrowed each time = $98

Step 3: Annual interest rate $= \dfrac{\text{Annual interest paid}}{\text{Amount borrowed each time}} = \dfrac{\$36.50}{\$98.00} = 37.2\%$

On day 11

Step 1: Annual interest paid $= \dfrac{365}{1} = 365 \times \$2 = \$730$

Step 2: Amount borrowed each time = $98

Step 3: Annual interest rate $= \dfrac{\text{Annual interest paid}}{\text{Amount borrowed each time}} = \dfrac{\$730}{\$98} = 744.89\%$

Effective Annual Interest Rate on Trade Credit Self-Quiz Problem

Assume that a hospital makes $150 purchase on the first day of the month and must pay a $5 late fee if it doesn't pay within the first 15 days. What is the annual interest rate if the hospital pays on day 16? On day 30?

FUTURE VALUE

Future Value Practice Problem

XYZ Sleep Disorder Clinic invests $106,944 for five years to retire a debt. Assuming the clinic can invest at 7 percent compounded annually, how much is the debt XYZ needs to retire?

Future Value Practice Problem Solution

$$FV = PV(1 + i)^n$$

$$FV = \$106{,}944(1 + .07)^5$$

$$FV = \$149{,}994.49$$

HB 10BII solution, compounded annually

Keys	Display	Description
1 ⬤ (P/YR)	1.00	Sets compounding periods per year to 1
5 (N)	5.00	Stores the number of compounding periods (1 x 5)
7 (I/YR)	7.00	Stores the interest rate
−106,944 (PV)	−106,944	Stores the present value
(FV)	$149,994.49	Calculates the future value

Future Value Self-Quiz Problem

Your hospital wants to invest $1 million at 5 percent compounded quarterly. How much will the investment be worth after 10 years?

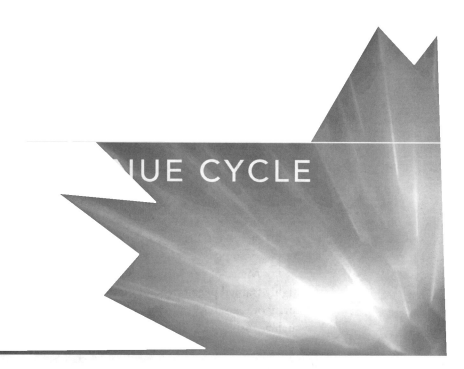

UE CYCLE

We urgently need to determine how to manage our costs yet still provide the high-quality care that patients expect and deserve; for an integrated delivery system, at least part of the solution is achieving true integration, and that's the real challenge.

Phyllis A. Cowling, FHFMA, CPA, former vice president
and CFO of Baptist St. Anthony's Health System, Amarillo, Texas

LEARNING OBJECTIVES

After completing this chapter, you should be able to do the following:

➤ Define and understand the importance of revenue cycle

➤ Explain the important elements of revenue cycle

➤ Identify methods of financing accounts receivable

➤ Describe the laws governing accounts receivable

➤ Discuss the ratios used to evaluate revenue cycle performance

INTRODUCTION

In most healthcare organizations, accounts receivable is the largest current asset and deserves special attention. Three factors set the healthcare industry apart from most other industries with regard to accounts receivable: the nature of the services provided, the cost of the services provided, and the method of payment for the services provided. Because many of the services provided by healthcare organizations are provided in an emergent nature, at least in the patient's mind, patients often do not have the time to raise the funds necessary to pay for the services they need or want.

Many of the services provided by healthcare organizations are services requiring highly trained personnel and high-tech equipment available 24 hours a day. Furthermore, many of the services provided by healthcare organizations are reimbursed by third parties, such as insurance companies.

DISTINGUISHING REVENUE CYCLE FROM ACCOUNTS RECEIVABLE

revenue cycle
A multidisciplinary approach to reducing the amount in accounts receivable by effectively managing the production and payment cycles.

Accounts receivable is money due to the organization from patients and third parties for services that the organization has already provided. **Revenue cycle** is a multidisciplinary approach to reducing the amount in accounts receivable by effectively managing the production and payment cycles, as illustrated in Exhibit 9.1.

During precare, the healthcare organization obtains from the patient all the information necessary to both treat and bill (Exhibit 9.2 provides a list of information to be collected during precare). The Healthcare Financial Management Association (HFMA 1998) says that inadequate or incorrect information gathered at this stage is the single greatest reason for not billing or collecting accounts receivable in a timely manner. According to HFMA, unless the care is emergent in nature, treatment should not begin until this stage is completed. From a legal perspective, the organization is not required to initiate treatment—absent an emergency—if the patient is unable to pay.[1] However, after the organization has initiated treatment, it cannot terminate treatment solely based on the patient's inability to pay.[2]

During care, the organization should post charges in a prompt and accurate manner. The medical record, which is in the hands of clinicians at this point, should document all phases of the patient's care. The medical record is the primary source of clinical data required for reimbursement from most third parties. Utilization review by the utilization review nurse or discharge planner ensures that the care provided to the patient is appropriate and is care that the patient or third party will reimburse. The organization should conduct utilization review during care, called concurrent review, as well as after care, called retrospective review.

During the care-completed phase, sometimes referred to as discharged but not final billed, the medical record is transferred from the clinicians to the medical record department. The patient's record is analyzed for completeness, abstracted, and coded.

EXHIBIT 9.1
Accounts
Receivable Cycle

Cycle	Patient Activity	Accounts Receivable Activity
Production cycle	Patient seeks care	
	Precare	Obtain demographic data
		Obtain insurance data
		Verify insurance coverage
		Obtain authorizations
		Obtain deductibles
		Obtain copays
	Care	Record charges
		Maintain medical record
		Review utilization
	Care completed	Transfer medical record
		Analyze medical record
		Abstract medical record
		Code medical record
		Transcribe dictation
Payment cycle*		Print bill
		Submit bill
		Follow up bill
		Collect bill, or bill resolution

* The payment cycle usually begins when the medical record is complete for billing purposes. However, in organizations where the medical records department reports to the chief financial officer (CFO), the payment cycle may begin at patient discharge owing to the fact that the CFO is responsible for the processing time in medical records.

gross receivable
The full amount a healthcare organization charges.

net receivable
The gross receivable minus any negotiated discounts.

The medical record department adds transcriptions from the physician, including final diagnosis.

On completion of the medical record, the payment cycle begins. In the bill print phase, a claim form is completed. Any previously agreed-on discounts, such as contractual discounts with the insurance company, are applied at this time, which changes the figure from a **gross receivable** to a **net receivable**. In the bill submission phase, a claim is sent from the organization to the patient and/or third-party payer.

EXHIBIT 9.2
Patient Information
Collected During
Precare

- Patient name and other identifiers, including Social Security number, gender, date of birth, place of birth, and race
- Patient address and telephone number
- Patient occupation, employer, employer address, and phone number
- Resident status of all foreign-born patients
- Name, address, and telephone numbers of next of kin
- Name, address, and telephone numbers of person responsible for bill
- Name, address, telephone numbers, and certificate numbers of all third-party payers
- Benefits to which the patient is entitled
- Name, address, and telephone number of primary care physician
- Name, address, and telephone number of attending physician
- Preliminary diagnosis
- Date of most recent previous outpatient services or admission
- Accident information
- Financial resources information for self-pay patients
- Authorizations and precertifications
- Consent for medical treatments and admissions
- Assignments of insurance benefits from the patient to the provider

Source: Adapted from Healthcare Financial Management Association (HFMA). 1998. *HFMA Core Certification Exam Self-Study Manual,* 1–16. White Plains, NY: The MGI Management Institute.

The bill collection phase also applies to bills that were not paid on time. The organization makes additional efforts to collect the bill, such as phone calls or letters, and if those don't work, it can submit the account to a collection agency. The organization's credit-and-collection policy and relevant federal and state laws should cover the extent to which the organization and collection agency should seek payment. The organization's board should also play a role in deciding how aggressively to pursue overdue bills. If a patient does not pay even after these efforts, the organization may decide to write off the bill as a bad debt. The Affordable Care Act of 2010 (ACA) has new regulations that direct how aggressively a nonprofit hospital can collect bills of patients who meet the hospital's financial assistance policy.

IMPORTANCE OF ACCOUNTS RECEIVABLE

The amount of current assets tied up in accounts receivable (accounts receivable can be as much as 75 percent of the current assets) can vary significantly among organizations, as can the associated costs. This variance is often attributed to the credit-and-collection policies of the board and to management methods used to reduce accounts receivable. Costs associated with accounts receivable include a **carrying cost**, a routine **credit-and-collection cost**, and a **delinquency cost**.

Carrying costs associated with accounts receivable are the costs incurred by the organization for extending credit to the patient after the organization has provided services. If patients paid at the time of service, the organization would have the funds on hand to either invest or pay current liabilities. Thus the carrying costs are the amount of money the organization would have earned had it been able to invest that money at a given interest rate, or the amount of money the organization must pay in interest to borrow funds to pay current liabilities.

Routine credit-and-collection costs are the costs incurred by the organization for billing and collecting during the organization's average payment cycle. If patients paid at the time of service, the organization would generate only one bill per patient. When the organization extends credit, it incurs the cost of sending additional bills and reminders.

Delinquency costs are the costs incurred by the organization for the patient not paying on time. These costs can include the costs associated with turning the account over to a collection agency or with writing off the account to bad debt.

MANAGEMENT OF THE REVENUE CYCLE

The extension of credit for most healthcare organizations is a necessary evil because of the nature and cost of the services provided, and the preponderance of third-party payment. However, the organization's credit-and-collection philosophy should treat the extension of credit as the exception to the rule, and not the rule itself. The rule should be to collect as much money as possible at the time of service and to extend credit to creditworthy patients only when necessary. The objective of managing the revenue cycle is to reduce the **collection period**, which is the number of days between the time of service and the time of payment. An obvious way to reduce the collection period is to collect as much money as possible as soon as service is provided.

POLICIES AND PROCEDURES

The first step in managing the revenue cycle is to have policies and procedures for the registration and admission of all patients. All patients who are not emergent in nature should go through a preregistration/preadmission process so the organization can obtain the information listed in Exhibit 9.2. At that time, deductibles, copayments, and deposits

carrying cost
The cost incurred by the organization for extending credit to the patient after the organization has provided services.

credit-and-collection cost
The cost incurred by the organization for billing and collecting during the organization's average payment cycle.

delinquency cost
The cost incurred by the organization for the patient not paying on time. These costs can include the costs associated with turning the account over to a collection agency or with writing off the account to bad debt.

collection period
The number of days between the time of service and the time of payment.

should also be collected. Organizations are much more likely to obtain information and payments prior to providing services than afterward because organizations cannot hold patients against the patient's will to obtain payment or information (see Showalter [2011] on false imprisonment).

Many healthcare organizations offer preregistration/preadmission, in which the patient completes the paperwork and other tasks before arriving for care. This process can be done in person, over the phone, or online. Not only does this speed things up for the patient, but it reduces wait times for everyone, and wait times are a key indicator of quality, according to patient surveys.

ACCOUNTING SYSTEM

internal auditor
Staff member who monitors the effectiveness of an accounting system by verifying the system's internal control.

The second step in managing the revenue cycle is to have an accounting system that provides prompt and accurate recording of charges. Not having such a system has been a problem in healthcare for decades and continues to be a problem. **Internal auditors** often play a role in determining the effectiveness of the accounting system by verifying the system's **internal control**. Internal control consists of accounting systems and supporting procedures that provide systematic, automatic safeguards to protect the integrity of the accounting information (Herkimer 1993). Internal controls also (Marrapese and Titera 1989):

internal control
Accounting systems and procedures that protect the integrity of an organization's accounting information.

◆   provide management with information that is up to date, reliable, and accurate;

◆   reduce the risk of losing assets through errors or misappropriations;

◆   promote operational efficiency by, among other things, reducing the likelihood of errors; and

◆   give employees direction through policies and procedures.

Exhibit 9.3 provides typical questions that an internal auditor may ask in relation to internal control of accounts receivable.

MEDICAL RECORD SYSTEM

The third step in managing the revenue cycle is to have a medical record system that allows for prompt and accurate recording of clinical information. With the advent of Medicare prospective payment in 1983, hospital health information management (HIM) departments had significant pressure to process medical records in a timely fashion so that the physician could attest to the final diagnosis, which was required prior to bill submission.

EXHIBIT 9.3
Internal Audit
of Accounts
Receivable
Questions

1. Do registration/admission procedures exist and ensure that complete and accurate accounts receivable and collection information is gathered, including such documents as signed authorization forms, patient billing information, and insurance assignments?

2. Do procedures exist and ensure that services rendered to patients are medically necessary?

3. Is a complete medical record prepared, including physician discharge summaries and physician statements attesting to the principal diagnosis and other clinical information?

4. Do procedures exist and ensure that amounts due from third-party payers are properly supported?

5. Do procedures exist and ensure that cash receipts are properly recorded?

6. Do procedures exist and ensure that charity care balances are identified and deducted from gross revenues?

7. Do procedures exist and ensure that detailed accounts receivable records are routinely compared to general ledger control accounts and third-party payer logs?

8. Do reviews exist and ensure that allowances for bad debts and contractuals are adjusted periodically to ensure that receivables are reported at estimated net realizable amounts?

9. Do procedures exist and ensure that medical records personnel are properly trained and supervised to provide appropriate coding?

10. Do procedures exist and ensure prompt coding of Medicare and other similar medical records data?

11. Do procedures exist and ensure independent coding reviews, primarily for Medicare patients?

Source: Adapted from Herkimer, A. G. 1993. *Patient Financial Services*, 288–89. Chicago: HFMA/Probus Press.

Traditionally, HIM departments were not involved with the medical record until after discharge. With the advent of Medicare prospective payment, hospitals needed a preliminary diagnosis-related group (DRG) assignment at patient admission; needed to monitor use during the patient stay; and needed to interface the patient billing system with the medical record system to determine cost per DRG. The resulting interfaced information systems are shown in Exhibit 9.4.

EXHIBIT 9.4
Patient Billing
System/Medical
Record System
Interface

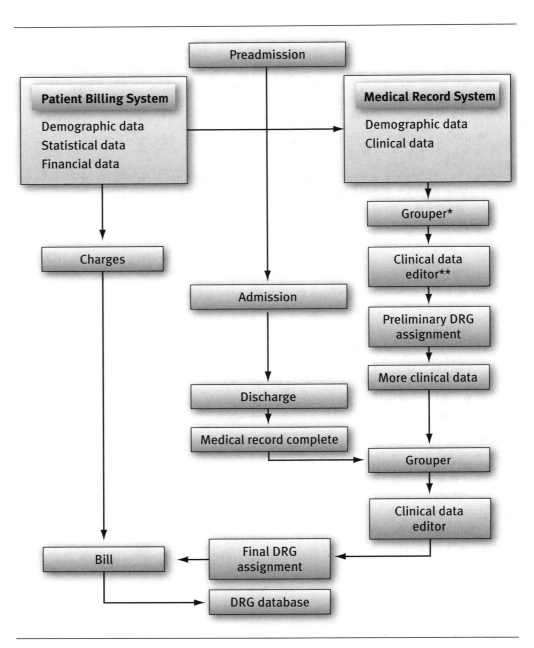

*Grouper: software package that assigns DRG.

**Clinical data editor: software package that edits clinical data by checking for coding errors.

Completing the medical record in a timely fashion is still important, particularly for Joint Commission accreditation. The penalty for delinquent medical records—limits on or suspension of medical staff privileges—has always been difficult to enforce because of the financial effect on the hospital caused by limiting physician privileges. However, from the accounts receivable perspective, emphasis has changed from promptness to accuracy of medical records.

Some of the pressure to complete the medical record in a timely fashion has diminished with the increase in fixed payments, such as DRGs. Also, hospitals are no longer required to have a signed physician attestation before submitting a Medicare claim. Finally, as electronic medical records become more common, medical records turnaround time is expected to improve.

HIM departments have experienced increased pressure for accuracy in medical records. Coding errors can delay payment until corrected and can initiate federal investigations and resulting fines. Since the passage of the 1986 False Claims Act amendments, the federal government has recovered more than $27 billion in false or erroneous claims to the Medicare program (OIG 2013).[3] Unfortunately, accurate coding is less objective than federal investigations and court cases might imply. For instance, current procedural terminology (CPT) codes were developed to identify physician services and often do not work well in hospital outpatient departments; therefore, they result in coding problems. Coding problems are often identified by fiscal intermediaries during routine focused medical reviews.

The most effective way for healthcare organizations to avoid fraud and abuse investigations and minimize the effects of investigations if they do occur is to have a comprehensive compliance plan that includes a coding compliance plan (see Chapter 5 for more information on compliance plans). A coding compliance plan provides the framework for effective internal controls, and is one way to defend against charges of reckless disregard. Under the provisions of the False Claims Act, the federal government does not need to prove intent to defraud but only reckless disregard for a claim's validity.

According to Russo and Russo (1998), a coding compliance plan should ensure that the HIM department is

- using the right coding resources,

- documenting all advice from fiscal intermediaries,

- supplying sufficient coding resources to coders,

- checking on computerized encoders,

- requiring periodic training for all coders,

- staying current on all International Classification of Diseases and CPT changes,

- developing and revising coding policies,

◆ contracting for and documenting annual external coding audits, and

◆ performing and documenting regular internal coding audits.

CREDIT-AND-COLLECTION POLICY

The fourth step in managing accounts receivable is to have a board-approved credit-and-collection policy that directs the organization's management regarding extending credit and collecting accounts. Organizations vary considerably in how aggressively they collect accounts receivable, but the credit-and-collection policy should address the following issues.

Charity Care

The discussion of charity care (as distinguished from bad debt) should include a discussion on eligibility criteria.

Bad Debt

The discussion of bad debt should address at what point and under what circumstances the organization turns accounts over to a collection agency and at what point and under what circumstances the organization writes off accounts as bad debts.

Self-Pay

Self-pay should include provisions for financial counseling to determine how the services provided will be reimbursed.

Financial counseling is the process of extending credit to self-pay patients. Because of this process, the organization should better understand the patient's ability or inability to pay the organization for services rendered, and the patient should better understand her financial responsibilities to the organization. Financial counseling should do the following:

1. Tell the patient about the organization's credit-and-collection policies and how the policies pertain to the patient.

2. Investigate the patient's credit history and determine to what extent the patient can pay for anticipated services.

3. Help the patient evaluate alternative payment options, including, but not limited to,

- credit cards;

- bank loans, including home equity loans;

- credit union loans;

- cash from sale of assets; and

- extended payment plans, with or without interest.

- Organizations should be willing to significantly discount their charges to obtain payments at time of service.

4. Follow up and resolve any pending financial transactions.

To the extent possible, money due from the patient (deductibles and copays) should be collected at time of service. In a 2004 study published by Zimmerman & Associates, best-performing hospitals collected only 31 percent of revenue due them from patients at time of service, while the national average was 16 percent. The study listed the reasons most often stated by the hospital for not collecting money due from the patient at time of service (respondents in the survey could provide more than one answer) (Runy 2004):

1. Too hard and inaccurate to prorate patient account (copays), 36 percent

2. Patient liability unknown at time of service, 34 percent

3. Lack of automated method of prorating claims, 26 percent

4. Hospital policy does not allow it, 20 percent

5. Poor public relations, 20 percent

6. Staff uncomfortable asking for money, 14 percent

7. Not a significant amount of money, 4 percent

Third-Party Insurance Relationships

The discussion of third-party insurance relationships should include provisions for **coordination of benefits**, which is the process of determining the order of insurance company liability when multiple insurance companies are involved; assignment of benefits, which is the process of transferring insurance benefits from patients to the healthcare organization; and third-party audits.

coordination of benefits
Step in the billing process during which the order of insurance company liability is identified for accounts that have multiple insurance companies.

Billing Procedures

The credit-and-collection policy should also discuss billing procedures, including provisions for

- bill cutoffs, which is the point at which the organization determines the bill is complete and ready for submission;

- methods for encouraging prompt payment, such as interest assessment on late payments; and

- follow-up billing, including both the format (i.e., how aggressive the language should be) and timing (i.e., how often the organization should mail reminders, called dunning notices).

Deposit Procedures

lock box
A system in which payments from patients are mailed directly to a bank, which credits the healthcare organization's account more quickly than if the check had been mailed to the organization.

The section of the credit-and-collection policy on deposit procedures should include provisions for a **lock box** and **electronic data interchange** (EDI) and other aspects of processing and posting payments. When an organization uses a lock box, payers mail their payments directly to the bank, which deposits the money and forwards the accompanying paperwork, along with a copy of the check, to the organization for processing. When using EDI, large payers such as Medicare wire the payment directly to the bank or organization and then forward accompanying paperwork via wire or mail. EDI reduces claims completion time substantially while reducing the administrative costs associated with processing the claim.

electronic data interchange
A method of payment in which the payer, such as Medicare, wires payment to the healthcare organization's bank, and transmits related information to the organization.

FROM ACCOUNTS RECEIVABLE MANAGEMENT TO REVENUE CYCLE MANAGEMENT

The Health Insurance Portability and Accountability Act (HIPAA) transaction standard provides a unique opportunity for healthcare organizations to improve their revenue cycle performance. Revenue cycle management conceptualizes the accounts receivable process as a continuum rather than as a set of isolated events (Laforge and Tureaud 2003) and incorporates the use of multidisciplinary teams, including clinicians, to improve performance. Any healthcare organization whose key financial measures lie outside the industry benchmarks should review its revenue cycle practices. Key benchmarks include the following (Guyton and Lund 2003):

- Outstanding revenues that exceed the industry average of about 50 days

- More than 15 percent of receivables exceeding 90 days

- High management turnover in revenue-related areas

◆ Evidence of cash-flow problems

◆ Declining net-to-gross ratios

Opportunities for improved revenue cycle management are usually found in the following five key areas:

1. Denials management—virtually all denials of payment by third-party payers are the result of administrative problems or clinical problems

2. Follow-up on unpaid claims

3. Patient payments of copays and deductibles at point of service and enhanced methods of patient payments

4. Third-party payment compliance to ensure that payment received was the correct amount

5. Vendor contract coordination to ensure a broad-based evaluation of contract terms in relation to coordination of benefits

> You were hired as charge analyst a few months ago at Bryant Hospital. Due to lack of proper training, you have steadily fallen behind in billing for hospital services to patients, and patients are now complaining about receiving late bills, even after they have made payments. The hospital is suffering from both a collections standpoint and a public relations standpoint because of late billings, and the hospital is now facing an internal audit.
>
> What problems will the internal audit discover? How will the hospital address these problems?
>
> What can the hospital do to process the bills in a timely manner? Are you the sole reason for the late billing? Who else should be held accountable? Are the patients still responsible for the late billing? What if they refuse to pay because the hospital was not upfront about the costs?

FINANCING ACCOUNTS RECEIVABLE

Sometimes healthcare organizations can convert outstanding accounts receivable into cash to meet short-term cash demands. There are two ways to do this: **factoring receivables** and **pledging receivables**. When an organization factors its accounts receivable, it sells the accounts at a discount to a bank or other agent, which then attempts to collect (and keeps the money). The advantage of factoring is that the organization receives the cash immediately, albeit at a discount. The disadvantage of factoring is that the organization loses control of the collection process, and the collection methods used by the bank or other agent may reflect poorly on the organization.

When an organization pledges its receivables, it uses the receivables as collateral for a loan. The advantage of pledging accounts receivable is that the organization maintains control of the collection process. The disadvantage of using receivables to secure a loan is that the resulting interest rate on the loan is usually higher than the rate for other conventional loans.

factoring receivables
The practice of selling accounts receivable to a third party at a discount. The third party attempts to collect the accounts and keeps the money.

pledging receivables
The practice of using accounts receivable as collateral for a loan.

FEDERAL LAWS GOVERNING ACCOUNTS RECEIVABLE

Four federal laws govern accounts receivable: the Fair Debt Collection Practices Act, the Truth in Lending Act, the Fair Credit Reporting Act, and the ACA.

FAIR DEBT COLLECTION PRACTICES ACT

The Fair Debt Collection Practices Act applies only to third-party collectors. As long as the healthcare organization collects its own debts, the act does not apply. If the organization contracts with a collection agency, or operates a collection agency under another name, the act does apply. The act deals with four key bill-collecting practices:

1. *Skiptracing:* Governs how the debt collector communicates with consumers owing the debt and under what conditions a debt collector can communicate with others regarding the debt

2. *Collector communication:* Governs when debt collectors can communicate with consumers

3. *Harassment:* Identifies certain behaviors and actions by debt collectors that may be considered harassment and are therefore prohibited

4. *Deceptive or false representations:* Prohibits misleading representation designed to intimidate the consumer

skiptracing

Provision of the Fair Debt Collections Practices Act that governs whom collection agencies can communicate with other than the consumer owing the debt and how the agency can communicate with those people.

TRUTH IN LENDING ACT

The Truth in Lending Act establishes disclosure rules for sales involving consumer credit. It requires a written agreement and four or more installments. In addition, the lending organization must disclose the following under Regulation Z:

- Annual percentage rate
- Amount of the finance charge
- Amount of the principal
- Amount of payments
- Number of payments
- Total of all payments
- Late charge arrangements

◆ Prepayment arrangements

◆ An opportunity for the debtor to receive an itemization of how the payments are to be applied

FAIR CREDIT REPORTING ACT

The Fair Credit Reporting Act governs the permissible uses of credit reports. The act lists the ways credit reports can be obtained, including by court order, by permission of the consumer, and by legitimate business need. Information that must be removed from credit reports and the time at which that information must be removed follows (HFMA 1998):

◆ Bankruptcies after ten years

◆ Judgments after seven years or when the statute of limitations expires, whichever is longer

◆ Paid tax liens after seven years

◆ Collection accounts or those charged to profit and loss after seven years

◆ Arrests, indictments, or convictions after seven years

◆ Other adverse items after seven years

AFFORDABLE CARE ACT

The ACA imposes new requirements on tax-exempt hospitals regarding billing and collections. Hospital financial assistance policy requirements must be adopted, implemented, and publicized, including

◆ Criteria for granting financial assistance to patient

◆ The basis for calculating the amount charged to patients and limitations on charges to patients eligible for financial assistance, including charging no more than the lowest amount charged to insured patients

◆ A method for applying for assistance

◆ Debt collection actions, including the avoidance of extraordinary collection efforts until eligibility for financial assistance is determined

◆ Availability of emergency care regardless of the patient's ability to qualify for financial assistance

EVALUATING REVENUE CYCLE PERFORMANCE

average collection period
A financial ratio that shows the average time a healthcare organization takes to collect money owed to it.

When evaluating accounts receivable performance, **average collection period** (also called days in accounts receivable) is most often used. Average collection period is the average amount of time it takes for an organization to collect a bill; the term is formally defined as the number of days of operating revenue that an organization has due from its patient billings after deducting for contractual allowances, bad debt, and charity care. The average collection period median for all hospitals reporting to Optum (2014) from 2012 audited financial statements was 50.4 days.

Average Collection Period

$$\frac{\text{Net accounts receivable}}{\text{Net patient services revenue} / 365}$$

The objective of managing the revenue cycle is to reduce the average collection period; the collection period does show direction; a smaller number is always better. One way to reduce the average collection period is to write off accounts as bad debt. However, writing off accounts prematurely may not be in the organization's best interest.

CHAPTER KEY POINTS

➤ *Accounts receivable* refers to the money due to the organization by patients and third parties for services already provided.

➤ *Revenue cycle* refers to a multidisciplinary effort to reduce the amount in accounts receivable by managing both the production cycle and the payment cycle.

➤ The objective of managing the revenue cycle is to reduce the collection period by reducing the amount of receivables.

➤ The four steps of managing the revenue cycle include having policies and procedures regarding admission and discharge, having an accounting system that records charges promptly and accurately, having a prompt and accurate medical record system, and having a credit-and-collection policy.

➤ Revenue cycle management views the accounts receivable process as a continuum.

➤ The Fair Debt Collection Practices Act, the Truth in Lending Act, the Fair Credit Reporting Act, and the Affordable Care Act are four federal laws that govern accounts receivable.

➤   The best way to evaluate the management of the revenue cycle is the average
    collection period ratio.

DISCUSSION QUESTIONS

1. What is the definition of *accounts receivable*? What are some primary reasons
    patients are sometimes not billed in a timely manner?

2. Distinguish the accounts receivable from the revenue cycle.

3. Describe what happens when an organization extends credit to patients.

4. What are the steps in managing accounts receivable? Explain each step.

5. Discuss the methods used to collect accounts receivable.

6. How can an organization improve its revenue cycle management?

7. What are the advantages and disadvantages of the two methods used to convert
    accounts receivable to cash?

8. Explain the four laws that govern accounts receivable.

9. What is the best way to evaluate revenue cycle management performance?

NOTES

1. From a legal perspective, the contract between the patient and the healthcare
    organization does not begin until treatment begins (see *Childs v. Weiss*, 440 S.W.2d
    104). The organization's tax status, as well as the organization's ethics as reflected in
    its credit-and-collection policy, may dictate otherwise, however.

2. Generally speaking, healthcare organizations cannot terminate treatment solely
    based on the inability to pay (see Holder [1973] on abandonment).

3. Between 2008 and 2012, the federal and state governments recovered $18.3
    billion from lawsuits and criminal cases claiming healthcare providers overbilled.
    Most cases were filed under the federal False Claims Act. Abusive billing occurs
    when products or services are billed to a public program and are not supported by
    documentation, are not medically necessary, are not covered by the public program,
    or other conditions of payment are not met. Significant abusive billing occurs in
    the following areas: hospital postacute discharges and transfers; hospital claims
    for mechanical ventilation; hospital claims for canceled elective surgeries; hospital
    inpatient and outpatient claims in risk areas; outpatient therapy services; medical
    equipment and/or supplies related to diabetes and lower limb prosthetics; and
    Medicare Part B drugs and Part B ambulance services (OIG 2013).

CHAPTER 10

MANAGING MATERIALS

Change, and the threat or the possibility of it, produces uncertainty and can result in conflict. The role of management in these circumstances is to recognize the inevitability of change and to help the organization (and the individuals within it) to deal with uncertainty while still moving towards its overall goals.

Sir Liam Donaldson, former chief medical officer of the
National Health Service, England

LEARNING OBJECTIVES

After completing this chapter, you should be able to do the following:

➤ Define and understand the importance of materials management

➤ Discuss methods of valuing inventory

➤ Identify costs related to inventory

➤ Discuss the ratios used to evaluate inventory performance

INTRODUCTION

In most healthcare organizations, materials, including supplies and pharmaceuticals, is the largest nonlabor cost in the operating budget and therefore deserves special attention. One of the problems associated with the cost of supplies and pharmaceuticals is the changing demand for healthcare services and the ability of organizations to manage that change. Proper management of materials can have a significant effect on operating costs and, as a result, the net income of the organization.

DEFINITION OF MATERIALS AND INVENTORY MANAGEMENT

Materials management is defined more broadly than inventory management: materials management is the management and control of inventory, services, and equipment from acquisition to disposition. Organizations further classify items into two major categories: patient care and administration. Items in patient care include medical supplies, surgical supplies, drugs, linens, and food. Items in administration include housekeeping supplies, office supplies, and other supplies not used for direct patient care.

The primary objective of materials management is to minimize the total cost associated with materials while ensuring that the proper materials, meaning in both quality and quantity, are readily available for patient care and administration.

Inventory management is the management and control of inventory, or items that have an expected useful life of less than 12 months.

materials management
The management and control of inventory, services, and equipment from acquisition to disposition.

inventory management
The management and control of items that have an expected useful life of less than 12 months.

IMPORTANCE OF MATERIALS MANAGEMENT

PATIENT CARE

Why are materials and, more specifically, inventory so important? First and most important, an organization must have the right kind and the right amount of supplies on hand for patient care. The right kind of supplies can be determined by the materials manager with the help of a user committee. The right amount of supplies can be more difficult to project for three reasons: time, uncertainties, and discontinuities.

Time

The time element refers to the fact that, for most supplies, a lag time exists between ordering and receiving the supplies.

Uncertainties

The demand for supplies fluctuates with volume and kind of patient; therefore, the demand for most healthcare supplies is uncertain. Because of uncertain demand, the materials manager must meet with each department manager to determine the actual necessity of every supply item. If the supply item is a life-saving drug used in emergencies, for example, the materials manager will stock the item at a high level to ensure that the organization never runs out. This procedure is called a stock-out. If the supply in question is a seldom-used office supply, the materials manager will stock the item at a low level, if at all. This method of classifying inventory is the ABC inventory method, where items in category A represent 80 percent of the inventory value, but only 20 percent of the items in inventory; category B represents 15 percent of the inventory value, but 30 percent of the items in inventory; and category C represents only 5 percent of the inventory value, but 50 percent of the items in inventory.

If the organization is large or has sufficient influence over its vendors, the organization may use **just-in-time (JIT) inventory** for some of its inventory items, meaning the supply item is delivered immediately prior to use. JIT means the organization has no, or very little, inventory on hand.

just-in-time inventory method
Inventory method in which supply items are delivered immediately prior to use.

Discontinuities

Discontinuities also affect the amount of supplies on hand. Discontinuities are disruptions to the inventory process, such as a new model of the supply or a missed delivery. The organization must have enough stock on hand to deal with possible discontinuities.

discontinuities
Disruptions to the inventory process, such as the introduction of a new version of a product.

Cost

The second reason materials management is so important is cost. Inventory, like accounts receivable, is a nonproductive asset; it does not grow or produce income. In fact, both accounts receivable and inventory lose value over time. For accounts receivable, the more time an account spends in receivables, the more likely it will become an uncollectible. The more time an item spends in inventory, the more likely it will become stolen, expired, or lost. For that reason, organizations seek to reduce inventory holdings and increase cash, marketable securities, and other assets that produce income.

Inventory Valuation

Costs related to inventory appear in two places on the healthcare organization's financial statements. First, inventory appears as a current asset on the organization's balance sheet. In this case, inventory, expressed as a dollar amount, represents the unused portion of inventory on hand for a given accounting period.

Second, inventory appears as expense items on the organization's statement of revenues and expenses. In this case, inventory, expressed as supplies, food, and drugs, represents the portion of inventory used for a given accounting period. The value of inventory on the balance sheet is based on the cost paid for the items in inventory. During the year, however, identical items of inventory will be purchased at different prices. Furthermore, some inventory items are expensed as the organization uses them. How does the materials manager determine which inventory items and related costs have been expensed and which inventory items and related costs are still in inventory? There are four commonly accepted methods of valuing inventory: first-in, first-out (FIFO); last-in, first-out (LIFO); weighted average; and specific identification. Each will produce a different value and each has advantages and disadvantages.

◆ **First-in, first-out (FIFO):** The first item put into inventory is the first item taken out of inventory. FIFO produces an inventory of newer items. The total cost of inventory is determined by multiplying the unit cost of the newest items in inventory by the number of units in inventory.

◆ **Last-in, first-out (LIFO):** The last item put into inventory is the first item taken out of inventory. LIFO produces an inventory of older items. The total cost of inventory is determined by multiplying the unit cost of the oldest items in inventory by the number of units in inventory.

◆ **Weighted average:** Determines the average cost of items placed in inventory and then multiplies the average cost by the number of units in inventory.

◆ **Specific identification:** Determines the actual cost of each item in inventory. Specific identification is used when inventory items are easy to identify and when the cost of each inventory item is high.

The organization's management must determine which method is best for the organization. Problem 10.1 demonstrates how each inventory method works.

MANAGEMENT OF INVENTORY

COSTS OF INVENTORY

To minimize the total costs of inventory, the materials manager must have a good understanding of inventory costs.[1] Inventory costs are reflected in the following issues:

◆ How much of an item to order each time

◆ When to order the item

◆ The cost of the item

first-in, first-out (FIFO)
An inventory valuation system that assumes that the first items put into inventory will be the first taken out. Thus, the value of the remaining inventory is based on the cost of the latest additions to inventory.

last-in, first-out (LIFO)
An inventory valuation system that assumes that the last items put into inventory will be the first taken out. Thus, the value of the remaining inventory is based on the cost of the earliest additions to inventory.

weighted average
An inventory valuation system that uses an average of the costs of inventory items to determine the value of inventory.

specific identification
An inventory valuation system that determines the actual value of each inventory item.

PROBLEM 10.1
Inventory Valuation

ABC Outpatient Clinic purchased surgical dressing trays at the following dates and amounts.

	Units	Price	Total
January 1 beginning balance	100	$10	$1,000
March 1 purchase	400	12	4,800
May 1 purchase	400	13	5,200
July 1 purchase	300	14	4,200
September 1 purchase	200	14	2,800
November 1 purchase	100	15	1,500
Total	1,500		19,500
Ending inventory on Dec. 31	150		

Using FIFO, LIFO, and weighted average, what is the ending cost of inventory?

FIFO (ending inventory is composed of the most recent 150 trays purchased)

	Units	Price	Total
November 1 cost	100	$15	$1,500
September 1 cost			
(apply 50 trays)	50	14	700
Ending inventory	150		2,200
			or $14.67 per tray

LIFO (ending inventory is composed of the earliest 150 trays purchased)

	Units	Price	Total
January 1 cost	100	$10	$1,000
March 1 cost			
(apply 50 trays)	50	12	600
Ending inventory	150		1,600
			or $10.67 per tray

(continued)

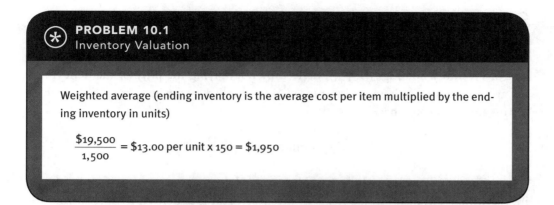

PROBLEM 10.1
Inventory Valuation

Weighted average (ending inventory is the average cost per item multiplied by the ending inventory in units)

$$\frac{\$19,500}{1,500} = \$13.00 \text{ per unit} \times 150 = \$1,950$$

Purchasing Cost

Purchasing cost (PD) is the total cost paid to vendors for a specific item during an accounting period, or year. Purchasing cost is derived by multiplying the price of the item (P) per unit paid to the vendor, by the demand (D) (i.e., the annual amount of the item used):

$$\text{Purchasing cost} = PD$$

Ordering Cost

Ordering cost (O) is the administrative cost associated with placing a single order for the inventory item. Ordering cost includes the costs of

◆ writing specifications;

◆ soliciting bids;

◆ evaluating and awarding bids;

◆ preparing and signing the contract;

◆ preparing the purchase order;

◆ receiving the items; and

◆ accounting for and paying the invoice.

Total ordering cost associated with an inventory item is dependent on the number of orders placed for the item. The number of orders is derived by dividing demand by the size of a single order, called quantity (Q). Total ordering cost for an item in inventory is then derived by multiplying the number of orders per year by the ordering cost:

$$\text{Total ordering costs} = (D/Q)\, O$$

Carrying Cost

Carrying cost is the cost of holding an inventory of items. When an organization holds items in inventory, carrying costs include an opportunity cost at least equal to the average cost of inventory holdings ($[P][\frac{Q}{2}]$), derived by multiplying the price of the item (P) by the average number of items in inventory ($\frac{Q}{2}$), multiplied by the interest rate (I) at which the organization could have invested:

$$\text{Opportunity cost} = IP\frac{Q}{2}$$

Carrying cost also includes a holding cost. Holding cost includes the costs of storing, securing, and insuring the items in inventory, and it is derived by multiplying the holding cost per unit (H) by the quantity ordered each time (Q):

$$\text{Holding costs} = HQ$$

Therefore, carrying costs can be derived by adding holding costs (HQ) and opportunity costs ($[IP]\frac{Q}{2}$):

$$\text{Carrying costs} = HQ + IP\frac{Q}{2}$$

Stock-Out Cost

Stock-out cost (S) is the cost associated with having insufficient inventory holdings to meet demand (i.e., running out of the item in inventory). Stock-out cost includes the purchasing costs and ordering costs associated with a stat (immediate) order, and the intangible costs of loss of goodwill among the organization's medical staff and patients. If the stock-out results in injury or death for the patient, the stock-out cost would include the cost associated with this liability. The stock-out cost is derived on a case-by-case basis.

Overstock Cost

Overstock cost (L) is the cost associated with having more than enough inventory holdings to meet demand. Overstock cost includes the carrying cost associated with stocking items for additional accounting periods until the organization uses and expenses the items.

Total Cost

The total cost (TC) formula produces the minimum costs associated with keeping a specific item in inventory for a period of one year, and it is derived by adding purchasing cost (PD), total ordering cost ($\frac{D}{Q}$ O), carrying cost (HQ + IP[$\frac{Q}{2}$]), stock-out cost (S), and overstock cost (L):

$$\text{Total costs} = PD + \left(\frac{D}{Q}\right) O + \left(HQ + IP \left[\frac{Q}{2}\right]\right) + S + L$$

The total cost formula can provide a basis for different real-world situations the manager may face. For instance, a vendor offers a manager a 10 percent discount on price if the vendor can reduce the number of deliveries per year to four. In this situation, the total cost (TC) formula changes based on the new information: price (P) becomes P – 10 percent, and quantity (Q) becomes $\frac{D}{4}$. After reworking the TC formula, if adjusted total cost is less than the original total cost, the manager should accept the vendor's offer.

Here's another example. If the manager has $10,000 budgeted for an inventory item and must ask the vendor for a discount on price, TC is $10,000, and the unknown variable is price (P). But before calculating the total cost formula in this example, the economic order quantity (Q_e) must be calculated.

ECONOMIC ORDER QUANTITY AND REORDER POINT

The **economic order quantity** (EOQ or Q_e) is the quantity of items that should be ordered each time to result in the minimum total inventory costs associated with the item. The Q_e formula is

$$Q_e = \sqrt{\frac{2DO}{IP + 2H}}$$

economic order quantity
The quantity of items that should be ordered each time to result in the minimum total inventory costs.

The Q_e model makes the following assumptions:

◆ Demand is fixed and constant during the year.

◆ Lead time for placing orders is constant.

◆ No discounts are offered for quantity orders.

◆ No stock-out or overstock costs exist.

These assumptions may be unrealistic in most healthcare organizations. However, in organizations where demand fluctuates weekly, the fluctuations tend to cancel out so that seasonal demand, or annual demand, appears constant (Siegel and Shim 2006). Calculation of the reorder point (RP) requires knowledge of the lag time in receiving orders, or how many days occur between ordering an item and receiving the item. Thus, the reorder point in units is the demand during the lag time and the reorder point in days is the lag time.

Problem 10.2 demonstrates the total cost (TC) formula, the economic order quantity (Q_e) formula, and the reorder point.

⊛ PROBLEM 10.2
Economic Order Quantity (EOQ), Total Cost, and Reorder Point

Find the EOQ, the total cost, and the reorder point in units given:

Price (P)	= $10
Annual demand (D)	= 10,000 units with a constant daily demand
Order cost (O)	= $10 per order
Interest (I)	= 7 percent
Holding cost (H)	= $.10 per unit
Lag time	= 5 days

Find the EOQ.

$$Qe = \sqrt{\frac{2DO}{IP+2H}}$$

$$Qe = \sqrt{\frac{2(10,000)\,(10)}{(.07)(10)+(2)(.10)}}$$

$$Qe = 471 \text{ units}$$

Find the total cost.

$$TC = PD + \frac{D}{Qe}O + (HQe + IP\frac{Qe}{2})$$

$$TC = (10)(10,000) + \frac{10,000}{471}\,(10) + \left[(.10)(471) + (.07)(10)\left(\frac{471}{2}\right)\right]$$

$$TC = \$100,424$$

Find the reorder point in units.

$$RP = \frac{D}{365} \times 5, \text{ or } RP = \frac{10,000}{365} \times 5, \text{ or } RP = 137 \text{ units}$$

Find the number of orders to be placed in a year.

$$\text{Orders per year} = \frac{D}{Q} \text{ or } \frac{10,000}{471}, \text{ or } 21.2$$

(continued)

PROBLEM 10.2
Economic Order Quantity (EOQ), Total Cost, and Reorder Point

Find the number of days between orders.

Days between orders = $\dfrac{365}{\text{Orders per year}}$, or $\dfrac{365}{21.2}$, or 17.2

Find the carrying cost.

Carrying cost = $HQe + IP\dfrac{Qe}{2}$, or $\left[(.10)(471) + (.07)(10)\left(\dfrac{471}{2}\right)\right]$, or \$211.95

Find the holding cost.

Holding cost = HQe, or \$47.10

Find the opportunity cost.

Opportunity cost= $IP\dfrac{Qe}{2}$, or $(.07)(10)\dfrac{471}{2}$, or \$164.85

Find the cost of the average inventory.

Average inventory cost = $P\dfrac{Qe}{2}$, or $(10)\dfrac{471}{2}$, or \$2,355

Find the volume of the average inventory.

Volume of the average inventory = $\dfrac{Qe}{2}$, or $\dfrac{471}{2}$, or 235.5 units

The vendor offers a 10 percent discount on price if he can make equal monthly deliveries. Should his offer be accepted?

Price (P) = \$9.00

Quantity (Q) =, $\dfrac{10,000}{12}$ or 833 units

TC2 = $(9)(10,000) + \dfrac{10,000}{833}(10) + (.10)(833) + (.07)(9)\left(\dfrac{833}{2}\right)$

TC2 = \$90,465

Yes, because \$90,465 is less than \$100,424.

MANAGING INVENTORY WHEN UNCERTAIN DEMAND EXISTS

In Problem 10.2, demand is constant. Each day the organization used the same amount of the product; daily demand was $10,000 \div 365 = 27.4$ units. A constant demand is unlikely in most healthcare organizations. Given an uncertain demand, the probability of stock-outs and overstocks increases, as shown in Exhibit 10.1. Measuring the costs associated with stock-outs and overstocks is admittedly difficult, but assume that stock-out cost is \$7.50 per unit and overstock cost is \$2.00 per unit in Problem 10.2.

EXHIBIT 10.1
Inventory Demand

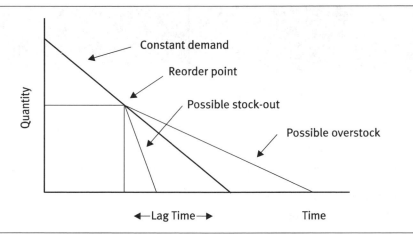

Source: Adapted from Berman, H. J., S. F. Kukla, and L. E. Weeks. 1994. *The Financial Management of Hospitals*, 8th ed., 287. Chicago: Health Administration Press.

You are the administrator of a 15-physician group practice. After completing a physical inventory, you have concluded that the practice has about three times more inventory than is needed based on current demand. You need to meet with the physicians and prove that they have excess inventory. What would you include in your presentation?

To determine the reorder point (RP) under conditions of uncertain demand, the organization needs to know the costs associated with stock-outs and overstocks, and the probability of a stock-out based on the history of the inventory item (see Problem 10.3). By multiplying the stock-out or overstock cost by the probability of occurrence, the projected cost can be calculated for each reorder point. For example, at a reorder point of 135 units and a demand of 136 units, one additional unit is needed at a stock-out cost of $7.50, which is then multiplied by the chance of that happening (0.25) for a cost in that specific cell of $1.88. In Problem 10.3, the low-cost solution is to establish a reorder point at 138 units, which will minimize the stock-out and overstock costs associated with an uncertain demand (Berman, Kukla, and Weeks 1994).

EVALUATING INVENTORY PERFORMANCE

inventory turnover
A ratio that measures how many times an organization turns over its inventory relative to its operating revenue.

The ratio most often used to evaluate inventory performance is the **inventory turnover,** which measures the number of times an organization turns over its inventory relative to operating revenue. The average inventory turnover median for all hospitals reporting to Optum (2014) from 2012 audited financial statements was 54.7.

PROBLEM 10.3
Reorder Point Under Conditions of Uncertainty

Find the reorder point under conditions of uncertainty, given the following information:
  Stock-out cost = $7.50 per item
  Overstocked cost = $2.00 per item

	Potential Demand					
	135	136	137	138	139	
Probability	.10	.25	.30	.25	.10	
Reorder Point						**Cost**
135	.00	1.88	4.50	5.63	3.00	$15.01
136	.20	.00	2.25	3.75	2.25	8.45
137	.40	.50	.00	1.88	1.50	4.28
138	.60	1.00	.60	.00	.75	2.95
139	.80	1.50	1.20	.50	.00	4.00

Answer: The low-cost reorder point under conditions of uncertainty is 138 units at $2.95.

Source: Adapted from Berman, H. J., S. F. Kukla, and L. E. Weeks. 1994. *The Financial Management of Hospitals*, 8th ed., 290. Chicago: Health Administration Press.

Inventory Turnover

$$\frac{\text{Total operating revenue} + \text{Other income}}{\text{Inventory expense}}$$

Low values indicate overstocking and thus an inappropriate investment in nonproductive assets. This ratio does show directionality; higher values are considered to be better. Because of their size, healthcare systems enjoy considerable purchasing power and often receive medical supplies on consignment. This means that the vendors do not charge the system until the supply item is used, so inventory value is very low. The inventory turnover ratio median from all hospitals reporting to Optum (2014) for 2012 audited financial statements was 54.69.

CHAPTER KEY POINTS

➤ Materials management is the control of inventory, services, and equipment from acquisition to disposition.

➤ Inventory management is the management and control of inventory, or items that have an expected useful life of less than 12 months.

➤ Inventory management is important to provide patients with high-quality supplies at the right time at the least possible cost.

➤ Inventory is valued using FIFO, LIFO, weighted average, and specific identification.

➤ The economic order quantity, the total cost, and the reorder point are calculated using formulas.

➤ The best way to evaluate inventory management is the inventory turnover ratio.

DISCUSSION QUESTIONS

1. What is the definition of inventory management?

2. Why is proper inventory management important?

3. Explain the different methods used to value inventory.

4. How can an organization reduce the value of inventory and the number of items in inventory?

5. What does an economic order quantity, or EOQ, tell management?

6. What does the total cost formula tell management?

7. What is the reorder point?

8. What is the best way to evaluate inventory management performance?

NOTE

1. Several formulas are used to determine inventory costs. This book uses the formula and cost descriptions from Berman, Kukla, and Weeks (1994) because of the level of detail.

Recommended Readings—Part III

Baker, J., and R. W. Baker. 2014. *Health Care Finance: Basic Tools for Nonfinancial Managers,* 4th ed. Boston: Jones & Bartlett Learning.

Berger, S. 2008. *Fundamentals of Healthcare Financial Management,* 3rd ed. San Francisco: Jossey-Bass.

Finkler, S. A. 2009. *Financial Management for Public Health and Non-Profit Organizations.* Upper Saddle River, NJ: Prentice Hall.

Gapenski, L. C. 2011. *Healthcare Finance: An Introduction to Accounting and Financial Management,* 5th ed. Chicago: Health Administration Press.

Gapenski, L. C., and G. H. Pink. 2010. *Understanding Healthcare Financial Management,* 6th ed. Chicago: Health Administration Press.

McLean, R. A. 2002. *Financial Management in Health Care Organizations,* 2nd ed. New York: Delmar Publishers.

Optum. 2014. *2014 Almanac of Hospital Financial and Operating Indicators.* Salt Lake City: Optum.

Zelman, W. N., M. J. McCue, N. D. Glick, and M. S. Thomas. 2014. *Financial Management of Health Care Organizations,* 4th ed. San Francisco: Jossey-Bass Publishers.

INVENTORY VALUATION

Inventory Valuation Practice Problem

XYZ Central Billing Office purchased magnetic storage disks on the following dates and amounts.

	Units	Price	Total
LiFo January I beginning balance	10	$15	$150
LiFo March I purchase	30	14	420
May I purchase	40	14	560
July I purchase *FiFo*	10	13	130
FiFo September I purchase	20	12	240
FiFo November I purchase	10	12	120
Total	120		$1,620
Ending inventory on Dec. 31	35		

Using FIFO, LIFO, and weighted average, what is the ending cost of inventory?

Inventory Valuation Practice Problem Solution

FIFO (ending inventory is composed of the most recent 35 disks purchased)

	Units	Price	Total
November 1 costs	10	$12	$120
September 1 costs	20	12	240
July 1 purchase (apply 5 disks)	5	13	65
Ending inventory	**35**		**$425**

or $12.14 per disk

LIFO (ending inventory is composed of the earliest 35 disks purchased)

	Units	Price	Total
January 1 costs	10	$15	$150
March 1 costs (apply 25 disks)	25	14	350
Ending inventory	**35**		**$500**

or $14.29 per disk

Weighted average (ending inventory is composed of the weighted average cost per disk times the ending inventory in units)

$$\frac{\$1,620}{120} = \$13.50 \text{ per unit} \times 35 = \$472.50$$

Inventory Valuation Self-Quiz Problem

Your radiology department purchased film on the following dates and amounts:

	Units	Price	Total
January 1 beginning balance	10	$150	$1,500
July 1 purchase	10	155	1,550
December 1 purchase	20	160	3,200
Total	**40**		**$6,250**
Ending Inventory	**25**		

Using FIFO, LIFO, and weighted average, what is your ending cost of inventory?

ECONOMIC ORDER QUANTITY

Economic Order Quantity Practice Problem

Find the economic order quantity (EOQ) and total cost (TC), assuming the following:

Price (P) = $100
Annual demand (D) = 1,000
Order cost (O) = $10
Interest (I) = 5%
Holding cost (H) = $.50
Lag time = 5 days

$6.00 P

5.00 D

$$Qe = \sqrt{\frac{2DO}{IP + 2H}}$$

$$TC = PD + \frac{D}{Qe}O + (HQe + IP\frac{Qe}{2})$$

Given a constant demand for the product, how many orders will be made in 1 year?

Given a constant demand and a lag time of 5 days between order and receipt, how many units will be in stock when you place an order?

Given a constant demand, how many days are between orders?

= 156.25
40

Economic Order Quantity Practice Problem Solution

$$EOQ = Qe \sqrt{\frac{2\,(1{,}000)\,(10)}{(.05)\,(100) + 2\,(.5)}} = 58 \text{ units}$$

$$TC = (100)\,(1{,}000) + \frac{1{,}000}{58}\,(10) + (.5 \times 58 + (.05)\,(100)\,\frac{58}{2}$$

$$TC = \$100{,}346$$

Demand $\dfrac{1{,}000}{58} = 17.24$ orders per year
Qe

$$\frac{1{,}000}{365} \times 5 = 13.70 \text{ units on the shelf}$$

$$\frac{365}{17.24} = 21.17 \text{ days between orders}$$

Economic Order Quantity Self-Quiz Problem

Find the EOQ and TC, assuming the following:

$$Qe = \sqrt{\frac{2DO}{IP + 2H}}$$

P = $5
D = 20,000
O = $10
I = 10%
H = $.75

$$Qe = \sqrt{\frac{2DO}{IP + 2H}}$$

$$TC = PD + \frac{D}{Qe} O + (HQe + IP\frac{Qe}{2})$$

Given a constant demand for the product, how many orders will be made in 1 year?

Given a constant demand and a lag time of 5 days between order and receipt, how many units will be in stock when you place an order?

Given a constant demand, how many days are between orders?

What is the carrying cost?

What is the opportunity cost?

What is the cost of the average inventory?

What is the volume of the average inventory?

The hospital has only $90,000 budgeted for the product. What is the new price the hospital must negotiate with the vendor to make budget?

REORDER POINT UNDER CONDITIONS OF UNCERTAINTY

Reorder Point Under Conditions of Uncertainty Practice Problem

Find the low-cost reorder point under conditions of uncertainty given the following information:

Stock-out cost = $5.00 per item
Overstocked cost = $1.00 per item

Probability of	.10	.25	.30	.25	.10
meeting demand	100	101	102	103	104

Reorder Point Under Conditions of Uncertainty Practice Problem Solution

		Potential Demand					
		100	101	102	103	104	
	Probability	**.10**	**.25**	**.30**	**.25**	**.10**	
Reorder Point							**Cost ($)**
100		.00	1.25	3.00	3.75	2.00	10.00
101		.10	.00	1.50	2.50	1.50	5.60
102		.20	.25	.00	1.25	1.00	2.70
103		.30	.50	.30	.00	.50	1.60
104		.40	.75	.60	.25	.00	2.00

Conclusion: The low-cost reorder point under conditions of uncertainty is 103 units at $1.60.

Reorder Point Under Conditions of Uncertainty Self-Quiz Problem

Find the low-cost reorder point under conditions of uncertainty given the following information:

Stock-out cost = $6.00 per item
Overstocked cost = $1.00 per item

Probability of	.10	.25	.30	.25	.10
meeting demand	100	101	102	103	104

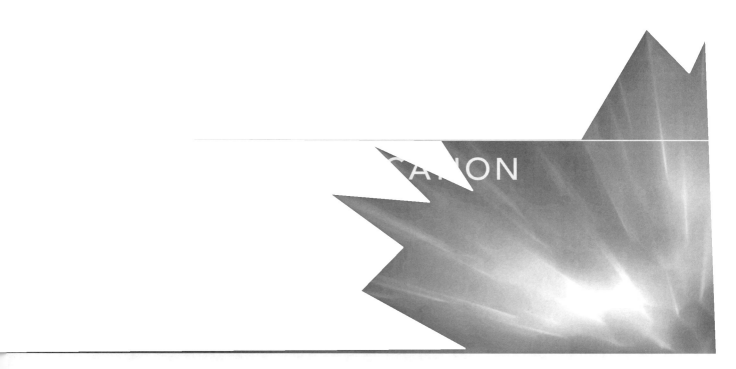

CANON

CHAPTER 11

STRATEGIC AND OPERATIONAL PLANNING

One fundamental misperception is that strategic planning outside of healthcare (in for-profits) is financially driven, but in not-for-profit healthcare it isn't because we're not sophisticated. The reality is that although there is more financial integration with strategic planning outside of healthcare, it's not the case that 'they do it right' and 'we don't.' And healthcare organizations are making good progress in linking financial planning and strategic planning and closing whatever gap that may still exist.

Alan Zuckerman, healthcare industry strategist

LEARNING OBJECTIVES

After completing this chapter, you should be able to do the following:

➤ Define and understand the importance of planning

➤ Identify the prerequisites to the planning process

➤ Explain the types of planning

➤ Compare and contrast strategic and operational planning

➤ List, in order, and explain each step in the planning process

➤ Discuss the methods used to evaluate the planning process

INTRODUCTION

Everyone agrees that planning—especially strategic planning—is critical for economic survival in today's turbulent environment. However, planning is a management function often neglected by healthcare managers. In a 2006 survey of 138 Texas hospitals, 13 percent did not have a strategic plan; for the hospitals that did have a strategic plan, 50 percent did not delegate the responsibility for the plan to the CEO. The average board member involvement was rated at 4.86 on a 7.0 scale. All three characteristics—existence of a strategic plan, delegation of plan responsibilities to the CEO, and board member involvement in the development of the strategic plan—had a statistically significant effect on higher financial performance (Kaissi and Begun 2008).

DEFINITION OF PLANNING

Planning as a management function is the process of deciding in advance what must be done in the future. Planning consists of establishing the goals, objectives, policies, procedures, methods, and rules necessary to achieve the purposes of the organization. Planning precedes, and serves as a framework for, the other management functions of organizing, staffing, influencing, and controlling. Effective planning is a continuous process; managers are responsible for planning for the appropriate use of resources in their areas of responsibility in concert with the operational and strategic direction of the organization. In the absence of effective planning, managers would engage in random activities. In healthcare organizations where customers demand a high degree of predictable outcomes, such random activities on the part of managers would have a disastrous effect (Dunn 2010).

PREREQUISITES TO PLANNING

Before effective planning can begin, the organization must meet certain requirements. First, the organization must have a sound organizational structure that ensures management accountability for the planning process. Second, the organization must have a well-defined chart of accounts that corresponds with the organizational structure. Third, the organization must have a prompt and accurate accounting system that ensures financial accountability for the planning process. Fourth, the organization must have a comprehensive management information system that captures nonfinancial information for each department (Berman, Kukla, and Weeks 1994).

TYPES OF PLANNING

Planning can be classified by planning horizon, management approach, and design characteristics.

PLANNING HORIZON

Planning horizon is the length of time management is looking into the future. Strategic plans look three to ten years into the future. Operating plans look one year into the future.

MANAGEMENT APPROACH

Planning can also be classified by management approach, or top-down versus bottom-up planning. These approaches correspond closely with top-down and bottom-up budgeting, as discussed in Chapter 12. In top-down planning, senior management, which includes the division heads or vice presidents, develops the plan with little or no input from subordinates. The advantage of such a design is that senior management may be in the best position to objectively view the future. The disadvantage of the top-down design is that plan implementation may be difficult if subordinates have little or no input.

In bottom-up planning, subordinates develop the plan and submit it to senior management for approval. The advantage to bottom-up planning is the commitment to the plan by those who developed it. The disadvantage is that subordinates may not be in the best position to view the future.[1]

In most cases, a combination of the top-down and bottom-up designs is used, with senior management deciding on plan parameters and subordinates submitting plans within those parameters.

DESIGN CHARACTERISTICS

Planning can also be classified by design characteristics, which also correspond closely with the design characteristics of budgeting, as discussed in Chapter 12.

Incremental Versus Zero-Base Planning

Incremental planning requires planning only for changes, such as new equipment, new positions, and new programs. Incremental planning assumes that all current operations, including positions and equipment, are essential to the continued mission of the organization, and that all current operations are working at peak performance. The advantages are the ease of incremental planning, the minimal time commitment required to plan, and the support of a bigger organizational culture. The principal disadvantage of incremental planning is the assumption that all current operations are essential in a healthcare environment that is changing so rapidly. Conversely, **zero-base planning** takes nothing for granted and requires rejustification for existing equipment, positions, and programs, as well as justification for new equipment, positions, and programs. Therein lies the principal advantage of zero-base planning: in a rapidly changing environment where reimbursement is moving away from cost-based approaches toward prospective payment per case or per enrollee, zero-base planning can eliminate unnecessary programs and improve operations. Disadvantages include the large time commitment required, employee fear and anxiety, and significant administrative and communication requirements (Person 1997).

Comprehensive Versus Limited-in-Scope Planning

Comprehensive planning integrates the strategic plan and the operational plan into one document. The advantage is the recognition that short-term objectives affect long-term goals. Limited-in-scope planning segregates the plans. Most organizations integrate the plans at the board and executive management level of the organization, but the issue is the level at which the plans should be segregated.

Fixed Versus Flexible Planning

Fixed plans assume that volumes, and related revenues and variable expenses, remain constant during the year. Fixed plans are easy to project, but they are unrealistic for healthcare organizations, whose volumes fluctuate during the year and whose variable expenses, which are dependent on volumes, account for more than half of an organization's operating expenses.

Flexible plans take into account fluctuations in volumes, at least within ranges expressed as probabilities, and adjust variable expenses accordingly.

Discrete Versus Continuous Planning

Discrete plans apply to a fixed period of time, usually a year. At the end of the year, a new plan begins. Discrete plans are relatively easy to prepare, but it can be difficult to plan things in 12-month increments because circumstances often change. Furthermore, discrete plans can be challenging to some managers who know if they exceed objectives at the end of the year they will receive new, more rigorous objectives for the coming year.

Continuous plans, sometimes referred to as rolling plans, are updated continuously so that year end never occurs. Department managers who manage wisely roll over their efforts to the next month.

CORPORATE PLANNING

Most healthcare organizations have moved away from facility planning—planning based on their own needs—which was popular under retroactive, cost-based reimbursement. They have adopted a business planning approach based on market needs, called corporate planning. Corporate planning consists of four major stages (see Exhibit 11.1):

Exhibit 11.1
Corporate Planning
Process

Stage	Planning Horizon
Strategic Planning	3–10 years out, revised annually
1. Validate mission and strategic interpretations	
2. Assess external environment	
3. Assess internal environment	
4. Formulate vision	
5. Establish strategic thrusts	
6. Identify critical success factors	
7. Develop primary, or core, objectives	
8. Develop strategic financial plan	
Operational Planning	1 year out
9. Develop secondary, or department, objectives	
10. Develop policies	
11. Develop procedures	
12. Develop methods	
13. Develop rules	
Budgeting	1 year out
14. Project volumes	
15. Convert volumes into revenues	
16. Convert volumes into expenses	
17. Adjust revenues and expenses as necessary	
Capital Budgeting	1–3 years out
18. Identify and prioritize requests	
19. Project cash flows	
20. Perform financial analysis	
21. Identify nonfinancial benefits	
22. Evaluate benefits and make decisions	

1. *Strategic planning:* determines the organization's overall direction in the next three to ten years

2. *Operational planning:* converts the strategic plan into next year's objectives

3. *Budgeting:* converts the operating plan into budgets for revenues, expenses, and cash

4. *Capital budgeting:* converts the operating plan into budgets for capital expenditures

STRATEGIC PLANNING

strategic planning
Long-range planning that anticipates where an organization will be in three to ten years.

Strategic planning forces managers to anticipate where they want the healthcare organization to be in three to ten years; to identify the resources that will be necessary to get there; and to preview the provision of healthcare services at the end of the planning horizon. Strategic planning also provides the starting point for the operating plan and budget.

The governing board has the overall responsibility for strategic planning for the organization, but it should actively seek input from the organization's stakeholders, which are those constituents with a vested interest in the organization. Certainly, the community (which may be represented by the board members), the medical staff, and organization employees should provide input. While a strategic plan is mandated by both Medicare and The Joint Commission, healthcare organizations sometimes offer excuses for not fully engaging in the planning process. Excuses range from a lack of time to a rapidly changing future. Paradoxically, if organizations spent more time planning, they would end up having more time to execute the plans. Organizations with serious planning processes position themselves to control the turbulent future, rather than simply react to it. Often financial management, including the chief financial officer (CFO), is not involved in the planning process until the budgeting stage. The CFO might be viewed as an impediment to the vision needed for the strategic plan to work. However, the CFO is necessary to provide input to the strategic financial plan—or the ability of the organization to fund the capital and operating costs necessary to make the strategic plan successful.

THE PLANNING PROCESS

STEP 1: VALIDATE MISSION AND STRATEGIC INTERPRETATIONS

The first step in the planning process is for the executive management team, which includes the governing body and the chief executive officer (CEO), to validate the organization's mission. The mission is a broad statement of organizational purpose that can be easily communicated throughout both the organization and the community. Because mission statements are broad, organizations should not need to change them frequently; mission statements should survive to the end of the planning horizon. A study of more than 200 *Fortune* 500 companies identified common characteristics of effective mission statements (Pearce and David 1987). The mission statements

- ◆ target customers and markets,

- ◆ indicate the principal services delivered by the organization,

- ◆ specify the geographic area in which the organization intends to operate,

- ◆ identify the organization's philosophy,

- ◆ confirm the organization's self-image, and

- ◆ express the organization's desired public image.

Because organizations want the mission statements to play well to the communities they serve, mission statements do not always accurately reflect the true purposes of the organization. Strategic interpretations, however, should reflect those true purposes.

Strategic interpretations provide the means for executive management to interpret the mission statement by recognizing the changing character of the healthcare industry and the changing needs of the community. Strategic interpretations may also prioritize organizational purposes when the mission statement includes multiple purposes that might conflict when operationalized. Strategic interpretations are seldom directly stated in any form and are more often represented in the actions of executive management. For instance, executive management may show a preference for one purpose over another through the budget allocation process.

STEP 2: ASSESS THE EXTERNAL ENVIRONMENT

The second step in the planning process is to assess the external environment, including factors that might have an effect on present or future performance. To maintain objectivity and guard against vested interests, a governing body or outside consultants should be responsible for assessing both the external and internal environments. The first part of the assessment should include a determination on the direction of the industry as a whole by investigating national trends. Some of the current national trends for the healthcare industry include

- ◆ decreasing reimbursement from federal and state health programs as government tries to slow rising healthcare costs;

- ◆ increasing popularity of managed care programs (and capitation), especially among payers including employers;

- ◆ increasing consolidation as a result of competition;

◆   continuing expansion into businesses outside the traditional healthcare industry;

◆   increasing growth in outpatient care, preventive care, and innovative alternative delivery systems;

◆   declining numbers of rural and public teaching hospitals; and

◆   decreasing numbers of uninsured and bad debt as the Affordable Care Act (ACA) is implemented and more people are insured.

The second part of the external environment assessment should determine the direction of the local market and should investigate the following elements:

◆   Demographic and socioeconomic characteristics of the primary and secondary service areas and their effect on present and future utilization patterns

◆   Key economic and employment indicators and their effect on present and future utilization patterns

◆   Patient migration patterns, to determine from where patients and potential patients come

◆   Market share statistics for key competitors, to determine market strengths and weaknesses

◆   Competitor profiles, including strengths and weaknesses, use by service, use by payer, exclusive and other managed care contracts, extent of horizontal and vertical integration, potential expansion plans, and cost comparisons

◆   Managed care profile, to determine present and future managed care penetration

◆   Physician profile, to determine numbers, ages, and specialists available in the market

Any significant difference between national trends identified in the first part of the external environment assessment and the local trends identified in the second part of the external environment assessment should be thoroughly analyzed to determine the reasons for the differences.

STEP 3: ASSESS THE INTERNAL ENVIRONMENT

The third step in the planning process is for the governing body or outside consultants to assess the internal environment, including factors that might have an effect on performance either now or in the future. The first part of the assessment should determine the direction of the organization by investigating organizational trends. Some of the organizational trends for analysis might include

◆ patient composition, including utilization patterns (i.e., patient days, outpatient visits, admissions, discharges, lengths of stay, age, payer, patient origin);

◆ medical staff composition, including use patterns by specialty, age, practice (solo versus group), admissions, lengths of stay, and board certification;

◆ agreements with payers and managed care organizations;

◆ financial assistance policy readily available to the public;

◆ financial ratios, including liquidity, profitability, activity, capital structure, and operating ratios (see Chapter 14); and

◆ Joint Commission status and quality indicators, including rate-based indicators and sentinel event indicators.

Some organizations use a SWOT (strengths, weaknesses, opportunities, and threats) analysis to assess the internal environment. A SWOT analysis forces the organization to identify its strengths and weaknesses during internal assessment. Then the organization identifies opportunities for additional market penetration with existing or new programs and threats from competitors that might reduce the organization's chances for success (Dunn 2010).

The ACA requires tax-exempt hospitals to complete a community health needs assessment every three years and to make the assessment, along with audited financial statements, available to the public. The assessment must include a treasurer review of community benefits and explain why certain community health needs are not being addressed. The presumption is that community health needs should be met and financed with the difference between tax savings and the cost of providing community benefits.

STEP 4: FORMULATE THE VISION

The fourth step in the planning process is for the executive management team to formulate a vision—a view of the future that they think gives the organization the best chance of accomplishing its mission. Executive management bases its vision on the information obtained from assessing the external and internal environments. It must communicate its vision throughout the organization. Effective vision statements have certain characteristics in common (Peters 1988). They should

◆ be inspiring first of all to employees, but also to customers;

◆ be clear, challenging, and about excellence;

◆ make sense to the community, be flexible, and stand the test of time;

◆ be stable, but change when necessary;

◆ provide direction in a chaotic environment;

◆ prepare for the future while honoring the past; and

◆ be easily translated into action.

STEP 5: ESTABLISH STRATEGIC THRUSTS

strategic thrusts
Broad statements of significant results that an organization wants to achieve related to its vision. Also called *goals*.

The fifth step in the planning process is for executive management to establish **strategic thrusts** or goals, which are broad statements of significant results that the organization wants to achieve related to the vision. Strategic thrusts should be limited in number, stable and enduring, and, taken together, comprehensive to the point that they provide meaningful results for all components of the organization's mission (Dunn 2010).

STEP 6: IDENTIFY CRITICAL SUCCESS FACTORS

The sixth step in the planning process is for executive management to identify critical success factors that will measure progress toward achieving the plan. The assessment of the environment should introduce both strategic thrusts and critical success factors. Critical success factors are organization specific, but most healthcare organizations will include critical success factors from the following areas:

◆ Inpatient use and market share

◆ Outpatient use and market share

◆ Managed care use and market share

◆ Medical staff profiles and activity levels

◆ Accessibility indicators

◆ Cost-effectiveness indicators

◆ Efficiency indicators

◆ Quality indicators

STEP 7: DEVELOP CORE OBJECTIVES

The seventh step in the strategic planning process is for executive management to develop primary, or core, objectives that support the strategic thrusts or goals. Primary objectives should encompass the entire organization. Organizations have several primary objectives; the real challenge lies in balancing them. See Exhibit 11.2 for a sample strategic plan.

EXHIBIT 11.2
Simple Not-for-Profit Nursing Home Strategic Plan

Mission

- Our mission is to be the nursing home of choice in our community by providing high-quality, competitively priced skilled nursing services.

Interpretation

- To provide a skilled nursing facility to those living in our community in a cost-effective manner to ensure financial survival.

Vision

- Our vision is to expand our services in the next five years to include a residential care facility and a hospice facility while maintaining a high-quality, cost-effective skilled nursing facility.

Strategic Thrusts

1. To provide high-quality skilled nursing care
2. To provide cost-effective skilled nursing care
3. To expand service without harming quality or increasing cost

Critical Success Factors

1. Continued accreditation
2. Continued licensure
3. Continued favorable physician relations
4. Cost increases not to exceed 3 percent per year
5. Residential care facility and hospice to open within five years

Primary Objectives

1. Initiate total quality management program
2. Initiate patient satisfaction surveys
3. Initiate physician satisfaction surveys
4. Initiate reengineering program to improve processes and reduce cost
5. Build residential care facility
6. Build hospice facility

Step 8: Develop the Strategic Financial Plan

The eighth and last step in the planning process is for the governing body and CEO to develop the strategic financial plan. The strategic financial plan is the link between the strategic plan, which looks three to ten years out, and the operating plan, which looks one year out. In essence, the strategic financial plan is the quantification of a series of strategic planning policy decisions that will answer whether the organization can make progress toward accomplishing its strategic plan over the next ten years. These decisions are based on the answers to the following questions regarding the five-year planning horizon (Berger 2007):

◆ How much cash should the organization have five years from now (days cash-on-hand ratio)?

◆ How much debt can the organization afford to take on five years from now (debt service coverage ratio)?

◆ What profitability targets are necessary to meet the cash and debt metrics identified above (operating margin and excess margin ratios)?

◆ What is the required level of operating change necessary to meet the profitability targets identified (projected increases in net revenues and decreases in operating expenses)?

◆ What are the organization's strategic capital requirements over the next five years (five-year capital spending projection)?

◆ What is the financing method for the capital necessary to meet the capital requirements identified (debt, equity, lease, or philanthropy)?

All of the industry ratios identified earlier can be obtained by rating agencies, which might rate the hospital in the future if part of the financing will be dependent on bonds. Progress toward these ratios is also an excellent way for the governing board to evaluate the CEO on an annual basis (Nowicki 2004).

Value of Strategic Planning

The value of strategic planning lies in its systematic approach to dealing with an uncertain future. Many organizations become disillusioned with strategic planning when their plans are not met. These plans often have too narrow a focus—the more narrow the focus, the less likely an organization is to accomplish the plan. Strategic planning that establishes the organization's overall direction without attempting to be specific has the following benefits:

◆ It integrates mission, vision, strategic thrusts, and primary objectives with the secondary objectives, policies, procedures, methods, and rules of the operating plan.

♦ It provides a process and time frame for making strategic decisions.

♦ It provides a framework for the operating plan, budget, and capital budget.

OPERATIONAL PLANNING

For the strategic direction of the organization to be useful, the organization's managers must translate the strategic direction into small, measurable steps to be taken during the next year. **Operational planning** is the process of translating the strategic plan into a year's objectives. Budgeting is the process of expressing the operating plan in monetary terms and is covered in Chapter 12. Many organizations have difficulty determining where strategic planning ends and operational planning begins, and where operational planning ends and budgeting begins.

Three characteristics distinguish strategic planning from operational planning:

operational planning
The process of translating the strategic plan into a year's objectives.

1. *Planning horizon:* Strategic planning is for the next three to ten years, and operational planning is for the next year.

2. *Principal participants:* The governing body and executive management develop the strategic plan; the department managers develop or have significant input in the operational plan.

3. *Objectives:* Strategic planning lists primary objectives common to the entire organization, and the operating plan lists secondary objectives by division or department.

STEP 9: DEVELOP SECONDARY, OR DEPARTMENT, OBJECTIVES

In the ninth step in the corporate planning process—the first step in the operational planning process—department managers develop secondary, departmental objectives to support the strategic plan of the organization (Berman, Kukla, and Weeks 1994; Dunn 2010).

♦ Department objective-setting should be participative. Meaningful employee participation in planning improves both morale and the chances of meeting objectives.

♦ Department objectives should be rigorous but attainable. The department will not progress if the objectives are easily attainable, and the department may not attempt objectives that seem too difficult.

♦ Department objectives should be verifiable and/or measurable to ensure progress and to reward those responsible for the progress. For Joint Commission purposes, the manager and subordinates should discuss desired outcomes and their indicators (see Chapter 1).

One method of developing department objectives is Peter Drucker's management by objectives (MBO), introduced during the 1950s. In a nutshell: (1) the manager provides subordinates with a general overview of the work to be accomplished in the coming year, (2) the subordinates propose objectives, and (3) the objectives are negotiated until final agreement. Reported advantages of MBO include directing work activity toward organizational goals, reducing conflict and ambiguity, providing clear standards for control and performance appraisals, and improving motivation. MBO is not without disadvantages, including burdensome procedures and paperwork; overemphasis on quantitative objectives at the possible expense of qualitative objectives; suboptimization of performance; and illusionary participation, which means that managers give the perception of participation, but the participation lacks meaningful substance, often because the subordinates sense that decisions have already been made.

STEP 10: DEVELOP POLICIES

The tenth step in the planning process and the second step in the operational planning process is for department managers to develop policies (i.e., broad guides to thinking) that provide subordinates with general guidelines for decision making. Policies are the most common type of plan at the department level (Dunn 2010). Good policies have the following characteristics (Ivancevich, Donnelly, and Gibson 1989):

◆ They have been thoroughly discussed in advance and are consistent with primary and secondary objectives.

◆ They are flexible, so managers can apply them to normal and abnormal circumstances.[2]

◆ They are communicated, understood, and accepted by subordinates. For subordinates to accept the policy, they must view it as reasonable, legitimate, and fair. Subordinates will resist or ignore policies that appear to show favoritism to selected groups or appear to be arbitrary and have no clear purpose. Policy statements should therefore be in writing and should start with a clear statement of purpose or intent.

◆ Policies are consistent with each other. Inconsistency between policies or in the application and enforcement of policies will hurt subordinates' morale and will likely detract from accomplishing objectives. Inconsistencies frequently occur in the enforcement of organizational policies between departments, and they can have dire consequences.[3]

◆ Policies are continuously reevaluated and changed if necessary.

STEP 11: DEVELOP PROCEDURES

The eleventh step in the planning process and the third step in the operational planning process is for department managers and supervisors to develop procedures, which are guides to action. Procedures are derived from policies, but they are considerably more specific. Procedures identify in a step-by-step fashion how to accomplish the policy. Good procedures are the result of a detailed analysis of how best to accomplish the intent of the policy. Good procedures provide the manager or supervisor with a consistent and uniform performance appraisal.

STEP 12: DEVELOP METHODS

The twelfth step in the planning process and the fourth step in the operational planning process is for department managers and supervisors to develop methods to accomplish the procedures (methods are detailed, uniform actions with specific instructions and predictable outcomes).

STEP 13: DEVELOP RULES

The thirteenth step in the planning process and the fifth step in the operational planning process is for department managers to develop rules, which are statements that either require or forbid an action or inaction. The manager or supervisor has some flexibility in the application and enforcement of policies, procedures, and methods, but not rules. Good rules are those that everyone sees as clearly necessary for the proper order and functioning of the department.

EVALUATING PLAN PERFORMANCE

The governing body of the organization should review the strategic plan on an annual basis and evaluate the CEO based on progress in accomplishing primary objectives. Likewise, executive management should review the operating plan, probably on a monthly or quarterly basis. It should also evaluate department managers on the basis of their progress in accomplishing secondary objectives and compliance with policies, procedures, methods, and rules. The Joint Commission requires that hospitals have a planned, systematic, hospital-wide approach to process design and performance measurement, assessment, and improvement. The relevant standard requires leaders to "establish priorities for performance improvement" (Joint Commission 2013):

1. Leaders set priorities for performance improvement activities and patient health outcomes.

2. Leaders give priority to high-volume, high-risk, or problem-prone processes for performance improvement activities.

3. Leaders prioritize performance improvement activities in response to changes in the internal or external environment.

Budgeting, the next step in the corporate planning process, begins once the strategic and operating plans have been approved; budgeting consists of converting the operating plan into monetary terms.

CHAPTER KEY POINTS

➤ Planning is the process of deciding in advance what must be done in the future.

➤ Planning can be classified several different ways: by planning horizon, by management approach, and by design characteristics.

➤ Corporate planning has replaced facility planning for most healthcare organizations.

➤ Corporate planning consists of four major stages: strategic planning, operational planning, budgeting, and capital budgeting.

➤ Strategic planning looks three to ten years into the future and consists of several sequential steps: validating the mission and strategic interpretations; assessing the external environment; assessing the internal environment; formulating the vision; establishing strategic thrusts; identifying critical success factors; developing core objectives; and developing a strategic financial plan.

➤ The value of strategic planning lies in its systematic approach in dealing with an uncertain future.

➤ Operational planning is the process of translating the strategic plan into next year's objectives and consists of several sequential steps: developing secondary, or department, objectives; developing policies; developing procedures; developing methods; and developing rules.

➤ The governing body of the healthcare organization is responsible for evaluating the progress of the strategic plan; the executive management of the healthcare organization is responsible for evaluating the progress of the operating plan.

DISCUSSION QUESTIONS

1. What is the definition of planning? Of strategic planning? Of operational planning?

2. What are the different ways to classify planning?

3. Explain the different management approaches to planning.

4. Identify in order and explain each step in the strategic planning process.

5. Identify in order and explain each step in the operational planning process.

6. What is the value of strategic planning? Imagine what organizations look like that do not engage in meaningful strategic planning.

7. Who is responsible for evaluating the progress of the strategic plan and the operational plan?

NOTES

1. Strategic planning for the organization is the responsibility of the governing board, who often contracts the preparation of the plan to outside consultants rather than organization employees. With a planning horizon of three to ten years, employees would be likely to produce plans with vested interests, rather than a clear picture of where the organization is going. For instance, how many employees would plan to diminish or eliminate their functions, even if that seemed like the right thing to do?

2. Managers must be cautious about indiscriminately granting exceptions to policy. Although a manager wants to treat subordinates and patients with mercy, the manager must also seek justice, or fair play. The following two questions may help managers resolve the frequently faced dilemma of mercy versus justice: Can the manager afford to grant everyone with similar extenuating circumstances an exception? How can the manager make sure that the other subordinates or patients know about the exception, are encouraged to apply for the exception if circumstances warrant, and are supportive of the manager's decision to grant the exception? (See Nowicki 1998.)

3. In *St. Mary's Honor Center v. Hicks* (1993), Melvin Hicks, a black prison guard, sued a Missouri prison for civil rights violations. Mr. Hicks, who had been fired for exceeding the prison's absenteeism policy, claimed other guards who were white had exceeded the absenteeism policy, but had been given exceptions. While Mr. Hicks lost in a 5 to 4 decision (the majority felt that Mr. Hicks had not proven intentional discrimination and the action could have been the result of poor management), the case had a chilling effect on the indiscriminate granting of policy exceptions.

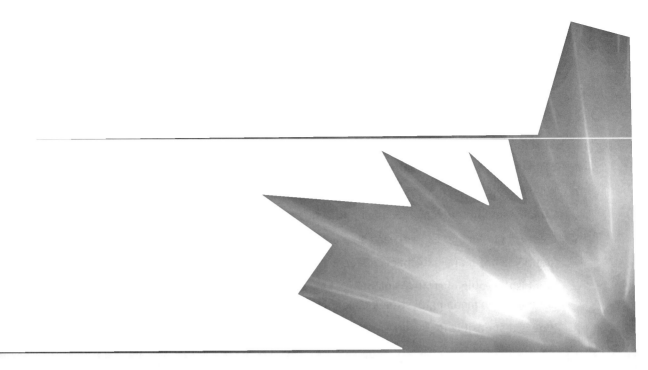

In healthcare today, a mission that focuses only on quality is only half a mission.

Richard L. Clarke, president of the Healthcare Financial
Management Association, 1986–2012

LEARNING OBJECTIVES

After completing this chapter, you should be able to do the following:

➤ Define and understand the importance of budgeting

➤ Identify the prerequisites to the budgeting process

➤ Explain the types of budgeting

INTRODUCTION

In *The Zero-Base Hospital*, Person emphasizes the need for budget skills for every management position in the healthcare organization:

> To function effectively in the healthcare industry in the foreseeable future, managers will need to develop specific financial skills. They will need to acquire an appreciation of volume, expense, and revenue relationships. They will need to become familiar with cost-containment strategies for their particular corner of the market. Most of all, they will need to cultivate an intimate knowledge of the details that define their operations and drive their costs, such as utilization statistics, seasonal trends, staffing models, productivity analysis, supply alternatives, inventory management, make/lease/buy options, physician practice patterns, and rate setting (Person 1997, 67).

In short, healthcare managers must learn how to budget. Considering that most managers in healthcare organizations are specialists in fields other than financial management, and that, as specialists, they have little or no formal education in budgeting, their records of accomplishment to date have been commendable. However, with healthcare costs and rapidly changing demographics at the center of public debate, and with prospective payment limiting the ability of organizations to "just raise rates" to cover expenses, tomorrow's healthcare managers clearly must do more work with fewer resources.

DEFINITION OF BUDGETING

Budgeting is the process of converting the operating plan into monetary terms. In addition to converting the operating plan into monetary terms for planning purposes, budgets are an important way for managers to exert the control function. Budgets become a control standard against which superiors can easily measure the performance of subordinates. Budgeting is also an excellent opportunity for the financial staff to educate the nonfinancial department managers about the relationship of revenues, expenses, and capital expenditures to the overall financial well-being of the organization.

Sequentially, budgeting occurs after the steps in operational planning have been completed. Budget information therefore does not bias operating information, especially in not-for-profit healthcare organizations. Department managers should prioritize objectives in the operating plan based on community need, not organizational profitability.

PREREQUISITES TO BUDGETING

Before effective budgeting can begin, the organization must meet several prerequisite requirements, the first four of which were introduced in Chapter 11 related to planning (Berman, Kukla, and Weeks 1994; Herkimer 1988):

1. A sound organizational structure that ensures management accountability for the budgeting process

2. A well-defined chart of accounts that corresponds with the organizational structure

3. Prompt and accurate accounting systems that ensure financial responsibility for the budgeting process

4. A comprehensive management information system that captures nonfinancial information for each department

5. A budget director who is responsible for coordinating the budget process and who serves as chair of the budget committee

6. A budget committee that is responsible for establishing a budget manual and a budget calendar and assisting department managers to develop their department budgets. Budget committees usually consist of senior managers who represent the department managers in their divisions.

7. A budget manual that includes necessary strategic planning information; the organizational structure; the chart of accounts; a list of budget committee members who can assist department managers; budget forms and instructions; budget assumptions regarding items such as anticipated growth, inflation, and employee raises; and a budget calendar with important completion dates

8. The previous year's data regarding volumes, revenues, and expenses

TYPES OF BUDGETS

Budgeting can be classified by management approach and design characteristics. Many of these classifications also apply to planning and were introduced in Chapter 11.

MANAGEMENT APPROACH

Budgets can be classified by management approach, either with top-down or bottom-up budgeting. In top-down budgeting, as in top-down planning, senior management develops the budget with little or no input from department managers. The advantage of this design is that senior management may be in the best position to objectively view the future; the disadvantage is that budget implementation may be difficult if subordinates have little or no input.

In bottom-up budgeting, subordinates develop the budget and submit it to senior management for approval. The advantage to bottom-up budgeting, as with bottom-up planning, is the commitment to the budget by those who developed it. The disadvantage is that subordinates may not be in the best position to view the future.

In most cases, a combination of top-down and bottom-up designs is used—senior management decides on budget parameters and subordinates submit plans within those parameters.

DESIGN CHARACTERISTICS

Budgeting can also be classified by design characteristics; these characteristics also apply to the design characteristics of planning (see Chapter 11).

Incremental Versus Zero-Base Budgeting

Incremental budgeting requires budgeting only for changes such as new equipment, new positions, and new programs. **Incremental budgeting** assumes that all current operations, including positions and equipment, are essential to the continued mission of the organization and that all current operations are working at peak performance. The advantages of incremental budgeting are its ease, the minimal time commitment required to prepare the budget, and the support of a bigger organizational culture. The main disadvantage is the assumption that all current operations are essential in a healthcare environment that is changing rapidly.

Conversely, **zero-base budgeting** takes nothing for granted and requires rejustification for existing equipment, positions, and programs, as well as justification for new equipment, positions, and programs.[1] Therein lies the principal advantage of zero-base budgeting: In a rapidly changing environment where reimbursement is moving away from cost-based approaches and moving toward prospective payment per case or per enrollee, zero-base budgeting can eliminate unnecessary costs and improve margins. Disadvantages are numerous and include the large time commitment, employee fear and anxiety, and the administrative and communication requirements (Person 1997).

Comprehensive Versus Limited-in-Scope Budgeting

Comprehensive budgeting integrates all the budgets into one document. The advantage is the recognition that capital affects operations. The limited-in-scope approach segregates the budgets. Most organizations integrate the budgets at the executive management level of the organization, but the issue is at what level of the organization the budgets should be integrated. For instance, many healthcare organizations do not show department managers revenue information because they feel that the department managers will not understand the difference between billed revenue and collected revenue, or that the organization uses department revenue to cover expenses in departments that do not generate revenue.

incremental budgeting
Budgeting only for changes, such as new equipment. The assumption in incremental budgeting is that current budget is already optimal.

zero-base budgeting
Budgeting that requires all operations to be justified anew; nothing in the current budget is assumed to be already optimal.

Another reason department managers might not be shown revenue information is because department managers cannot effect changes in revenue, which is a function of volumes ordered by the physicians multiplied by rates set by the chief financial officer. A similar case can be made regarding whether department managers should be shown indirect expenses.

Fixed Versus Flexible Budgeting

Fixed budgets assume that volumes, related revenues, and variable expenses remain constant during the year. Fixed budgets are easy to project, but they are unrealistic for healthcare organizations whose volumes fluctuate during the year and whose variable expenses, which are dependent on volumes, account for more than half of an organization's operating expenses.

Flexible budgets take into account fluctuations in volumes, at least within ranges expressed as probabilities, and adjust variable expenses accordingly.

Discrete Versus Continuous Budgeting

Like discrete plans (discussed in Chapter 11), discrete budgets apply to a fixed period of time, usually a year. At the end of the year, a new budget begins. Discrete budgets are relatively easy to prepare, but budgeting in 12-month increments can be difficult because circumstances often change. Furthermore, discrete budgets can be challenging to some managers who know that if they are efficient and spend less than originally budgeted, they may receive less money in the following year's budget.

Continuous budgets, sometimes called rolling budgets, are updated continuously so that year end never occurs. Department managers who manage wisely roll over their efforts to the next month.[2]

STEPS IN THE BUDGETING PROCESS

The budgeting process is an extension of the planning process discussed in Chapter 11.

STEP 14: PROJECT VOLUMES

The fourteenth step in the planning process and the first step in the budgeting process is to project volumes for the budget year. This step is often called the statistical budget, and it is sometimes part of the operating plan. Typically, the budget committee will give its projections of the organization's production units to department managers in the budget manual. Department managers use the organization's production units to calculate department production units that are specific to each department. For instance, the radiology department manager must be able to determine how many radiology procedures are generated for every 100 admissions.

Production units are the best measures of what an entity is producing. For example, hospitals produce patient days and admissions (both of which are called production units), but neither reflects severity of illness or the volume of outpatient work produced by the hospital. The unit used to show severity of illness, a factor that affects resource consumption, will vary—many hospitals have adopted diagnosis-related groups (DRGs) or another severity index.[3] Regarding the volume of outpatient work produced by the hospital, either outpatient work needs to be captured separately as outpatient visits and with the related revenues and expenses, or the inpatient production unit must be adjusted to reflect outpatient work produced.[4] Regardless of which production units are chosen by the organization, the units must be reported by payer to project both gross and net revenues by payer.

Each department should have a production unit that best measures what the department is producing. Radiology, for example, produces radiology procedures. However, this production unit, like patient days for the hospital, does not reflect the complexity of the procedure and the related resource consumption.[5] To show complexity of the procedure, most departments have developed a relative value unit (RVU) that reflects relative complexity and related resource consumption (refer to Chapter 7 for information on developing RVUs). If the hospital can tell the radiology department manager how many of each DRG they are projecting, the radiology manager should be able to project the number and type of procedures. In addition to serving as a basis for projecting volumes for budgeting purposes, department production units are used (Herkimer 1988b)

◆ to measure and evaluate department productivity,

◆ to measure and evaluate employee productivity,

◆ to serve as the basis for calculating the cost of each procedure (see Chapter 6),

◆ to serve as the basis for calculating the charge for each procedure, and

◆ to serve as the basis for determining staffing requirements and staffing schedules.

To project future volumes under conditions of uncertainty, most managers rely on forecasting, which is the process to determine what alternative scenarios are likely to occur in the future, given what managers know about the past and present. To forecast, the manager must first prepare the forecast content, which is a description of the specific situation in question. Next, the manager must prepare the forecast rationale, which is an explanation of how the situation will evolve from its current state to its forecasted state (Reeves, Bergwall, and Woodside 1979).

In preparing the forecast content, the manager first identifies content items, which are descriptions of important occurrences, such as admissions, patient days, and outpatient visits. Next, the manager must measure the current status of content items. The final step

production units
The best measures of what an entity is producing. For example, patient days and admissions are both considered production units for a hospital.

of the forecast content is to identify the expected state of the content items in the future budget period. Although forecast content often produces quantifiable data, the manager also must consider the effect of the following subjective factors on the forecast content (Reeves, Bergwall, and Woodside 1979):

- Political factors

- Social factors

- Economic factors

- Technologic factors

- Personal health factors

- Environmental health factors

A manager may use several different forecasting techniques to prepare the forecast content, including the use of experts, causal models, and time-series methods.

The use of experts depends on the manager's ability to identify and secure the services of appropriate experts. Then, she must consider the advantages and disadvantages of using experts in preparing the forecast. Using experts is usually quick and relatively inexpensive. However, different experts may develop different, yet valid, opinions about the future. Which expert is correct? To address this disadvantage, managers can choose a variety of models to obtain their opinion (Reeves, Bergwall, and Woodside 1979):

- A task force brings together several experts who provide collective input.

- The Delphi technique gathers information from a group of dispersed experts with anonymity and limited interaction.

- The Delbecq technique, or nominal group process, is similar to the Delphi technique, except that the group of experts meets face to face for discussion and to present and defend their forecasts.

- Questionnaires are used to gather responses to questions from a large group of experts.

- Permanent panels maintain a group of experts who can be used for several forecasts over time.

- Essay writing obtains opinions from experts in a format that can be used for preparing the forecast rationale.

- Computer-facilitated group processes can reveal and "parallel process" more contributions from a greater number of participants than is possible using manual facilitation techniques alone.

In addition to relying on expert opinion regarding the future, a manager may apply probability statistics to the expert opinion. Another derivative of using expert opinion is the program evaluation and review technique (PERT). This technique requires estimates of optimistic (O), pessimistic (P), and most likely (ML) future scenarios. These three estimates are weighted to calculate an expected value that equals

$$\frac{(O + P + 4ML)}{6}$$

The manager may use causal models when the forecast variable is dependent on a causal, or independent, variable. The most common statistical method used in causal models is regression analysis. Regression analysis mathematically describes an average relationship between a forecast variable and one or more causal variables. For instance, the manager can use a regression line based on past volumes over time to predict future volumes. Problem 12.1 demonstrates the use of regression lines.

The coefficient of determination, symbolized by R^2, indicates the proportion of the variance of the forecast variable that is explained by the regression statistic. When given a choice between two or more regression statistics, the manager should select the statistic that maximizes the coefficients of determination. The causal variables in regression may include time, leading economic indicators, demographic factors, or any other variables that might exhibit a causal relationship with the forecast variable.

A measure of the statistical contribution of a causal variable to regression's causal power is the beta coefficient, which indicates the relative importance of each of the causal variables in explaining or predicting changes in the forecast variable. In multiple regression, the manager can use beta coefficients to decide which causal variables to retain and

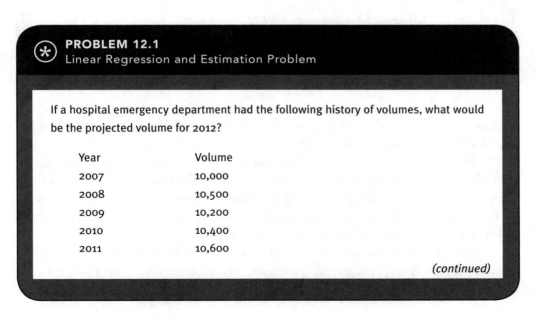

PROBLEM 12.1
Linear Regression and Estimation Problem

If a hospital emergency department had the following history of volumes, what would be the projected volume for 2012?

Year	Volume
2007	10,000
2008	10,500
2009	10,200
2010	10,400
2011	10,600

(continued)

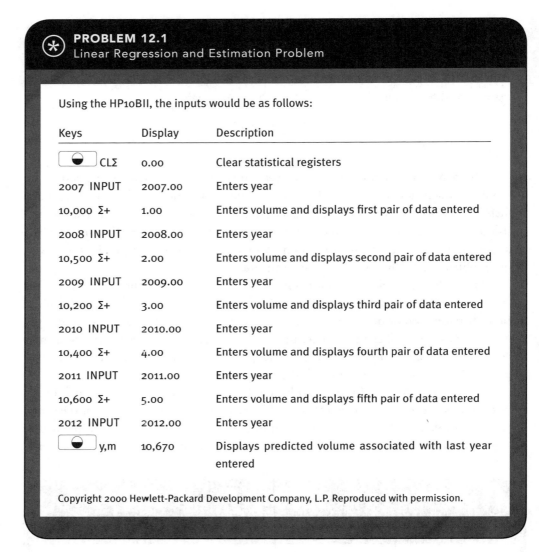

PROBLEM 12.1
Linear Regression and Estimation Problem

Using the HP10BII, the inputs would be as follows:

Keys	Display	Description
⬤ CLΣ	0.00	Clear statistical registers
2007 INPUT	2007.00	Enters year
10,000 Σ+	1.00	Enters volume and displays first pair of data entered
2008 INPUT	2008.00	Enters year
10,500 Σ+	2.00	Enters volume and displays second pair of data entered
2009 INPUT	2009.00	Enters year
10,200 Σ+	3.00	Enters volume and displays third pair of data entered
2010 INPUT	2010.00	Enters year
10,400 Σ+	4.00	Enters volume and displays fourth pair of data entered
2011 INPUT	2011.00	Enters year
10,600 Σ+	5.00	Enters volume and displays fifth pair of data entered
2012 INPUT	2012.00	Enters year
⬤ y,m	10,670	Displays predicted volume associated with last year entered

which to exclude. The manager should be cautioned regarding one flaw in multiple regression: multicollinearity, which is the phenomenon that occurs when causal variables relate to each other in addition to the relationship to the forecast variable.[6]

The manager may use time-series methods when the past behavior of a variable is available to predict the future behavior of the variable. Time-series methods do little to account for causal relationships; rather, they attempt to identify historic patterns that are likely to be repeated in the future. The manager may use regression for long-term forecasts and time-series methods for forecasts of less than one year.

Many series of data collected over time will exhibit trend, seasonal, cyclical, and random patterns. A trend pattern exists when the value of the variable consistently increases or decreases over time. A seasonal pattern exists when the value of the variable fluctuates according to a seasonal influence, such as hour of the day, day of the week, week of the month, or month of the year. A cyclical pattern is similar to a seasonal pattern; however, the length of each cycle is longer than one year and cycles vary in length. Horizontal patterns exist when the variable's value does not change over time. Random patterns exist when the variable's value changes, but in no predictable way (Bittel and Bittel 1978).

> You are the new chief executive officer at Memorial Hospital. Memorial is a nonprofit hospital with 300 beds and is located in a busy metropolitan area directly adjacent to a large university. Memorial is the only hospital within a 20-mile radius of campus, but construction on a new, competing hospital has just started within five miles. Identify three forecast content items. How will they be measured and what is the expected status of the content items in the future? Which forecasting techniques should you use? Why?

After preparing the forecast content, the manager must prepare the forecast rationale, which is an explanation of how the situation will evolve from its current state to its forecasted state. The forecast rationale clarifies the result of the forecasting process, provides a basis for evaluating the forecasting process, and provides a basis from which future forecasts can be made (Reeves, Bergwall, and Woodside 1979).

STEP 15: CONVERT VOLUMES INTO REVENUES

The fifteenth step in the planning process and the second step in the budgeting process is to convert volumes into patient revenues. Managers must consider whether the organization should budget revenues before or after the expense budget is completed. Historically, healthcare organizations have determined their expense budgets first and then set rates in their revenue budgets to cover the expenses, which is called **cost-led pricing**. However, healthcare organizations that are facing increasing proportions of fixed payment arrangements, such as prospective payment and premium payment (which essentially dictate the rate to the organization) may decide to calculate revenue first, which is called **price-led costing**. The organization then must adjust expenses to match the projected patient revenues.

> **cost-led pricing**
> Setting prices after costs have been projected.

To project gross patient services revenues, projected production units are classified by payer and then multiplied by the projected charge that, at this point, usually includes a projected increase. Next, net patient services revenue is determined by deducting contractual allowances and charity care allowances and bad debt, if the organization recognizes significant portions of patient revenues at the time of service, even though the organization does not assess the patient's ability to pay at time of service. To project total revenues from operations, net patient services revenue is added to premium revenue, other revenue (e.g., parking, catering), and net assets released from restrictions and used for operations. Other projected changes in net assets that would be reported at the bottom of the statement of operations may also be available for operations (see Statement of Operations in Chapter 14).

> **price-led costing**
> Reducing costs after prices, or effective prices meaning collections, have been determined by the payers.

STEP 16: CONVERT VOLUMES INTO EXPENSE REQUIREMENTS

The sixteenth step in the planning process and the third step in the budgeting process is to convert volumes into expense requirements: labor expense with benefits, nonlabor expense, and overhead expense. Department managers should have budget histories that indicate labor expense with benefits per production unit. They should also have budget histories for nonlabor expense per production unit, which includes supplies, travel, and repairs. The budget director should have budget histories for overhead expense for the organization.

Department managers should review the labor expense with benefits per production unit to determine if they can reduce expenses. Senior management determines the benefits package (approximately 32 percent of wages for a full-time employee),[7] but department managers can reduce benefit expenses by using part-time and temporary workers. Part-time employees usually receive benefits in proportion to the number of hours worked (approximately 16 percent of wages for a half-time employee), and temporary workers usually receive only the benefits required by law (approximately 12 percent of wages). Department managers must decide on the appropriate mix of full-time, part-time, and temporary workers. Part-time and temporary workers are less expensive to the department manager, but continuity of patient care may suffer if the manager uses too many part-time and temporary workers. Many department managers staff their minimum needs with full-time workers, moderate needs with part-time workers, and maximum needs with temporary workers (see Exhibit 12.1).

Staffing mix is the mix of full-time, part-time, and temporary workers and should be reviewed by the department manager; department **skill mix**, which is the mix of skilled positions, should also be reviewed by managers. Most departments have a variety of tasks requiring a variety of skills performed by a variety of positions paid a variety of wages. The department manager's job is to match the tasks to the positions in the most cost-effective manner possible.

staffing mix
The mix of full-time, part-time, and temporary employees in a department.

skill mix
The mix of different skilled positions in a department.

EXHIBIT 12.1
Staffing Mix

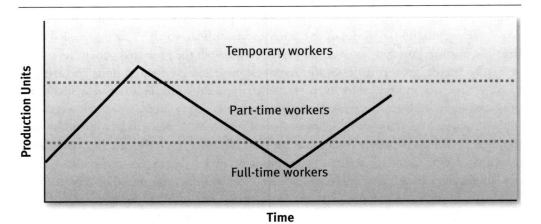

After the department managers have reviewed staffing mix and skill mix and have made any necessary changes, they must consider the effect of employee raises on their expense budget. The budget committee should provide department managers with information regarding cost-of-living raises, merit raises, and bonuses. Cost-of-living raises are designed to protect employees from inflation. The use of these raises is declining because inflation has been low and employee spending is not all inflation prone. However, if the organization uses a cost-of-living raise, the raise is administered to all employees at the same time. The effect of cost-of-living raises on the department budget depends on the effective date of the raise. For instance, if the effective date is the first day of the new budget year, the department budget will realize the full effect of the raise. If the effective date of the raise is three months into the new budget year, the department will realize 75 percent of the effect of the raise.

Merit raises are designed to motivate employees toward, and reward employees for, meritorious performance. Merit raises as a motivator are dependent on the amount of the raise and the likelihood that superiors will judge performance meritorious. Merit raises are expensive for organizations because the amount of the raise is built into the employee's base pay for future years.

Organizations typically give merit raises in conjunction with employee performance appraisals on employment anniversaries. Assuming that employment anniversaries occur in equal distribution throughout the year, the effect on the department budget will be 50 percent of the total amount for merit raises, and the budget should be adjusted accordingly. For instance, if the department manager can give 7 percent raises to meritorious employees on their employment anniversaries, and all the department's employees are meritorious, the annual effect on the department will be 3.5 percent, assuming that 50 percent of the employment anniversaries are in the first half of the budget year and 50 percent of the employment anniversaries are in the second half of the budget year.

Bonuses are designed to motivate employees in much the same way as merit raises. However, using bonuses as a motivator is dependent on the amount of the bonus, the likelihood that superiors will judge performance bonus-worthy, and the proportion of employees receiving the bonus. For instance, if all employees receive bonuses, motivation resulting from the bonus will be low because everyone receives a bonus. If 1 out of 100 employees receives a bonus, motivation will be low because the chance of being rewarded for bonus-worthy performance is low. However, if one out of seven employees receives a bonus, motivation as a result of the bonus will be maximized because the chances of receiving a bonus are realistic. Organizations typically award bonuses at the end of the budget year, and the funds come from the organization, not the department; budgeting the effect of bonuses, therefore, is relatively easy.

After budgeted department wages have been adjusted for changes in staffing mix, skill mix, and employee raises, department managers multiply the budgeted wages and benefits per production unit by the number of production units projected for the budget year to determine the total budgeted wages and benefits for the department.

Department managers should have budget histories that indicate nonlabor expense per production unit and should review those figures to determine if they can reduce expenses. Managers should review supply use to ensure that generic supplies are used whenever possible. The pharmacy manager should provide information on the use of generic medicines and work with the pharmacy committee to maintain a formulary with as many generics and as few brand-name pharmaceuticals as possible. The pharmacy manager should also establish security measures to ensure that narcotics are secure. Department managers should review travel expenses and bring training programs to the organization whenever possible to reduce travel expense. Department managers should review repair expense and maintenance agreements, and replace equipment when feasible. The manager of materials management should provide department managers with an estimate of anticipated cost increases in supplies, repairs, and travel as a result of contract renewals or inflation. After department managers have reduced nonlabor expense wherever possible, department managers multiply the nonlabor expense per production unit by the number of production units projected for the budget year to determine the total budgeted nonlabor expense for the department.

Largely, overhead expenses for the organization, such as depreciation, heating and cooling, insurance premiums, and so on, do not fluctuate with production units. Therefore, the budget committee determines the overhead expenses for the budget year after reviewing historic data to determine if adjustments are necessary.

STEP 17: ADJUST REVENUES AND EXPENSES AS NECESSARY

The seventeenth step in the planning process and the fourth step in the budgeting process is for the budget committee to determine if budgeted net revenues are adequate to cover budgeted expenses. If budgeted expenses exceed budgeted net revenues, the budget committee may recommend to executive management ways to generate additional revenues or ways to reduce expenses. To cover the budget shortfall, executive management must decide whether to generate additional revenues and consider the possible effect of such action on expenses; whether to reduce expenses and consider the possible effect on quality and patient access; or whether to release funds from unrestricted net asset accounts to cover the loss.

EVALUATING BUDGET PERFORMANCE

The governing body of the organization should review the budget annually and evaluate the CEO on the basis of organizational compliance to the budget. Likewise, the CEO should review senior management quarterly and evaluate senior managers based on divisional compliance to budget. Senior management should review department managers monthly and evaluate departmental compliance to budget.

The most common method of evaluating budget performance is **variance analysis**, which compares budgeted production units, revenues, and expenses to actual production units, revenues, and expenses, typically monthly. Labor variance analysis, including hours and expense, may be completed every two weeks in conjunction with payroll. The variance is the amount of the difference between the actual and budgeted:

$$\text{Variance} = \text{Actual} - \text{Budgeted}$$

For production units and revenue, positive variances are favorable and negative variances are unfavorable:

$$\text{Revenue variance} = \text{Actual revenue} - \text{Budgeted revenue}$$

For expenses, negative variances are favorable and positive variances are unfavorable:

$$\text{Expense variance} = \text{Actual expense} - \text{Budgeted expense}$$

Variance analysis ensures accountability by requiring managers responsible for the variances to explain why the variances occurred and what actions are being taken to ensure that favorable variances reoccur and negative variances do not reoccur.

Once the budget has been reviewed and approved, the healthcare organization can begin the capital budgeting process. Problem 12.2 demonstrates the budgeting steps in a radiology department.

> **variance analysis**
> An examination of the differences (variances) between budgeted and actual amounts; variance analysis requires managers to explain why budgeted and actual amounts do not match.

(✳) PROBLEM 12.2
Budgeting Exercise

The radiology department is developing a budget for DRG 250: Fracture, Sprain, Strain, and Dislocation of Forearm, Hand, and Foot. This year the department saw 1,100 admissions for DRG 250 analyzed in the following way: 50 percent of the admissions were for a hand X-ray (which takes 5 minutes), 20 percent for a foot X-ray (which takes 15 minutes), and 30 percent for a forearm X-ray (which takes 30 minutes). The budget committee is projecting a 9.1 percent increase in DRG 250 for next year analyzed in the same proportions. The controller states that the charges for a hand X-ray will be $75, for a foot X-ray will be $285, and for a forearm X-ray will be $450. The controller also projects the payer analysis for DRG 250 to be 45 percent Medicare (DRG rate is 80 percent of charges), 35 percent Medicaid (DRG rate is 85 percent of charges), 15 percent managed

(continued)

care (discount is 30 percent of charges), and 5 percent self-pay (self-pay patients pay full charges, but 10 percent of self-pay patients don't pay their bills and their fees are recorded as charity care).

DRG 250 accounts for 25 percent of the radiology department's labor, supply, and overhead expenses. The department's labor expenses are $225,000—labor expenses are expected to increase 5 percent next year due to raises. The department's nonlabor expenses are $185,000—nonlabor expenses are expected to increase 6 percent next year due to inflation. The department's overhead expenses are $375,000—overhead expenses are not expected to increase next year. Using the budgeting steps, calculate the volumes, collected revenues, expenses, and adjustments for DRG 250 in the radiology department.

Step 13: Project Volumes

1. Calculate the current volume for each X-ray procedure.

Procedure	Admissions	Volume
Hand X-ray	1,100 X .50	550
Foot X-ray	1,100 X .20	220
Forearm X-ray	1,100 X .30	330

2. Convert the current volumes to RVUs

Procedure	Minutes	Minutes/ * GCD	RVUs/ Procedure	Volume	Total RVUs
Hand X-ray	5	5/5	1	550	550
Foot X-ray	15	15/5	3	220	660
Forearm X-ray	30	30/5	6	330	1,980
					3,190

* GCD = greatest common denominator

3. Calculate the projected volume for each X-ray procedure (1,100 DRG 250 x 1.091 increase = 1,200 DRG 250)

Procedure	Admissions	Volume
Hand X-ray	1,200 X .50	600
Foot X-ray	1,200 X .20	240
Forearm X-ray	1,200 X .30	360

(continued)

PROBLEM 12.2
Budgeting Exercise

4. Convert the projected volumes to RVUs

Procedure	Minutes	Minutes/ GCD	RVUs/ Procedure	Volume	Total RVUs
Hand X-ray	5	5/5	1	600	600
Foot X-ray	15	15/5	3	240	720
Forearm X-ray	30	30/5	6	360	2,160
					3,480

Step 14: Convert Projected Volumes into Projected Revenues

1. Calculate projected gross and net revenues by payer

Medicare

Procedure	Projected Charge	Projected Volume	%	Gross Revenue	Rate	Net Revenue
Hand X-ray	$75	600	.45	$20,250	.80	$16,200
Foot X-ray	285	240	.45	30,780	.80	24,624
Forearm X-ray	450	360	.45	72,900	.80	58,320
				$123,930		$99,144

Medicaid

Procedure	Projected Charge	Projected Volume	%	Gross Revenue	Rate	Net Revenue
Hand X-ray	$75	600	.35	$15,750	.85	$13,388
Foot X-ray	285	240	.35	23,940	.85	20,349
Forearm X-ray	450	360	.35	56,700	.85	48,195
				$96,390		$81,932

Procedure	Projected Charge	Projected Volume	%	Gross Revenue	Rate	Net Revenue

Managed Care

Procedure	Projected Charge	Projected Volume	%	Gross Revenue	Rate	Net Revenue
Hand X-ray	$75	600	.15	$6,750	.70	$4,725
Foot X-ray	285	240	.15	10,260	.70	7,182
Forearm X-ray	450	360	.15	24,300	.70	17,010
				$41,310		$28,917

(continued)

PROBLEM 12.2
Budgeting Exercise

Self-Pay

Hand X-ray	$75	600	.05	$2,250	.90	$2,025
Foot X-ray	285	240	.05	3,420	.90	3,078
Forearm X-ray	450	360	.05	8,100	.90	7,290
				$13,770		$12,393
Total				$275,400		$222,386

Step 15: Convert Projected Volumes into Projected Expenses

1. Calculate current expenses per RVU

    $225,000 x .25 = 56,250 / 3,190 = 17.63 labor expense/RVU

    185,000 x .25 = 46,250 / 3,190 = 14.50 supply expense/RVU

    375,000 x .25 = 93,750 / 3,190 = 29.39 overhead expense/RVU

2. Calculate projected expenses per RVU

Projected labor expense	= 17.63 + 5%	=	18.51
Projected supply expense	= 14.50 + 6%	=	15.37
Projected overhead expense	= 29.39 + 0%	=	29.39
Total			$63.27

3. Calculate projected expenses per procedure

Procedure	Projected RVUs	Projected Expense/RVU	Total Projected Expense
Hand X-ray	600	$63.27	$37,962
Foot X-ray	720	63.27	45,554
Forearm X-ray	2,160	63.27	136,663
Total			$220,179

Step 16: Adjust Revenues and Expenses as Necessary

1. Determine initial gain/loss

Net Revenues	$222,386
Expenses	220,179
Gain/(Loss)	$2,207

(continued)

PROBLEM 12.2
Budgeting Exercise

2. If the initial determination is a loss, first investigate whether collected revenues can be increased through a rate increase or improvements in collection efforts. If collected revenues cannot be increased, investigate whether expenses can be reduced. Usually this involves investigating variable labor expenses and reviewing the mix of full-time to part-time to temporary as well as a review of skill mix. If collected revenues cannot be increased and expenses cannot be decreased, then management must decide whether to continue the service at a loss and how that loss is going to be covered by other profitable services.

Source: Neil Dworkin, PhD, Emeritus Associate Professor of Management, Western Connecticut State University. Used with permission.

CHAPTER KEY POINTS

➤ Budgeting is the process of converting the operating plan into monetary terms.

➤ Certain prerequisites need to be in place before budgeting can begin.

➤ Budgeting consists of several sequential steps: projecting volumes, converting volumes to revenues, converting volumes into expense requirements, and adjusting revenues and expenses as necessary.

➤ The governing body should review the budget annually, and each management level in the organization should be evaluated based on its performance to budget.

DISCUSSION QUESTIONS

1. What is the definition of budgeting?

2. What are the different ways to classify budgeting?

3. Explain the different management approaches to budgeting.

4. Identify in order and explain each step in the budgeting process.

5. Who is responsible for evaluating budget performance?

NOTES

1. For a compelling argument for zero-base planning, see Person's (1997) *The Zero-Base Hospital: Survival and Success in America's Evolving Healthcare System*. Person also provides a historic perspective by identifying the US Department of Agriculture as the first zero-base planner in 1964. Zero-base planning was abandoned at the Department of Agriculture, but it was successfully adopted at Texas Instruments in the late 1960s, as related by Pyhrr (1970). During the 1970s and 1980s, zero-base planning was used by a variety of organizations with a variety of success. Hospitals, according to Person, did not adopt it because of the financial security provided by retrospective, cost-based reimbursement.

2. Continuous budgets avoid the year-end "sucking sound"—the sound of year-end unnecessary spending of budgeted but not-yet-spent funds—that occurs in organizations using discrete budgeting.

3. DRGs measure severity of illness between DRGs, but they do not measure severity of illness within the same DRG. Eastaugh (1987, 1992) discusses several severity of illness (SOI) indices that do measure how ill a patient is within a specific DRG or condition: Horn's SOI index, Horn's computerized severity index, Western Pennsylvania Blue Cross patient management categories, and Brewster's MEDISGRPS.

4. As discussed in Appendix 1.3 after Chapter 1, adjusted patient days is used to reflect outpatient production with the following formula:

$$\text{Inpatient days} + \text{Outpatient visits} \times \frac{\text{Outpatient revenue per visit}}{\text{Inpatient revenue per day}}$$

5. Even after adopting an RVU schedule for the production unit, most departments maintain a procedure count as a basis for auditing charges (each procedure should generate a charge).

6. Multicollinearity was one of the weaknesses of the Herzlinger and Krasker (1987) study on for-profit hospitals, which is referenced in Chapter 3. Arrington and Haddock (1990) used discriminate analysis to avoid the multicollinearity problem in their follow-up study, which is also referenced in Chapter 3.

7. Benefits include not only payroll taxes and retirement and health insurance, but also sick leave (approximately 96 hours, depending on the organization's policy), holiday leave (approximately 84 hours), and vacation (approximately 80 hours). Full-time employees are paid for 2,080 hours per year (52 x 40), but are scheduled (or work, depending on the definition) approximately 1,820 per year.

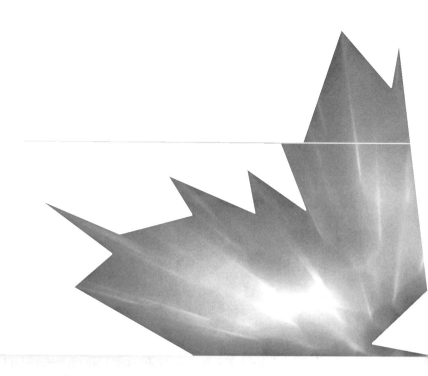

We live in a world of limited financial resources, so we have to make guns-versus-butter decisions all the time: capital decisions about whether we invest in x, y, or z or make cost reductions as we go through the budgeting process.

Joseph J. Filer, FHFMA, CPA, president and CEO,
Healthcare Financial Management Association

LEARNING OBJECTIVES

After completing this chapter, you should be able to

➤ Define and understand the importance of capital budgeting

➤ Explain the types of capital budgets

➤ List in order and explain each step in the capital budgeting process

➤ Describe the methods used to finance capital expenditures

➤ Discuss the methods used to evaluate the capital budgeting process

INTRODUCTION

Capital costs, which are generally defined as purchases of land, buildings, and equipment (see a more complete definition later in this chapter), are a relatively small percentage of total organization costs—in hospitals, they are 6 to 10 percent. However, their importance in terms of rising healthcare costs and dictating current trends in acquisitions, mergers, joint ventures, and closings cannot be overstated. Under cost-based reimbursement from 1966 to 1983 (cost-based reimbursement continued for capital costs until 1990), capital costs for new equipment (38 to 40 percent of capital costs) and plants exploded with little resistance from regulation or the market.

Two programs were enacted in 1974 in attempts to slow the growth in healthcare capital costs. Certificate-of-need legislation (PL 93-641 as the National Health Planning and Resources Development Act of 1974) and Section 1122 of the Social Security Amendments of 1974 both compelled hospitals to get permission from a government entity before major capital expenditures. However, these programs did little to slow capital growth (Eastaugh 1987).

The Social Security Amendments of 1983 introduced Medicare prospective payment, which was designed to slow Medicare costs by reimbursing hospitals and other healthcare providers on the basis of predetermined payments rather than reimbursing costs after the fact. However, those amendments did not affect capital costs, because until 1992 capital costs were reimbursed on the basis of cost, which meant that if Medicare approved a capital expenditure, it would pay its portion of the expenditure whether the piece of equipment was used or not. For example, if Medicare normally covered 30 percent of a hospital's costs and the hospital acquired a new X-ray machine, Medicare would pay for 30 percent of that X-ray machine even if it were never used.

Finally, in the mid-1980s to early 1990s, government efforts to slow capital costs paid off. The Tax Reform Act of 1986 lowered the tax deductibility for charitable gifts and restricted or increased the cost of acquiring capital through tax-exempt bond markets. The Omnibus Budget Reconciliation Act (OBRA) of 1990 moved capital costs to prospective payment over a ten-year implementation period. These acts slowed capital growth markedly, causing one investment banker to comment (Eastaugh 1987, 600):

Starting in 1988 [1990] the typical hospital should be viewed as a more risky venture, and will pay higher interest rates unless they can demonstrate DRG [diagnosis-related group] profitability. Hospitals shall no longer have government as a 'Sugar Daddy' paying the interest on their debt coupon by coupon. One thousand hospitals may close. We view such hospitals as 'cross-eyed javelin throwers' in that they will not win any rewards, but they will keep the attention of their fearful audience.

The Balanced Budget Act of 1997 also had a stifling effect on the access to capital, as many hospitals were forced to use funds earmarked for capital projects to subsidize operations because of reduced reimbursements from Medicare. Reflecting this effect, bond downgrades outnumbered bond upgrades by rating agencies during this time until 2005, when reimbursement began improving. This effect inspired a series of studies published by the Healthcare Financial Management Association beginning in 2003 and ending in 2006. The studies found that larger hospitals, newer hospitals, and hospitals that belonged to systems had broader access to capital than other hospitals. The following strategies were recommended to compete for capital (HFMA 2004):

- Be distinctive.

- Hold onto physicians.

- Focus on core service lines.

- Improve quality of care.

- Protect profits.

- Integrate strategic and financial plans.

- Establish/fine-tune policies regarding charity care.

The studies went on to predict that the major trends to affect capital in healthcare organizations in the future would be competition, payment, and technology. To afford technology in the future, hospitals must have operating margins that exceed 2 percent, the studies stated.

DEFINITION OF CAPITAL EXPENDITURES

Capital expenditures are defined by an organization in its capital expenditures policy, and as a result, the definitions vary. Generally speaking, capital expenditures are purchases of land, buildings, and equipment used for operations; are not for resale; have a useful life of more than one year; cost $500 or more; and are subject to depreciation, with the exception of land, which is not depreciated unless the use of the land harms the future use of the land. Capital expenditures are classified into the following categories:

capital expenditures
Purchases of land, buildings, and equipment used for operations.

- Land, including all costs associated with acquiring land and making it ready for use (the cost of the land itself cannot be depreciated unless the use of the land harms the future use of the land)

- Land improvements, including all costs associated with sidewalks, parking lots, driveways, and fencing

- Buildings, including all costs associated with constructing or buying buildings

- Fixed equipment, including all costs associated with equipment that is permanently attached to the building, such as the plumbing system, furnace, and air conditioners

◆ Major movable equipment that has a useful life of three years or more and has a unit cost of $5,000 or more

◆ Major repairs that benefit future periods and/or extend the useful life of the building or equipment (ordinary repairs are expensed)

TYPES OF CAPITAL EXPENDITURE BUDGETS

Healthcare organizations typically divide capital expenditure budgets into two broad categories: replacement and new. Budgets for replacement capital expenditures include requests to replace existing buildings and equipment that are made for a number of reasons:

◆ Scheduled replacement at the end of the useful life or when fully depreciated[1]

◆ Improved productivity

◆ Improved quality

◆ Required by regulation

Budgets for new capital expenditures include requests to add buildings and equipment for a number of reasons:

◆ Expanded services

◆ Improved safety conditions

◆ Reduced operating expenses

◆ Improved patient care

STEPS IN THE CAPITAL BUDGETING PROCESS

The capital budgeting process is an extension of the budgeting process discussed in Chapter 12. The budgeting process must be concluded to determine funds available for capital expenditures.

STEP 18: IDENTIFY AND PRIORITIZE REQUESTS

The eighteenth step in the corporate planning process and the first step in the capital budgeting process is for the budget committee to identify and prioritize all capital requests. Typically, the budget committee asks department managers, including the chief of medical staff services (included with department managers in this chapter discussion), to list

> ⚠ **CRITICAL CONCEPTS**
> The Trustees' Responsibility
>
> Allen County Clinic has been growing rapidly in the past few years. Many of the patients they see are women needing prenatal care and screening. To meet these needs, Allen County Clinic would like to open a new women's health clinic.
>
> Name three steps Allen County Clinic needs to take to ensure this is a viable option. Besides building an addition to the clinic, what costs must be considered? What are some advantages and disadvantages of building a new clinic? What are some options for the clinic to fund for this new addition?

the capital equipment and buildings needed and to justify the resources needed. After the department managers have provided a list,[2] the budget committee prioritizes the list on the basis of community need and compliance with the strategic plan as initial criteria.[3]

STEP 19: PROJECT CASH FLOWS

The nineteenth step in the planning process and the second step in the capital budgeting process is for the department managers to project, and the budget committee to confirm, cash flows for each capital expenditure request. In cases of replacement equipment, this is a relatively easy step in that revenues (Volumes × Charge per procedure), expenses (Volumes × Expense per procedure), and resulting cash flow (Revenues − Expenses) already exist.[4] However, the department manager must indicate any changes in revenue or expenses that will occur with the replacement equipment.

For new equipment, or equipment that the organization has never had before, revenues and expenses may be difficult to project. The department manager can obtain volumes in a number of ways. First, if the organization is currently using an outside service that will be replaced by the new equipment, the department manager can obtain volumes from accounts payable. If the organization is not currently using an outside service, the department manager can administer a questionnaire to potential users or complete a medical record review to determine how many patients would have used the new equipment had it been available. For expensive equipment like computed tomographic scanners, manufacturers will assist in the medical record review; however, the department manager should review manufacturer projections carefully, because manufacturers have a vested interest and may over-project volumes. The department manager can obtain charge information from neighboring facilities or insurance companies. The department manager can also obtain expense information from neighboring facilities or the manufacturer. If he obtains the information from the manufacturer, it is a good idea to confirm it with other organizations that use the same equipment—manufacturers should be willing to provide client lists.

For equipment that does not generate revenue, department managers can still project cash flow by using salary savings, utility savings, and so on.

Previously incurred costs, or sunk costs, and costs that would be incurred regardless of the budget outcome should not be included in cash-flow projections.

STEP 20: PERFORM FINANCIAL ANALYSIS

The twentieth step in the planning process and the third step in the capital budgeting process is for the budget committee or the chief financial officer (CFO) to perform financial analyses on the requests. Before Medicare stopped reimbursing capital at cost, few healthcare organizations performed any significant financial analyses on equipment because in the risk-free environment of cost-based reimbursement, healthcare organizations and their lenders were guaranteed a return on capital expenditures, whether they used the equipment or not. In a 1973 study of large hospitals, only 8 percent of the hospitals calculated the net present value of a capital expenditure before purchasing it (William and Rakich 1973). Some hospitals had two of everything in case the first broke (they preferred capital expense to labor and repair expenses).

As the Medicare reimbursement for capital costs was folded into the DRG formula during the 1990s as a result of the OBRA of 1990, healthcare organizations found themselves competing with other industries for limited capital funds. Healthcare organizations no longer had cost-based reimbursement to put up as collateral, and as a result, lending institutions required financial analyses to ensure that the capital expenditure would generate sufficient revenue to repay the loan. As a result, net present value and return on investment calculations are completed on most capital expenditures today.

This section defines and explains how to calculate several analyses that are used to measure the benefit to cost ratio. In theory, these analyses are benefit-cost analyses, which are based on the Pareto optimality, or a condition in which changes occur only if they improve the benefits more than increasing the costs. In benefit-cost analysis, both costs and benefits are variable, as opposed to cost-effectiveness analysis, where either costs or benefits are held constant (Reeves, Bergwall, and Woodside 1979). In their simplest forms, benefit-cost analysis is the ratio of discounted benefits to discounted costs, and cost-effectiveness analysis is the benefits obtained for a particular cost.

A federally qualified community health center is implementing an electronic medical record (EMR) costing $35,000 per physician provider. Identify benefits of the EMR and ways the benefits can be estimated to calculate a benefit-cost ratio.

The typical financial analyses for capital expenditures are **payback period** analysis, **net present value** (NPV) analysis, and **internal rate of return** (IRR) analysis.

PAYBACK PERIOD ANALYSIS

Payback period is the number of years necessary for cash flows to recover the original investment. Payback period analysis is easy to calculate (see Problem 13.1), but it is the least sophisticated of the three analyses because it does not take into account the effects of time on money.

NET PRESENT VALUE

NPV is a commonly used financial analysis for capital expenditures that relies on discounting cash flows. Where discounted payback period gives the manager an answer in years, NPV gives the manager an answer in dollars. An NPV of zero means that the capital expenditure is generating discounted cash flows just sufficient to repay the original investment. If the NPV is positive, the expenditure is generating discounted cash flows in excess of the amount necessary to repay the original investment. If the NPV is negative, the expenditure is generating discounted cash flows insufficient to repay the original investment.

NPV has some flaws (see Zelman, McCue, and Millikan 1998b)—the principal flaw seems to be determining the discount rate. Most theorists agree that NPV is superior to IRR as a method of evaluating capital expenditures (Brigham 1992). However, because IRR is a common method of evaluating capital expenditures in the real world, managers should be prepared to calculate both NPV and IRR.

After managers understand the concept of discounting, they can apply discounting to payback period analysis, NPV analysis, and IRR analysis. Discounted payback period is similar to payback period except that the manager discounts the projected cash flows by discount factors for the expenditure's discount rate (see Problem 13.2). Managers can find discount factors on a PV table (see Exhibit 13.1).

INTERNAL RATE OF RETURN

IRR analysis is the discount rate of a capital expenditure where the discounted cash flows equal the expenditure's original investment, or the discount rate where the NPV is zero. Discounted payback period analysis gives the manager an answer in years, and NPV analysis gives the manager an answer in dollars. IRR analysis gives the manager an answer in a percentage. Solving the NPV equation by hand is relatively simple, but solving the IRR is difficult without a calculator. Solving the IRR by hand using the equation necessitates a trial-and-error methodology—inserting discount factors representing different discount rates until the sum equals zero (Brigham 1992):

---

payback period
The number of years necessary for cash flows to recover the original investment.

---

net present value
The present value of the future cash flow of an investment. NPV takes into account the fact that future cash flows are "discounted" to determine their present value.

---

internal rate of return
The necessary net present value of an investment that, when added to the final market value of the investment, equals the current cost of the investment. In other words, the IRR is the minimum return one needs to break even on an investment.

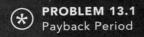

PROBLEM 13.1
Payback Period

ABC Day Surgery Center wants to buy equipment for $10,000 with projected cash flows (net revenues minus expenses) of $3,000 per year during the equipment's five-year useful life. What is the payback period?

Year	Cash Flow ($)	Cumulative Cash Flow ($)
cf0	(10,000)	($10,000)
cf1	3,000	(7,000)
cf2	3,000	(4,000)
cf3	3,000	(1,000)
cf4	3,000	2,000
cf5	3,000	5,000

Initial investment represented by cf0; cf = cash flow.

The day surgery center will recover the cost of the equipment sometime during year 4. Sometimes when comparing capital equipment requests it is necessary to use a value more exact than whole years. To determine exactly when during year 4 the equipment will break even, assuming an even distribution of cash flow during the year:

Payback period

$$= \text{Year before recovery} + \frac{\text{Unrecovered cost at beginning of year}}{\text{Cash flow during year}}$$

$$= 3 + (1{,}000 / 3{,}000)$$

$$= 3.33 \text{ years}$$

The primary disadvantage of payback period analysis is that it does not take into account the effects of time on money.

$$cf_0 = \frac{cf_1}{(1+\text{IRR})^1} + \frac{cf_2}{(1+\text{IRR})^2} + \cdots \frac{cf_n}{(1+\text{IRR})^n} = 0$$

Problem 13.3 shows how the healthcare manager can use a calculator to find NPV and IRR.

PROBLEM 13.2
Calculating the Present Value

Discounting is used to compare capital expenditures that will generate future cash flows. Discounting is a way of looking at a future amount of money, called future value (FV), and calculating the present value (PV) of the money using the following formula:

$$PV = FV / (1 + i)^n$$

What is the PV of $100,000, discounted at 5 percent annually for five years?

$$PV = \frac{FV}{(1+i)^n} = \frac{100,000}{(1+.05)^5} = \frac{100,000}{1.2763} = \$78,351.48$$

Note: This answer is formula driven. Use of a calculator or spreadsheet may alter the answer slightly because of rounding or how interest is calculated (at the end of the period versus during the period).

HP 10BII Solution to Problem 13.2

Keys	Display	Description
1 [●] P/YR	1.00	Sets compounding periods per year to 1
5 N	5.00	Stores the number of compounding periods
5 I/YR	5.00	Stores the interest rate
−100,000 FV	−100,000.00	Stores the future value as an annuity (−)
PV	78,352.62	

After managers understand the concept of discounting, they can apply discounting to payback period analysis, NPV analysis, and IRR analysis. Discounted payback period is similar to payback period except that the manager discounts the projected cash flows by discount factors for the expenditure's discount rate (see Problem 13.3). Managers can find discount factors on a PV table (see Exhibit 13.1).

STEP 21: IDENTIFY NONFINANCIAL BENEFITS

The twenty-first step in the planning process and the fourth step in the capital budgeting process is for the department manager requesting the capital expenditure to identify nonfinancial benefits for the request. Examples of nonfinancial benefits could include community need or medical staff politics. Even if the organization is buying equipment

EXHIBIT 13.1
Present Value Table

Discount Rate (%)					
	10	20	30	40	50
Year 1	0.909	0.833	0.769	0.714	0.667
Year 2	0.826	0.694	0.592	0.511	0.444
Year 3	0.751	0.579	0.455	0.364	0.296
Year 4	0.683	0.482	0.351	0.261	0.198
Year 5	0.621	0.402	0.269	0.186	0.132
Year 6	0.564	0.335	0.207	0.133	0.088
Year 7	0.513	0.279	0.159	0.095	0.059
Year 8	0.467	0.233	0.123	0.068	0.039
Year 9	0.424	0.194	0.094	0.048	0.026
Year 10	0.385	0.162	0.073	0.035	0.017

to please a valuable physician, the organization should still complete a financial analysis to determine the equipment's loss, which will need to be subsidized elsewhere.

STEP 22: EVALUATE BENEFITS AND MAKE DECISIONS

The twenty-second and last step in the planning process and the fifth and final step in the capital budgeting process is for the budget committee to evaluate the financial and nonfinancial benefits for each request and make decisions. The budget committee can use

EXHIBIT 13.2
Decision Matrix for
Capital Budget

Request	Financial Analysis	Community Need	Cost Containment	Physician Relations	Total
	40	20	30	10	
A	30	20	25	10	85
B	40	10	20	05	80
C	35	05	10	10	60
D	20	20	05	10	55

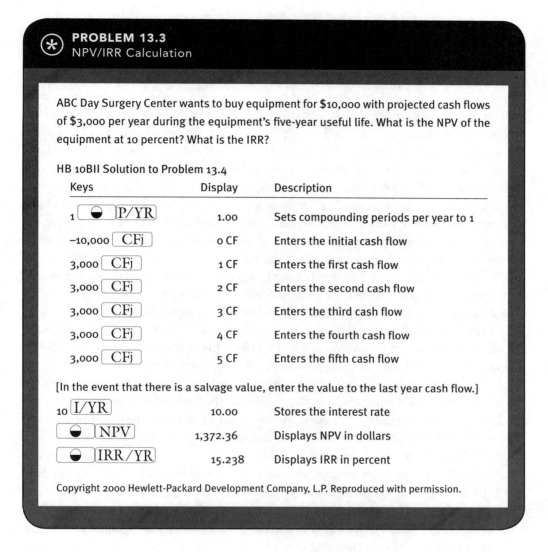

PROBLEM 13.3
NPV/IRR Calculation

ABC Day Surgery Center wants to buy equipment for $10,000 with projected cash flows of $3,000 per year during the equipment's five-year useful life. What is the NPV of the equipment at 10 percent? What is the IRR?

HB 10BII Solution to Problem 13.4

Keys	Display	Description
1 ⊖ P/YR	1.00	Sets compounding periods per year to 1
–10,000 CFj	0 CF	Enters the initial cash flow
3,000 CFj	1 CF	Enters the first cash flow
3,000 CFj	2 CF	Enters the second cash flow
3,000 CFj	3 CF	Enters the third cash flow
3,000 CFj	4 CF	Enters the fourth cash flow
3,000 CFj	5 CF	Enters the fifth cash flow

[In the event that there is a salvage value, enter the value to the last year cash flow.]

Keys	Display	Description
10 I/YR	10.00	Stores the interest rate
⊖ NPV	1,372.36	Displays NPV in dollars
⊖ IRR/YR	15.238	Displays IRR in percent

a decision matrix with weighted criteria similar to that shown in Exhibit 13.2. Implicit in the decision-making process is an evaluation of the decision. Many healthcare organizations use their internal audit departments to review capital expenditure decisions and the justifications of the department managers to determine their accuracy. Internal auditors can review the actual volumes, revenues, and expenses to determine whether the projections used to support the decisions were accurate.

FINANCING CAPITAL EXPENDITURES

Healthcare organizations can use cash generated from philanthropy, funded depreciation, operating surpluses, and debt to finance capital expenditures. Generally speaking, the organization should use funded depreciation to finance replacement equipment and philanthropy, operating surpluses, or debt to finance new equipment.

The Tax Reform Act of 1986 limited the tax deduction individuals were able to take for donations; as a result, philanthropy to healthcare organizations declined. The decline in philanthropy paralleled an increase in debt financing because of two federal government policies. First, Medicare reduced the risk associated with debt financing by reimbursing 100 percent of the interest on debt used for capital expenditures (which ended in 1992 when capital and interest associated with capital became part of the DRG formula). Second, the Nixon administration encouraged debt financing by allowing local governments to create taxing authorities that issued tax-exempt bonds. As a result of these two policies, hospitals and many other healthcare organizations have relied on debt financing significantly more than other industries have. Private industries finance 40 to 50 percent of their capital needs with debt, and public utilities finance about 60 percent of their capital needs with debt. Hospitals finance 80 to 90 percent of their capital needs with debt (Eastaugh 1987).[5]

Facing rising demand for capital caused by aging facilities, the need for expansion, and the introduction of new technologies, many healthcare organizations may not have access to the capital they need. In 2012, the American Hospital Association reported that, in Moody's credit outlook for hospitals, "the preponderance of credit factors facing the industry is unequivocally negative, and is expected to remain negative for at least the next several years" (AHA 2012). Likewise Standard & Poor's (2013) reported a negative outlook for hospitals in the near future.

One of the most significant factors affecting an organization's ability to access the capital markets is the organization's creditworthiness. The healthcare industry relies on rating agencies such as Standard & Poor's, Moody's, and Fitch to measure creditworthiness using both objective criteria and subjective assessments of organizations and the markets in which they operate.

Moody's downgraded a record amount of debt held by not-for-profit hospitals in 2012. In downgrading the debt, Moody's noted a challenging operating environment, increasing debt loads, declining liquidity, more competition, and management and governance issues. Historically, size has insulated large systems from downgrades; however, in 2012 the majority of the downgraded debt ($13 out of the $20 billion) belonged to just three large systems. In addition to size of system, the following characteristics have typically led to stronger bond ratings (Kutscher 2013):

◆   effective management and governance,

◆   improved and sustained operating performance,

◆   strong and liquid investment portfolios and management of debt structure risks,

◆   favorable market demographics and market share, and

◆   favorable change in organizational or legal structure.

With many hospitals at debt capacity, credit markets limiting the extension of credit, and operating and investment margins declining, many future capital expenditures will be financed through hospital consolidations, including mergers, acquisitions, and joint ventures (Grauman, Harris, and Martin 2010), which makes the planning and budgeting functions all the more important. Sometimes leasing is considered as another method of financing a capital expenditure.

LEASE VERSUS PURCHASE DECISIONS

Lease versus purchase decisions are made after the decision to acquire the equipment; therefore, the lease versus purchase decision is in fact a financing decision. Generally, there are two types of leases: operating leases and capital leases. Operating leases are for periods shorter than the equipment's useful life and are common for copy machines, desktop computers, and cars. Capital leases are for the equipment's approximate useful life and usually include provisions for the lessee to purchase the equipment at the end of the lease period.

Lease decisions have several advantages over purchase decisions and can provide the lessee with more flexibility, more financing options for other equipment, more protection from unexpected events such as changes in technology, and more and better maintenance. In the case of for-profit healthcare organizations, capital leases can provide the same tax advantages as equipment purchases.

Lease decisions have several disadvantages over purchase decisions—including penalties for early lease termination and the requirement that the property be maintained in good working condition—and leases are generally more expensive than the purchase decision because lessors must make a profit and cover their risk of loss.

Problem 13.4 gives a simple way of analyzing the costs associated with a nonprofit facility purchasing or leasing a $1.3 million magnetic resonance imaging machine by applying a PV of 10 percent to both decisions (a for-profit facility would have tax shields, or reductions in the amount of income taxes paid, due to the tax deductibility of depreciation and interest expense).

EVALUATING CAPITAL BUDGETING PERFORMANCE

When evaluating capital budgeting performance, several ratios are used to determine how much debt an organization can incur.

DEBT TO CAPITALIZATION RATIO

$$\frac{\text{Long-term debt}}{(\text{Long-term debt } + \text{ Net assets})}$$

PROBLEM 13.4
Lease Versus Purchase Decision Exercise

Purchase Considerations	Lease Considerations
Borrow $1.3 million at 10 percent on declining balance	Lease payments of $26,000 per month for 60 months (includes maintenance)
Depreciate straight line over five years	
Trade-in value of $130,000 at end of useful life	
Maintenance expense of $12,000 per year	

(Revenues, as well as labor and supply expenses, are the same for both decisions, and therefore are not included in the analysis.)

PURCHASE

Year	Principal Payment	Interest Payment	Maintenance Expense	Total Expense	PV Factor at 10%	PV Expense
1	260,000	130,000	12,000	402,000	0.909	365,418
2	260,000	104,000	12,000	376,000	0.826	310,576
3	260,000	78,000	12,000	350,000	0.751	262,850
4	260,000	52,000	12,000	324,000	0.683	221,292
5	260,000	26,000	12,000	298,000	0.621	185,058
Trade-in (130,000)					0.621	(80,730)
						1,264,464

LEASE

Year	Lease Payment	PV Factor at 10%	PV Expense
1	312,000	0.909	283,608
2	312,000	0.826	257,712
3	312,000	0.751	234,312
4	312,000	0.683	213,096
5	312,000	0.621	193,752
			1,182,480

Because the PV expense of the lease decision is less than the PV expense of the purchase decision, the financial merit supports the lease decision. However, other criteria mentioned in the advantages and disadvantages of the lease decision already mentioned should also be considered before making a final decision.

Debt to capitalization, or long-term debt to capitalization, is an indicator of the long-term debt divided by the long-term debt plus net assets. Higher values imply a greater reliance on debt financing as a percentage and may imply a reduced ability to carry additional debt. The debt-to-capitalization median for all hospitals reporting to Optum (2014) for 2012 audited financial statements was 26.3.

CAPITAL EXPENSE RATIO

$$\frac{(\text{Interest expense} + \text{Depreciation expense})}{\text{Total expense} \times 100}$$

Capital expense ratio provides an important indicator of operating leverage, which is a measurement of fixed costs to variable costs. Organizations with high fixed costs in proportion to variable costs are said to be highly leveraged. The capital expense median for all hospitals reporting to Optum (2014) for 2012 audited financial statements was 6.4.

AVERAGE AGE OF PLANT

$$\frac{\text{Accumulated depreciation}}{\text{Depreciation expense}}$$

Average age of plant provides an indicator in years of the age of a healthcare organization's fixed assets. Higher values reflect an older plant and equipment and indirectly may imply a difficulty in competing with "newer" healthcare organizations; lower values reflect a newer plant and equipment. The median average age of plant for all hospitals reporting to Optum (2014) for 2012 audited financial statements was 10.2.

CHAPTER KEY POINTS

➤ Capital costs are important because of rising healthcare costs and in dictating the trends of acquisitions, mergers, joint ventures, and closings.

➤ Capital expenditures are the purchases of land, buildings, and equipment for operations.

➤ *Replacement* and *new* are the two broad categories for capital expenditures.

➤ The capital budgeting process has five steps: identifying and prioritizing requests, projecting cash flows, performing financial analyses, identifying nonfinancial benefits, and evaluating benefits and making decisions.

➤ Funded depreciation should be used to finance replacement equipment, while operating surpluses, philanthropy, or debt should be used to finance new equipment.

➤ The decision to lease or purchase is a financial decision, and both have pros and cons.

➤ The debt-to-capitalization ratio, capital expense ratio, and average age of plant are three of the ratios used to evaluate capital budgeting performance.

DISCUSSION QUESTIONS

1. Why are capital costs such an important aspect of a healthcare organization's costs?

2. What two categories are capital expenditure budgets divided into? Provide real-world examples of both these categories.

3. Briefly explain the five steps involved in the capital budgeting process.

4. What are the three methods of financial analysis for capital expenditures? What are the formulas for each? Which of these three is the least sophisticated? Why?

5. Explain what led to an increase in debt financing. What result did the two policies have on healthcare organizations?

6. What factors do rating agencies look at when issuing bond ratings?

7. Why would an organization choose to lease equipment over purchasing it? Provide an example of when an organization would be better off purchasing equipment than leasing.

NOTES

1. Useful life is part of the depreciation controversy between providers and insurers regarding allowable cost for reimbursement purposes. The issues include what the useful life should be; whether the amount to be depreciated should be based on historic cost or replacement cost; and what method of computing depreciation (i.e., straight line, sum-of-the-years digits, or double declining balance—the latter two of which are accelerated) should be used.

2. In some cases, the budget committee may ask the medical staff or chief of the medical staff to prioritize the list of chief-of-service requests before submitting it to the budget committee. This avoids the problem of nonphysician department managers making decisions on physician-generated requests.

3. Most organizations prioritize replacement equipment that is fully depreciated ahead of new requests to avoid the snowball effect of not replacing assets on schedule.

Doing so is easy to justify because the need for the equipment is supportable with procedure logs; if the organization funded the equipment's depreciation properly, funds exist for the replacement. Some organizations prioritize new equipment ahead of replacement equipment to generate new streams of revenue. However, this strategy could result in long-term problems for the organization, especially if the organization uses funded depreciation to acquire the new equipment.

4. Usually the budget committee, CFO, or designee is responsible for converting gross revenue to net revenue by subtracting contractual adjustments, charity care adjustments, and bad debt adjustments. This can be accomplished in a fashion similar to that shown in Problem 4.1, Step 1, in Chapter 4.

5. Health economists agree that organizations with this kind of excessive debt have great difficulty with cyclical recessions or downturns in the economy. This helps explain the growing trend of not-for-profit organizations entering joint ventures or being acquired by for-profit organizations that have access to different capital markets.

RECOMMENDED READINGS—PART IV

Berger, S. 2007. *Fundamentals of Healthcare Financial Management,* 3rd ed. San Francisco: Jossey-Bass Publishers.

Cleverley, W. O., J. O. Cleverley, and P. H. Song. 2010. *Essentials of Health Care Finance,* 7th ed. Boston: Jones and Bartlett.

Kaufman, K. 2006. *Best Practice Financial Management: Six Key Concepts for Healthcare Leaders,* 3rd ed. Chicago: Health Administration Press.

McLean, R. A. 2003. "Budgeting and Variance Analysis." *Financial Management in Health Care Organizations.* New York: Cengage Learning.

Nowicki, M. 1998. "Beware the 'Slippery Slope' of Granting Exceptions." *Journal of Healthcare Resource Management* 16 (1): 20–22.

Optum. 2014. *Almanac of Hospital Financial and Operating Indicators.* Salt Lake City, UT: Optum.

Zelman, W. N., M. J. McCue, and N. D. Glick. 2014. *Financial Management of Health Care Organizations,* 4th ed. San Francisco: Jossey-Bass Publishers.

Zuckerman, A. M. 2012. *Healthcare Strategic Planning,* 3rd ed. Chicago: Health Administration Press.

PAYBACK PERIOD

Payback Period Practice Problem

XYZ Skilled Nursing Facility wants to buy equipment for $100,000 with projected cash flows of $22,000 per year during the equipment's five-year useful life. What is the payback period?

Payback Period Practice Problem Solution

Year	Cash Flow ($)	Cumulative Cash Flow ($)
cf_0*	(100,000)	(100,000)
cf_1	22,000	(78,000)
cf_2	22,000	(56,000)
cf_3	22,000	(34,000)
cf_4	22,000	(12,000)
cf_5	22,000	10,000

*cf_0 represents initial investment

By looking at the table, the skilled nursing facility will recover the cost of the equipment during year 5. Sometimes when comparing capital equipment requests it might be necessary to use a value more exact than whole years. To determine exactly when during year 5 the equipment will break even (assuming an even distribution of cash flows during the years), use the following formula:

$$\text{Payback period} = \text{Year before recover} + \frac{\text{Unrecovered costs at beginning of year}}{\text{Cash flow during year}}$$

$$= 4 + \frac{(\$)12,000}{(\$)22,000} = 4.55 \text{ years}$$

Payback Period Self-Quiz Problem

Your sleep disorder clinic wants to buy new software for $20,000 with projected cash flows (salary savings) of $12,000 per year during the software's three-year useful life. What is the payback period?

PRESENT VALUE

Present Value Practice Problem

What is the present value of $50,000, discounted at 7.5 percent annually for five years?

Present Value Practice Problem Solution

$$PV = \frac{FV}{(1 + i)^n}$$

$$PV = \frac{\$\,50{,}000}{(1 + .075)^5}$$

$$PV = \frac{\$50{,}000}{1.4356}$$

$$PV = \$34{,}829$$

HB 10BII Solution, compounded annually

Keys	Display	Description
1 ⬤ P/YR	1.00	Sets compounding periods per year to 1
5 N	5.00	Stores the number of compounding periods (1 × 5)
7.5 I/YR	7.50	Stores the interest rate
−50,000 FV	−50,000	Stores the future value
PV	$34,827.93	Calculates the present value

Present Value Self-Quiz Problem

What is the present value of $25,000, discounted at 3.5 percent annually for three years?

$$PV = \frac{25,000}{(1+3.5]^3} = 91.185$$

$$PV = \$274.35$$

Net Present Value/Internal Rate of Return

NPV/IRR Practice Problem

XYZ Skilled Nursing Facility wants to buy equipment for $100,000 with projected cash flows of $22,000 per year during the equipment's five-year useful life. What is the net present value at 10 percent with a salvage value of $10,000? What is the internal rate of return?

HB 10BII solution

Keys	Display	Description
1 (●) (P/YR)	1.00	Sets compounding periods per year to 1
−100,000 (CF$_j$)	0 CF	Enters the initial cash flow as an annuity (−)
22,000 (CF$_j$)	1 CF	Enters the first cash flow
22,000 (CF$_j$)	2 CF	Enters the second cash flow
22,000 (CF$_j$)	3 CF	Enters the third cash flow
22,000 (CF$_j$)	4 CF	Enters the fourth cash flow
32,000 (CF$_j$*)	5 CF	Enters the fifth cash flow

*In the event that there is a salvage value, enter the value to the last year cash flow

10 (I/YR)	10.00	Stores the interest rate
(●)(NPV)	10,393.48	Displays NPV in dollars
(IRR/YR)	6.05	Displays IRR in percent

Net Present Value/Internal Rate of Return Self-Quiz Problem

The physician's office that you manage wants to buy equipment for $20,000 with projected cash flows of $3,000 per year over the equipment's ten-year useful life. Calculate the NPV/IRR at 10 percent.

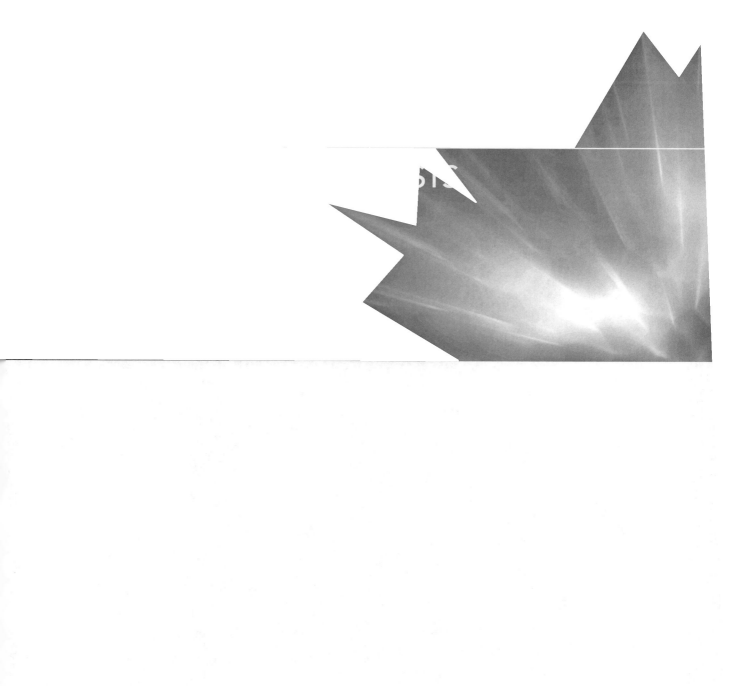

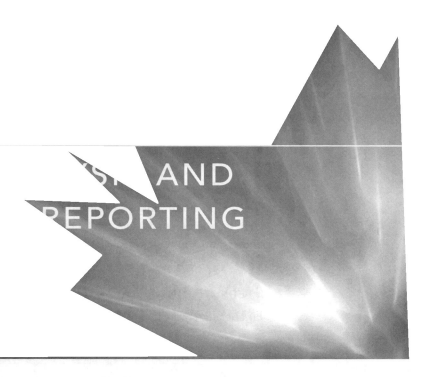

YSIS AND
REPORTING

There is much more cognizance and awareness of the capital aspects of the balance sheet and a better understanding of the credit markets so you can decide where to invest cash, how to eke out investment returns on excess cash, and how to position the organization for the future.

Robert Hemker, chief financial officer of Palomar Health,
San Diego, California

LEARNING OBJECTIVES

After completing this chapter, you should be able to

➤ Identify and understand the major components of financial statements
➤ List in order and explain each step in the financial analysis process
➤ Explain the principles in preparing good financial reports

INTRODUCTION

Financial analysis and management reporting are integral parts of the management functions of control and financial management. As introduced in Chapter 8, financial analysis includes methods used by investors, creditors, and management to evaluate the past, present, and future financial performance of a healthcare organization. On completion of the analysis, the information is reported to the appropriate stakeholders, inside and outside the organization, at which time the stakeholders take corrective action in the form of decisions.

STEPS IN FINANCIAL ANALYSIS

Financial analysis includes the following three steps (Berman, Kukla, and Weeks 1994):

1. Establish the facts about the organization.

2. Compare the facts about the organization over time and to facts about similar organizations.

3. Use perspective and judgment to make decisions regarding the comparisons.

Financial analysis by management can occur at any level—departmental, divisional, or organizational—within the organization.

At the organizational level, establishing the facts (the first step) usually relates to a review of the organization's key financial statements, including the balance sheet, statement of operations, statement of changes in net assets, and statement of cash flows. Healthcare organizations with permanent controlling financial interests in other healthcare organizations should prepare consolidated financial statements to properly report the relationship (AICPA 2012). Before they undertake financial analysis, investors and creditors may require that independent auditors review the financial statements to confirm their accuracy.

The second step, comparing the facts in the organization over time and to facts in other, similar organizations, includes ratio analysis, horizontal analysis, and vertical analysis. **Ratio analysis** evaluates an organization's performance by computing the relationships of important line items found in the financial statements. There are four kinds of ratios: liquidity, profitability, activity, and capital structure.

Horizontal analysis evaluates the trend in the line items by focusing on the percentage change over time. **Vertical analysis** evaluates the internal structure of the organization by focusing on a base number and showing percentages of important line items in relation to the base number. Once ratio analysis, horizontal analysis, and vertical analysis are complete, the organization can compare present ratios, trends, and percentages to its past ratios, trends, and percentages. The organization can also develop industry comparisons that compare the organization's present ratios, trends, and percentages to those of other, similar organizations.[1]

ratio analysis
Evaluation of an organization's performance by computing the relationships of important line items in the financial statements.

horizontal analysis
Evaluation of the trends in an organization's finances by focusing on percentage change over time.

vertical analysis
Evaluation of the internal structure of an organization by focusing on a base number and showing percentages of important line items in relation to the base number.

The third step of financial analysis, using perspective and judgment to make decisions, uses the information obtained in the first two steps, in addition to information derived from the decision maker's unique perspective and judgment, to make the decision. Decisions that may at first appear to be contrary to the information provided in the first two steps may make perfect sense based on pressures from internal and external constituents, including medical staff, employers, regulators, donors, and others.

The example of a fictional facility, Bobcat Hospital, will be used to illustrate the financial analysis concepts in this chapter.

BALANCE SHEET

The balance sheet shows the organization's financial position at a specific point in time, typically at the end of an accounting period (see Exhibit 14.1). The balance sheet presents the organization's assets, liabilities, and net assets (or shareholders' equity in for-profit organizations) and its relationships, which are reflected in the following accounting equation:

$$\text{Assets} = \text{Liabilities} + \text{Net assets}$$

Assets are economic resources that provide or are expected to provide benefit to the organization. **Current assets** are economic resources that have a life of less than one year (i.e., the organization expects to consume them within one year). Current assets are listed on the balance sheet in order of liquidity. Cash is money on hand and in the bank that the organization can access immediately. Temporary investments are money placed in securities with maturities up to one year, such as commodities and options. **Receivables, net,** or patient accounts receivable, net of allowances for contractual allowances, charity care, and bad debt, are money due to the organization from patients and third parties for services already provided. **Inventory** is the cost of food, fuel, drugs, and other supplies purchased by the hospital but not yet used or consumed. Prepaid expenses are expenditures made by the hospital for goods and services not yet consumed or used in hospital operations (sometimes referred to as deferred expenses).

Long-term investments are economic resources that the hospital owns, such as corporate bonds and government securities, and intends to hold for more than one year. **Plant and equipment, net** is economic resources, such as land, buildings, and equipment, minus the amount that has been depreciated over the life of the buildings and equipment (which is called accumulated depreciation).

Liabilities are economic obligations, or debts, of the organization. **Current liabilities** are economic obligations, or debts, that are due in less than one year. **Accounts payable** are amounts the hospital owes to suppliers and other trade creditors for merchandise and services purchased from them, but for which the hospital has not paid. **Accrued expenses payable** are liabilities for expenses that have been incurred by the hospital, but

---

assets
Economic resources that provide or are expected to provide benefit to the organization.

current assets
Economic resources that the organization expects to consume in less than one year.

receivables, net
Money due to the organization from patients and third parties for services already provided.

inventory
The cost of food, fuel, drugs, and other supplies purchased by the hospital but not yet consumed.

long-term investments
Economic resources that the hospital owns, such as corporate bonds and government securities, and intends to hold for more than one year.

plant and equipment, net
Economic resources, such as land, buildings, and equipment, minus the amount that has been depreciated over the life of the buildings and equipment.

EXHIBIT 14.1

Bobcat Hospital
Balance Sheet, as
of December 31
2013, 2012
(in thousands)

	2013	2012
ASSETS		
Current assets		
Cash	$ 124	$ 280
Temporary investments	45	30
Receivables, net	3,536	3,717
Inventory	175	140
Prepaid expenses	32	40
Total current assets	3,912	4,207
Noncurrent assets		
Property, plant, and equipment	6,980	6,580
Accumulated depreciation	−1,730	−1,660
Net property, plant, and equipment	5,250	4,920
Long-term investments	609	990
Other noncurrent assets	113	109
Total noncurrent assets	5,972	6,019
Total assets	9,884	10,226
LIABILITIES & NET ASSETS		
Current liabilities		
Accounts payable	$ 302	$ 370
Notes payable	345	335
Accrued expenses payable	871	408
Estimated third-party adjustments	147	239
Current portion of long-term debt	184	178
Total current liabilities	1,849	1,530
Noncurrent liabilities		
Long-term debt, less current portion	3,600	3,500
Total liabilities	5,449	5,030
NET ASSETS		
Unrestricted net assets	3,285	3,896
Temporarily restricted net assets	750	700
Permanently restricted net assets	400	600
Total net assets	4,435	5,196
Total liabilities and net assets	$9,884	$10,226

liabilities
Economic obligations,
or debts, of the
organization.

current liabilities
Economic obligations,
or debts, that are due
in less than one year.

accounts payable
Amounts the hospital
owes to suppliers and
other trade creditors
for merchandise and
services purchased
from them, but for
which the hospital has
not paid.

for which the hospital has not yet paid, such as compensation to employees. **Deferred revenue** is revenue received by the hospital but not yet earned by the hospital, such as premium revenue from managed care organizations.

    Long-term liabilities are economic obligations, or debts, that are due in more than one year. **Long-term debt, net of current portion** is an economic obligation, or debt, that is due in more than one year, minus the amount that is due within one year. **Net assets**[2] is the current American Institute of Certified Public Accountants (AICPA)–approved term for the difference between assets and liabilities in not-for-profit healthcare organizations. **Unrestricted net assets** include net assets that have not been externally restricted by donors or grantors, such as the excess of revenues to expenses from operations. Unrestricted net assets include net assets that are contractually limited by the governing body, such as proceeds of debt issues, funds deposited with a trustee and limited to use by an indenture agreement, and funds set aside under self-insurance arrangements and statutory reserve requirements. **Temporarily restricted net assets** include donor-restricted net assets that the organization can use for the donor's specific purpose once the organization has met the donor's restriction, such as the passage of time or an action by the organization. **Permanently restricted net assets** include donor-restricted net assets with restrictions that never expire, such as endowment funds.

    Shareholders' equity is the current AICPA-approved term for the difference between assets and liabilities in for-profit healthcare organizations; it represents the ownership interest of stockholders in the organization. Shareholders' equity is also called stockholders' equity, owners' equity, and net worth and comprises common stock and retained earnings. **Common stock** is money invested in the organization by its owners. **Retained earnings** is income earned by the organization from operations minus dividends (which are distributions of earnings paid to stockholders based on the number of shares of stock owned).

    Explanatory notes for the balance sheet and the other financial statements should identify extraordinary events, as well as certain required provisions, and should be presented following the financial statements.

STATEMENT OF OPERATIONS

The statement of operations, called the income statement for for-profit organizations, summarizes the organization's net revenues, expenses, and excess of net revenues over expenses (this is income before taxes in a for-profit organization) over a period of time (see Exhibit 14.2). The relationship of the statement of operations to the balance sheet can be best expressed by the expanded accounting equation:

$$\text{Assets} = \text{Liabilities} + \text{Net assets} + (\text{Net revenue} - \text{Expenses})$$

---

accrued expenses payable
Liabilities for expenses that have been incurred by the hospital, but for which the hospital has not yet paid, such as compensation to employees.

deferred revenue
Revenue received by the hospital but not yet earned by the hospital, such as premium revenue from managed care organizations.

long-term liabilities
Economic obligations, or debts, that are due in more than one year.

long-term debt, net of current portion
A debt that is due in more than one year, minus the amount that is due within one year.

net assets
The difference between assets and liabilities in a not-for-profit organization.

unrestricted net assets
Net assets that have not been externally restricted by donors or grantors, such as the excess of revenues to expenses from operations.

EXHIBIT 14.2
Bobcat Hospital
Statement of
Operations
(in thousands)
through December
31, 2013, 2012

*temporarily restricted
net assets*
Donor-restricted
net assets that the
organization can use
for the donor's specific
purpose once the
organization has met
the donor's restriction,
such as the passage of
time or an action by the
organization.

*permanently restricted
net assets*
Donor-restricted net
assets with restrictions
that never expire, such
as endowment funds.

shareholders' equity
The difference between
assets and liabilities
in for-profit healthcare
organizations; it
represents the
ownership interest of
stockholders in the
organization.

common stock
Money invested in the
organization by its
owners.

	2013	2012
REVENUES		
Patient services revenue	$13,031	$12,610
Provision for contractual allowances (non-GAAP)	− 4,209	− 4,083
Provision for charity care allowances (non-GAAP)	− 420	− 408
Provision for bad debt allowance	− 600	− 476
Net patient services revenue	7,802	7,643
Premium revenue	400	0
Other revenue	440	447
Total operating revenue	$8,642	$8,090
EXPENSES		
Salaries, wages, and benefits	4,980	5,278
Supplies, drugs, purchased services	3,080	2,956
Depreciation and amortization	471	443
Interest	113	109
Total operating expenses	8,644	8,786
Total operating income	− 2	− 696
NONOPERATING INCOME		
Investment income	$ 95	$ 85
EXCESS OF REVENUE OVER EXPENSES	93	− 611
CHANGES IN NET ASSETS		
Unrestricted net assets	3,285	3,896
Temporarily restricted net assets	750	700
Permanently restricted net assets	400	600
Total changes in net assets	4,435	5,196

where the permanent accounts of the balance sheet, which are accounts that carry balances forward to the next year, relate to the temporary accounts of the statement of operations, which are accounts that zero out at the end of each year. To zero out the net results of the statement of operations at the end of the year, the net results are transferred to unrestricted net assets on the balance sheet, or to retained earnings on the balance sheet of a for-profit organization.

Gross patient services revenues are the total amount of charges for patients utilizing the hospital, regardless of the amount actually paid. Deductions from gross patient services revenues include amounts deducted from total charges to account for contractual allowances and charity care. **Patient services revenue** is money generated by providing patient care minus the amount the organization will not collect as a result of discounting charges per contractual agreement and providing charity care. For financial reporting purposes, patient services revenue does not include provisions for charity care because charity care was never intended to result in cash flow. In 2006, several professional associations, including the Healthcare Financial Management Association, advised that healthcare organizations should be required to report the cost of providing charity care, and not the associated revenues, in the footnotes. This change in generally accepted accounting principles (GAAP) occurred in 2010 and included the requirement to include the organization's method of determining cost and the organization's charity care policy in the footnotes. **Net patient services revenue** is patient services revenue minus provisions for bad debt if the healthcare organization recognizes significant amounts of patient services revenue at time of service without assessing the patient's ability to pay. This change in GAAP occurred in 2012 and was partially the result of the patient's inability to pay deductibles for high-deductible health policies (previous to 2012, healthcare organizations showed bad debt as an operating expense, but only after the organization attempted to collect the deductible).

Premium revenue is money generated from capitation arrangements that must be reported separately from patient services revenue because premium revenue is earned by agreeing to provide care, regardless of whether care is ever delivered. **Other operating revenue** is money generated from services other than health services to patients and enrollees. This may include revenue from rental equipment and office space, sales of supplies and pharmaceuticals, cafeteria and gift shop sales, and so on. Often the test for whether revenue is operating revenue or nonoperating revenue is whether the revenue was generated in support of the organization's mission statement. Why is it important to distinguish between operating or nonoperating revenue? Because for a not-for-profit hospital, income derived from operations is not taxed, but income from unrelated businesses, such as the gift shop, may be taxed as unrelated business income. **Net assets released from restrictions used for**

retained earnings
Income earned by the organization from operations minus dividends.

gross patient services revenue
The total amount of charges for patients utilizing the organization, regardless of the amount actually paid.

patient services revenue
Money generated by providing patient care minus the amount the organization will not collect as a result of discounting charges per contractual agreement and providing charity care.

net patient services revenue
Patient services revenue minus the amount the organization will not collect as a result of bad debt.

premium revenue
Money generated from capitation arrangements that must be reported separately from patient services revenue.

(!) CRITICAL CONCEPTS
Not Required, But Done

Hospitals follow generally accepted accounting principles (GAAP) when they prepare their financials, but sometimes they go beyond what GAAP requires. For example, gross patient services revenues are not required by GAAP, nor are deductions from revenues. As these are not GAAP requirements, they are not included on statements intended for external audiences.

operations, while not reflected in Hopeful Hospital's statement of operations, is money previously restricted by donors that has become available for operations.

Operating expenses is money spent on operations to generate revenue in support of the organization's mission statement. These expenses can be listed by functional classification (organizational division), such as nursing department and support department, which is useful for internal purposes, or by natural classification (also called object-of-expenditure), such as wages or supplies, as is the case with Hopeful Hospital's statement of operations, which is useful for external purposes.

Depreciation and amortization reflects the expensing of long-term assets over time to show their declining value. **Interest** is the expense incurred with borrowed money. Bad debt is the accounting recognition of how much money the organization has billed but will not collect; the amount reported must be based on charges. Bad debt should not be confused with charity care. Bad debt expense reflects that the organization provided services with the expectation of payment. Charity care reflects services the organization provided with no expectation of payment. **Other operating expenses** are miscellaneous expenses that have not been reported elsewhere.

Operating income is the money earned from providing patient care services and includes the total revenue, gains, and other support minus the total expenses; **nonoperating or other income** is the money earned from non–patient care services, such as investment income. **Excess of revenues over expenses** (or net income in for-profit organizations) is the operating income plus the other income minus total expenses. For not-for-profit organizations, AICPA requires excess of revenues over expenses to be reported as the performance indicator that reflects the results of operations. Not-for-profit organizations must report the performance indicator in a statement of operations that also presents the total changes in unrestricted net assets. The notes to the financial statements should provide a description of the nature and composition of the performance indicator (AICPA 2012).

STATEMENT OF CHANGES IN NET ASSETS

The statement of changes in net assets, called equity in a for-profit organization, shows the reasons why net assets changed from the beginning of the statement period to the end of the statement period as reported in summary fashion on the balance sheet. Because AICPA requires not-for-profit organizations to report changes of unrestricted net assets on the statement of operations, many organizations also include changes in temporarily restricted and permanently restricted net assets on the statement of operations, which eliminates the need for a separate statement of changes in net assets. This statement is important in showing how the changes in the excess of revenues over expenses affect the net asset, or equity, position of the organization (see Exhibit 14.2).

Unrestricted net assets come directly from the statement of operations and have already been explained in that section. *Temporarily restricted net assets* present the changes in temporarily restricted net assets during the statement period. *Contributions for charity care* is money donated to the hospital for the provision of charity care. *Net realized and unrealized gains on investments* are an increase in the value of the investment (unrealized until sold) and an increase in cash (realized through dividends or interest). *Net assets released from restrictions* is money previously restricted by donors that has become available for use. *Increase (decrease) in temporarily restricted net assets* presents the total changes in temporarily restricted net assets during the statement period.

Permanently restricted net assets present the changes in permanently restricted net assets during the accounting period. *Contributions for endowment funds* is money received from donors with permanent restrictions on the principal and interest. *Net realized and unrealized gains on investments* are an increase in value of the investment and an increase in cash. The increase in net assets is the difference between total net assets at the beginning of the year and total net assets at the end of the year.

STATEMENT OF CASH FLOWS

The statement of cash flows shows the organization's cash flow, that is, the amounts of cash receipts and where they came from and the amounts of cash disbursements and where they went during the statement period (see Exhibit 14.3; notes for the statement are in Exhibit 14.4). In a not-for-profit organization, the statement is divided into cash flows from operations, cash flows from investments, and cash flows from financing, including restricted income and contributions. For-profit organizations do not divide the cash flows into categories, but the bottom line is the same—net increase (decrease) in cash.[3]

Cash flows from operating activities begins with the change in net assets (this figure comes from the statement of changes in net assets or is computed from the difference in total net assets between statement periods) and then includes the changes in cash between statement periods for providing patient care services. Information from the statement of operations was prepared using accrual accounting, as required by GAAP. This means that revenues were recorded when the services were billed, not when the bills were paid. Expenses were recorded when they contributed to operations, not when they were paid. Revenues and expenses must be adjusted as well as noncash events, such as depreciation. The remainder of this section of the statement of cash flows makes the necessary adjustments.

Cash flows from investing activities include the changes in cash between statement periods for investing in fixed assets, such as property and equipment, and for selling fixed assets. *Cash flows from financing activities* include the changes in cash between statement periods for financing activities—such as debts, endowments, grants, and transfers—to and from parent organizations. *Net increase (decrease) in cash and cash equivalents* is computed by adding the net cash from operating, investing, and financing activities.

Cash and cash equivalents, beginning of year corresponds with the cash and cash equivalents, end of year for the previous year. *Cash and cash equivalents, end of year* is

operating income
Money earned from providing patient care services; includes the total revenue, gains, and other support minus the total expenses.

nonoperating or other income
Money earned from non–patient care services, such as investment income.

excess of revenues over expenses
Operating income plus the other income minus total expenses.

EXHIBIT **14.3**
Bobcat Hospital
Statement of Cash
Flows, 2013
(in thousands)

	2013
Cash flow from operating activities	
Change in net assets	$ (384)
Adjustments to reconcile change in net assets to net cash provided by operating activities	
Extraordinary loss from extinguishment of debt	
Depreciation and amortization	471
Net realized and unrealized gains on investments	0
Transfer to parent	0
Provisions for bad debt	600
(Increase) decrease in:	
Patient accounts receivable	181
Trading securities	0
Other current assets	27
Other assets	47
Increase (decrease) in:	
Accounts and notes payable	−58
Accrued expenses payable	463
Estimated third-party settlements	−92
Other current liabilities	6
Other liabilities	100
Net cash flow from operating activities	1,361
Cash flow from investing activities	
Purchase of investments	
Capital expenditures	−1,413
Net cash flow from investing activities	−1,413
Cash flow from financing activities	
Transfers to parent	0
Proceeds from restricted contributions and restricted investments income	95
Payments on long-term debt	−184
Payments on capital lease obligations	0
Proceeds from issuance of long-term debt	0
Net cash flow from financing activities	−89
Net increase (decrease) in cash and cash equivalents	−141
Cash and cash equivalents at the beginning of the year	310
Cash and cash equivalents at the end of the year	169

EXHIBIT 14.4
Bobcat Hospital Notes to Financial Statements 2013

1. Organization and Nature of Operations

Bobcat Hospital is a 120-bed, nonprofit hospital offering the following services: inpatient, outpatient, emergency, long-term care, rehab, and home care.

2. Community Benefit and Charity Care

Changes in generally accepted accounting principles (GAAP) in 2010 require hospitals to report charity care at cost with the method of arriving at cost. Bobcat Hospital provides healthcare services through various programs that are designed to enhance the health of the community. Bobcat Hospital provides emergent and urgent care to persons who cannot afford health insurance because of inadequate financial resources. Bobcat Hospital's financial assistance policy provides care to patients regardless of their ability to pay, and all uninsured patients are eligible for discounts based on their income up to 400% of the federal poverty level. The amount of charity care provided is based on this policy and the cost of charity care is calculated based on the charges for such services multiplied by the hospital's cost-to-charges ratio (0.66334). The cost of charity care provided in 2013 was $134,400. Not included in this amount, but still considered a community benefit, is the loss to the Medicaid program.

3. Bad Debt

Changes in generally accepted accounting principles (GAAP) in 2011 require hospitals that recognize significant amounts of patient services revenue at time of service even though the hospital does not assess the patient's ability to pay shall present that portion of bad debt as a deduction from revenue. The amount of bad debt is based on this principle of revenue recognition and the amount recognized in 2013 was $600,000 based on charges.

4. Net Patient Services Revenue

Patient services revenue is reported at estimated net realizable amounts for services rendered. The amount is net of provisions for contractual allowances ($4,209,000) in addition to provisions for charity care ($420,000) and bad debt ($600,000). Provisions for contractual allowances recognized discounts provided based on agreements with Medicare, Medicaid, other government programs, and major insurance companies.

computed by adding the net increase (decrease) in cash and cash equivalents to the cash and cash equivalents, beginning of year, and corresponds to cash and cash equivalents on the balance sheet for the same statement period.

RATIO ANALYSIS

ratio
A comparison between two or more financial facts, such as income to assets or assets to liabilities.

Ratios are comparisons between two or more financial facts, such as income to assets or assets to liabilities. Ratios are useful because they help an organization compare a period's results to previous periods or to the results of other, similar organizations.

Ratios emerge from facts located on the financial statements, which report an organization's financial position at a point in time and its financial operations over a period of time. Investors and creditors analyze financial statements, primarily through ratio analysis, to predict future earnings and the ability to service debt. Managers use ratio analysis to predict the future and to plan strategies that will influence the future. Financial statement analysis concentrates on four classifications of ratios: liquidity, profitability, activity, and capital structure (see Exhibit 14.5 for Optum medians for all hospitals reporting in 2012).

LIQUIDITY RATIOS

liquidity ratio
Ratio that measures an organization's ability to meet short-term obligations.

Liquidity ratios are measures of an organization's ability to meet short-term obligations. Measuring an organization's liquidity is important in evaluating an organization's financial performance.

• **Current Ratio**

$$\frac{\text{Total current assets}}{\text{Total current liabilities}}$$

Current ratio is the basic indicator of financial liquidity, which is an organization's ability to meet its obligations. It is nondirectional; higher values mean better debt-paying capacity, but a ratio that is too high may mean the organization could invest excess current assets more wisely. The primary disadvantage of the current ratio is that it does not take into account the relative liquidity of the different current assets.

• **Collection Period**

$$\frac{\text{Net receivables}}{\text{Net patient services revenue}/365}$$

Exhibit 14.5
Selected Financial
Ratios, Optum
Medians 2012

Ratios	Optum Median 2012
Liquidity	
Current	2.15
Collection period	50.40
Days cash-on-hand, all sources	93.8
Days cash-on-hand, short-term sources	30.5
Average payment period	51.8
Profitability	
Operating margin (%)	1.16
Total margin (%)	3.40
Return on net assets (%)	5.570
Asset efficiency	
Total asset efficiency	1.0
Age of plant (years)	10.20
Fixed asset turnover	2.32
Current asset turnover	3.72
Inventory turnover	54.69
Capital structure	
Net asset financing (%)	56.50
Long-term debt to capitalization	26.30
Debt service coverage	3.02
Cash flow to debt (%)	21.70

Source: Adapted from Optum (2014). Used with permission.

The collection period is also called days in accounts receivable and is a measure of how long the average patient (or payer) takes to pay the bill after discharge. It is directional; higher values indicate the organization is collecting its bills slowly, and may indicate liquidity problems; lower values indicate more rapid collections, which lead to more available cash.

- **Days Cash on Hand, Short-Term Sources**

$$\frac{\text{Cash} + \text{Temporary investments}}{(\text{Total expenses} - \text{Depreciation expenses})/365}$$

- **Days Cash on Hand, All Sources**

$$\frac{\text{Cash} + \text{Temporary investments} + \text{Unrestricted long-term investments}}{(\text{Total expenses} - \text{Depreciation expenses})/365}$$

Days cash on hand is a measure of how long an organization could meet its obligations if cash receipts were discontinued. Higher values indicate liquidity.

- **Average Payment Period**

$$\frac{\text{Total current liabilities}}{(\text{Total expenses} - \text{Depreciation expenses})/365}$$

Average payment period is a measure of how long the organization takes to pay its obligations. Lower values indicate liquidity and are preferable.

PROFITABILITY RATIOS

profitability ratios
Ratios that measure an organization's ability to exist and grow.

Profitability ratios reflect an organization's ability to exist and grow by measuring the relationship of revenues to expenses. Profitability is a two-edged sword for not-for-profit healthcare organizations in that too much profit brings criticism from the community (and possibly the Internal Revenue Service) and too little profit brings criticism from the governing body.

- **Operating Margin**

$$\frac{\text{Operating income}}{\text{Total operating revenue}} \times 100$$

Operating margin is operating income divided by total operating revenue and reflects profits from only operations. Higher values indicate profitability.

- **Total Margin**

$$\frac{\text{Excess of revenues over expenses}}{\text{Total operating revenue}} \times 100$$

Total margin is the excess of revenues over expenses divided by total operating revenues and reflects profits from both operations and nonoperations (typically investment income). Higher values indicate profitability.

- **Return on Net Assets**

$$\frac{\text{Excess of revenues over expenses}}{\text{Net assets}} \times 100$$

Return on net assets (equity) is the basic measure of profit in relationship to investment. Higher values reflect profitability.

ASSET EFFICIENCY RATIOS

Asset efficiency ratios reflect an organization's ability to be efficient by measuring the relationship between revenue and assets. For purposes of these ratios, total revenue includes net nonoperating gains.

asset efficiency ratios
Ratios that measure efficiency by comparing revenue to assets.

- **Total Asset Turnover**

$$\frac{\text{Total operating revenue + Other income}}{\text{Total assets}}$$

Total asset turnover is the basic measure of how efficiently an organization is using its assets in relation to making revenue. Higher values usually indicate higher efficiency; however, older facilities with assets that are mostly depreciated may appear to be efficient because of a low numerator. Cleverley (2010) recommends calculating the age of plant ratio to determine whether efficiency or an older facility is causing a high total asset turnover ratio. The formula to determine the average age of a facility is

$$\frac{\text{Accumulated depreciation}}{\text{Depreciation expense}}$$

Lower values are preferable.

- **Fixed Asset Turnover**

$$\frac{\text{Total operating revenue + Other income}}{\text{Net fixed assets}}$$

Fixed asset turnover is a subset of the total asset turnover in that it measures how efficiently an organization is using its fixed assets (usually property, plant, and equipment) in relation to generating revenue. Higher values indicate higher efficiency.

- **Current Asset Turnover**

$$\frac{\text{Total operating revenue} + \text{Other income}}{\text{Current assets}}$$

Current asset turnover measures how efficiently an organization is using its current assets in relation to generating revenue. Higher values indicate higher efficiency and can be obtained by increasing revenue proportionately more than current assets or decreasing current assets proportionately more than total revenue.

- **Inventory Turnover**

$$\frac{\text{Total operating revenues} + \text{Other income}}{\text{Inventory}}$$

Inventory turnover measures the number of times an organization turns over its inventory relative to total operating revenue and other income. Low values usually indicate overstocking.

CAPITAL STRUCTURE RATIOS

capital structure ratios
Ratios that measure an organization's long-term liquidity by measuring a variety of relationships to capital.

Capital structure ratios reflect the organization's long-term liquidity by measuring a variety of relationships to capital. Capital structure ratios are used by banks and bond rating agencies to determine creditworthiness.

- **Net Asset Financing**

$$\frac{\text{Net assets}}{\text{Total assets}} \times 100$$

Net asset (equity) financing measures the relationship between assets owned by the organization (i.e., assets minus liabilities) and total assets. This is nondirectional; higher values are usually preferable. However, high-performing hospitals use debt financing, which lowers this ratio, but not excessively.

- **Long-Term Debt to Capitalization**

$$\frac{\text{Long-term debt}}{\text{Long-term debt} + \text{Net assets}} \times 100$$

Long-term debt to capitalization measures the relationship between long-term debt and assets owned by the organization. Lower values are preferable, whereas higher values imply a greater reliance on debt financing and may indicate a reduced ability to take on additional debt.

- **Debt Service Coverage**

$$\frac{\text{Excess of revenues over expenses + Depreciation expense + Interest expense}}{\text{Debt principal payment + Interest payments}}$$

Debt service coverage measures the ability to meet long-term debt obligations. Higher values indicate an organization's ability to meet long-term debt obligations. Because hospital profitability declined in 2007 and 2008, and as a result, debt service coverage also declined during that period, some hospitals were in violation of debt service coverage thresholds in their bond indentures. However, during 2009 hospital profitability and debt service coverage increased. Note: Principal payments are found as payments on long-term debt on the statement of cash flows.

- **Cash Flow to Debt**

$$\frac{\text{Excess of revenues over expenses + Depreciation expense}}{\text{Current liabilities + Long-term debt}} \times 100$$

Cash flow to debt measures the ability to meet both short-term and long-term obligations. Higher values indicate an organization's ability to meet both short-term and long-term obligations, and lower values indicate a possible problem in meeting long-term obligations. Cleverley (2010) indicates that the cash flow to debt ratio is one of the best predictors of financial failure in organizations.

OPERATING INDICATORS

In addition to ratio analysis using information found in the financial statements, management may also analyze the following operating indicators, which are important measures of financial performance in relation to operations. Operating indicator information is not usually found on the financial statements, but it should be readily available on a variety of reports used by management.

- **Average Length of Stay**

$$\frac{\text{Patient days}}{\text{Discharges}}$$

> ⚠ **CRITICAL CONCEPTS**
> Creating a Financial Analysis
>
> You are the financial manager of Clark Pediatrics Center and you have a meeting with the board of directors in a month. You need to create a financial analysis of the organization. You have also been asked to compare Clark Pediatrics to other pediatric healthcare organizations in the area to create a trend comparison. What must you do to complete a financial analysis? What information do you need for both horizontal analysis and vertical analysis? What sources can you use for comparison? What kind of decisions can be made regarding this information?

The average length of stay (ALOS) measures how long patients stay in the hospital on average. Because a high percentage of hospital patients either reimburse the hospital per case or are on a capitated arrangement, lower ALOSs that hold down costs are preferable. However, hospital management should be aware of the incremental costs associated with keeping patients longer before developing rigorous discharge policies to lower their ALOS. Median ALOS for all hospitals reporting to Optum (2014) for 2012 was 4.50. Hospital management should also be aware that ALOS varies for a variety of reasons, including case mix. Adjusted ALOS usually means that ALOS has been adjusted for case mix. Median ALOS adjusted for case mix for all hospitals reporting to Optum (2014) for 2012 was 2.7.

• **Occupancy Rate**

$$\frac{\text{Patient days}}{365 \times \text{Licensed beds}}$$

Occupancy rate measures capacity, or the percentage of the hospital that is being used. Higher values are typically preferable unless a large portion of the hospital's business is represented by capitation agreements. Median occupancy rate for all hospitals reporting to Optum (2014) for 2012 was 49.4. Hospital management should also be aware that occupancy rate varies for a variety of reasons, including the difference between licensed beds in the facility and staffed beds in the facility. Median occupancy rate for staffed beds for all hospitals reporting to Optum (2014) for 2012 was 55.7.

FINANCIAL ANALYSIS AND ANNUAL REPORTS

For-profit organizations prepare annual reports, which report financial and other information, and send them to their stockholders. Only recently have not-for-profit organizations begun preparing annual reports as a vehicle of communication and accountability to the community.

There are several principles for preparing good reports, including annual reports:

◆ *Audience and purpose:* Management should prepare reports with the audience and purpose as the central focus. Preparing reports that readers will not understand is always dangerous. For instance, executive management should use a different level of detail in preparing a report for department managers and preparing a report for the governing body. In addition to audience, management should always keep in mind the primary reason for the report. For instance, annual reports for for-profit organizations that have selling stock as a primary purpose will attract attention by using lots of color. Not-for-profit organizations, which must be more concerned about costs incurred, should provide an austere, yet functional, annual report.

◆ *Timeliness:* Reports designed to provide control within the organization, such as budget reports, must be prepared and distributed in a timely manner to maximize the effects of corrective action.

◆ *Accuracy:* Accuracy in reporting information is more important than timeliness. Reports with mistakes are detrimental to the organization because they create credibility problems.

◆ *Clarity:* Reports should be clear and concise to the audience and should leave little room for misinterpretation.

◆ *Comparability:* Reports should maintain formats to accommodate easy comparisons from statement period to statement period and among different organizations.

◆ *Commentary:* Reports should provide explanations when necessary. Even financial statements should provide explanations in the form of notes to the financial statements.

◆ *Meaningfulness:* Reports should be used for better decision making, which can only happen if the information is needed by the decision maker.

Annual reports provide accountability of the organization to the stockholders and act as a vehicle to sell more stock.

CHAPTER KEY POINTS

➤ Financial analysis includes three steps: establish the facts in the organization, compare facts in the organization over time and to facts in similar organizations, and use perspective and judgment to make decisions regarding the comparisons.

➤ The balance sheet represents the organization's assets, liabilities, and net assets.

➤ The statement of operations summarizes the organization's net revenues, expenses, and excess of net revenues over expenses.

➤ The statement of changes in net assets is the equity in a for-profit organization.

➤ The statement of cash flows categorizes an organization's cash flows.

➤ Ratio analysis compares facts over time of an organization and compares this information to similar organizations.

➤ Operating indicators measure the financial performance in relation to operations.

DISCUSSION QUESTIONS

1. Explain the three steps in financial analysis at the organizational level.

2. What is the purpose of creating a balance sheet? List the three general classifications of the balance sheet and possible categories under these classifications.

3. For the statement of operations, list the main classifications and the possible categories under the classifications.

4. What types of organizations use the statement of changes in net assets, and why?

5. What is the statement of cash flows? The statement is divided into three segments; list each category.

6. List the four classifications of ratios that the financial statement analysis focuses on.

7. Describe the operating indicators used to analyze the financial performance of an organization.

8. What must an annual report include to be considered a good report?

NOTES

1. Acquiring ratio, trend, and percentage data on specific competitors may be impossible. However, several services sell data in the aggregate for comparable organizations, and some data are published by Moody's Investors Service, Dun & Bradstreet, and Troy.

2. In the 1996 *AICPA Audit and Accounting Guide for Health Care Organizations,* the term "net assets" replaced the term "fund balance" in not-for-profit healthcare organizations for external reporting purposes. Prior to 1996, not-for-profit organizations established numerous self-balancing funds consisting of assets, liabilities, and fund balances. AICPA, and more specifically Financial Accounting Standards Board (FASB) Statement No. 117, concluded that some not-for-profit organizations did not always present information about the fund balances on external reports. Although the AICPA and FASB Statement No. 117 do not preclude not-for-profit healthcare organizations from using fund accounting for internal reporting purposes, since 1996 those organizations have been required to classify all fund balances into three broad categories and report the categories on the balance sheet.

3. Statements of cash flows can be prepared using either the indirect method or the direct method. The indirect method of computing cash flows is based on accrual accounting changes in various assets and liabilities. The direct method is based on the actual changes in cash accounts for revenues and expenses. The direct method, which is recommended by FASB Statement No. 95, focuses on the primary sources of cash, such as patients and third-party payers, and uses of cash, such as salaries and supplies. The computation of the direct method is a complex process because of the number of accruals in each line item.

RECOMMENDED READINGS—PART V

Berger, S. 2005. *The Power of Clinical and Financial Metrics: Achieving Success in Your Hospital.* Chicago: Health Administration Press.

———. 2008. *Understanding Nonprofit Financial Statements,* 3rd ed. Washington, DC: BoardSource.

Baker, J. J., and R. W. Baker. 2014. *Health Care Finance: Basic Tools for Nonfinancial Managers,* 4th ed. Burlington, MA: Jones & Bartlett Learning.

Brigham, E. F. 1992. "Analysis of Financial Statements." *Fundamentals of Financial Management,* 6th ed. New York: Dryden Press.

Cleverley, W., P. H. Song, and J. O. Cleverley. 2010. *Essentials of Healthcare Finance,* 7th ed. Burlington, MA: Jones & Bartlett Learning.

Finkler, S. A., T. Calabrese, R. Purtell, and D. L. Smith. 2012. *Financial Management for Public, Health, and Nonprofit Organizations,* 4th ed. Upper Saddle River, NJ: Prentice Hall.

Finkler, S. A., and D. M. Ward. 2006. *Accounting Fundamentals for Health Care Management.* Burlington, MA: Jones & Bartlett Learning.

Gapenski, L. C. 2011. *Healthcare Finance: An Introduction to Accounting and Financial Management*, 5th ed. Chicago: Health Administration Press.

Gapenski, L. C., and G. H. Pink. 2010. *Understanding Healthcare Financial Management*, 6th ed. Chicago: Health Administration Press.

McLean, R. A. 1996. "Organizational Diagnostics: Financial Statement Analysis." In *Financial Management in Health Care Organizations*. New York: Delmar Publishers.

Nowicki, M. 2006. *HFMA's Introduction to Hospital Accounting*, 5th ed. Chicago: Health Administration Press.

Zelman, W. N., M. J. McCue, and N. D. Glick. 2014. *Financial Management of Health Care Organizations*, 4th ed. San Francisco: Jossey-Bass Publishers.

RATIO ANALYSIS

Ratio Analysis Practice Problem

Using the financial statements for Bobcat Hospital in Chapter 14, calculate the following ratios for 2012:

Current ratio

Collection period ratio

Days cash on hand, short-term sources, ratio

Days cash on hand, all sources, ratio

Average payment period ratio

Operating margin ratio

Excess margin ratio

Return on net assets ratio

Total asset turnover ratio

Age of plant ratio

Fixed asset turnover ratio

Current asset turnover ratio

Inventory ratio

Net asset financing ratio

Long-term debt capitalization ratio

Debt service coverage ratio

Cash flow to debt ratio

Ratio Analysis Practice Problem Solution

Current ratio

$$\frac{\text{Total current assets}}{\text{Total current liabilities}} = \frac{\$4,207}{\$1,530} = 2.75$$

Collection period ratio

$$\frac{\text{Net receivables}}{\text{Net patient service revenue}/365} = \frac{\$3,717}{\$7,643/365} = 177.507$$

Days cash on hand, short-term sources, ratio

$$\frac{\text{Cash} + \text{Temporary investments}}{(\text{Total expenses} - \text{Depreciation expense})/365} = \frac{\$280 + \$30}{(\$8,786 - \$443)/365} = 13.562$$

Days cash on hand, all sources, ratio

$$\frac{\text{Cash} + \text{Temporary investments} + \text{Unrestricted long-term investments}}{(\text{Total expenses} - \text{Depreciation expenses})/365}$$

$$= \frac{\$280 + \$30 + \$85}{(\$8,786 - \$443)/365} = 17.281$$

Average payment period ratio

$$\frac{\text{Total current liabilities}}{(\text{Total expenses} - \text{Depreciation expense})/365} = \frac{\$1,530}{(\$8,786 - \$443)/365} = 66.935$$

Operating margin ratio

$$\frac{\text{Operating income}}{\text{Total operating revenue}} \times 100 = \frac{\$-696}{\$8,090} \times 100 = -8.603\%$$

Total margin ratio

$$\frac{\text{Excess of revenues over expenses}}{\text{Total operating revenue}} \times 100 = \frac{\$-61}{\$8,090} \times 100 = -7.553\%$$

Return on net assets ratio

$$\frac{\text{Excess of revenue over expenses}}{\text{Total net assets}} \times 100 = \frac{\$-611}{\$5,196} \times 100 = -11.759\%$$

Total asset turnover ratio

$$\frac{\text{Total operating revenue} + \text{Other income}}{\text{Total assets}} = \frac{\$8,090 + \$85}{\$10,266} = 0.799$$

Age of plant ratio

$$\frac{\text{Accumulated depreciation}}{\text{Depreciation expense}} = \frac{\$1,660}{\$443} = 3.747$$

Fixed asset turnover ratio

$$\frac{\text{Total operating reveune} + \text{Other income}}{\text{Net fixed assets}} = \frac{\$8,090 + \$85}{\$4,920} = 1.662$$

Current asset turnover ratio

$$\frac{\text{Total operating revenue} + \text{Other income}}{\text{Total current assets}} = \frac{\$8,090 + \$85}{\$4,207} = 1.943$$

Inventory turnover ratio

$$\frac{\text{Total operating revenue} + \text{Other income}}{\text{Inventory}} = \frac{\$8,090 + \$85}{\$140} = 58.393$$

Net assets financing ratio

$$\frac{\text{Total net assets}}{\text{Total assets}} \times 100 = \frac{\$5,196}{\$10,226} \times 100 = 50.812$$

Long-term debt to capitalization

$$\frac{\text{Long-term debt}}{\text{Long-term debt} + \text{Net assets}} \times 100 = \frac{\$3,500}{\$3,500 + \$5,196} \times 100 = 40.248\%$$

Debt service coverage ratio

$$\frac{\text{Excess of revenues over expenses} + \text{Interest expense} + \text{Depreciation}}{\text{Interest} + \text{Principal payments}}$$

$$= \frac{\$-611 + \$443 + \$109}{\$178 + \$109} = -0.206$$

Cash flow to debt ratio

$$\frac{\text{Excess of revenues over expenses} + \text{Depreciation}}{\text{Current liabilities} + \text{Long-term debt}} \times 100$$

$$= \frac{\$-611 + \$443}{\$1,530 + \$3,500} \times 100 = -3.340$$

Ratio Analysis Self-Quiz Problem

Using the financial statements for Bobcat Hospital in Chapter 14, calculate the following ratios for 2013 and indicate whether they are better or worse than the 2012 ratios. Indicate whether the 2013 ratios are better or worse than the benchmarks using the Optum medians for each ratio (see Exhibit 14.4):

Current ratio

Collection period ratio

Days cash on hand, short-term sources, ratio

Days cash on hand, all sources, ratio

Average payment period ratio

Operating margin ratio

Excess margin ratio

Return on net assets ratio

Total asset turnover ratio

Age of plant ratio

Fixed asset turnover ratio

Current asset turnover ratio

Inventory ratio

Net asset financing ratio

Long-term debt to capitalization ratio

Debt service coverage ratio

Cash flow to debt ratio

M:
AND FUTURE

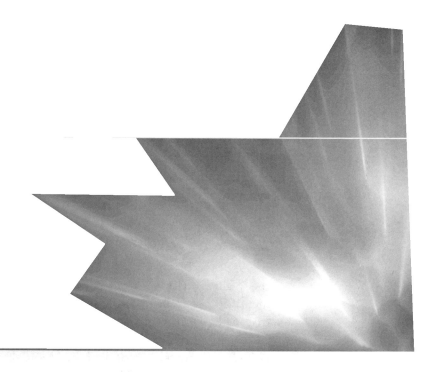

The bill I'm signing will set in motion reforms that generations of Americans have fought for and marched for and hungered to see. Today we are affirming that essential truth, a truth every generation is called to rediscover for itself, that we are not a nation that scales back its aspirations.

President Barack Obama, while signing the
Affordable Care Act on March 23, 2010

LEARNING OBJECTIVES

After completing this chapter, you should be able to do the following:

➤ Identify the need for healthcare reform

➤ Compare and contrast healthcare reform proposals

➤ Discuss the Affordable Care Act of 2010

➤ Explain the need for entitlement reform

➤ Discuss various state proposals for healthcare reform

HEALTHCARE REFORM

NEED FOR HEALTHCARE REFORM

The need for national healthcare reform has focused on three problems: quality, access, and cost.

QUALITY

In 1999, the Institute of Medicine (IOM) published *To Err Is Human,* which reframed the quality movement from improvement of quality to reduction of errors. The report identified the scope and extent of medical errors in American hospitals and concluded that medical errors kill between 46,000 and 98,000 Americans every year. An additional 1.2 million Americans suffer an adverse event caused by the hospital that results in an extended hospitalization or disability. More than half of the adverse events were reported as preventable (IOM 1999).

In 2001, the IOM published *Crossing the Quality Chasm,* which called for fundamental change in the delivery of healthcare to improve quality and reduce medical error. The report provided a set of six performance expectations for the twenty-first century healthcare system (safe, effective, patient-centered, timely, efficient, and equitable), a new framework to better align financial incentives with better practice (accountability), steps to promote evidence-based practice and clinical information systems, and ten new rules to guide patient–clinician relationships (IOM 2001).

ACCESS

One of the goals of the Healthy People 2020 program is to improve access to comprehensive, quality healthcare services. The percentage of persons who had health insurance increased from 84.3 percent in 2011 to 84.6 percent in 2012, or about 48 million (see Exhibit 15.1). While not statistically significant, there were increases in the percentage insured in every age cohort except 35 to 44 (DeNavas-Walt, Proctor, and Smith 2013).

The percentage of persons who had access to a usual primary care provider declined from 78.2 percent in 2001 to 76.8 percent in 2011 (HHS 2013).

Proponents of healthcare reform to ensure access argue that 17.2 percent of Americans, or approximately 55 million Americans, were without health insurance before reform. Many proponents feel that healthcare is the right of every American.

Opponents of healthcare reform argue that while 17.2 percent of Americans are without insurance, 82.8 percent of Americans have insurance. Opponents also argue that insurance coverage is available for many Americans in need: Medicare for the elderly, Medicaid for the poor and disabled, and Temporary Assistance for Needy Families (TANF) and Children's Health Insurance Program (CHIP) for children. Opponents argue that most of the uninsured represent the young (see Exhibit 15.1) whose risk for serious illness and

Exhibit 15.1
Insured by Age
Group, 2012

Age Group	% Insured
Overall	84.6
Under 19	91.1
19–25	72.8
26–34	72.8
35–44	78.9
45–64	83.8
65+	1.5

SOURCE: DeNavas-Walt, Proctor, and Smith (2013).

resulting large healthcare expenditures is small (see Exhibit 15.2). Opponents also argue that many of the uninsured are employed (85 percent) and earn more than the federal poverty level for Medicaid eligibility but refuse to purchase health insurance because it is too expensive (Scalise and Thrall 2002).

Cost

The argument for healthcare reform to reduce costs is far more compelling; employers, employees, taxpayers, and patients are seemingly all in agreement that healthcare costs are too high. Exhibit 15.3 shows the projected growth in healthcare expenditures, per capita

Exhibit 15.2
Health
Expenditures by
Age Group, 2009

Age Group	Total Personal Healthcare Expenditures per Person ($)
All ages	4,850
Under 6	2,711
6–17	1,941
18–44	3,285
45–64	6,266
65+	10,082

Note: Data compiled for persons with at least one healthcare expenditure during the year.
SOURCE: National Center for Health Statistics (2013).

healthcare expenditures, and healthcare expenditures as a percent of gross domestic product (GDP) since 2009 and projected through 2022.

The federal government is projected to account for 30 percent of the $3 trillion spent on healthcare in 2014, while state and local government will account for an additional 6.4 percent of total expenditures. Because professional providers and hospitals are the largest recipients of healthcare dollars (27.2 percent and 31.5 percent, respectively, projected in 2014), understanding the government's growing emphasis on reducing the rate of growth for expenditures for hospital and physician care is easy (Cuckler et al. 2013).

President Obama summarized the problem of rising healthcare costs in a speech to the joint session of Congress in 2010.

Then there's the problem of rising cost. We spend one and a half times more per person on health care than any other country, but we aren't any healthier for it. This is one of the reasons that insurance premiums have gone up three times faster than wages. It's

Exhibit 15.3
Projected Growth in Healthcare Expenditures, Total Expenditures, per Capita, and Percent of GDP

Year	Health Expenditures (in $ billions)	Per Capita ($)	Percent GDP*
1950	12.7	82	4.4
1960	26.9	146	5.3
1970	73.2	341	7.1
1980	247.3	1,052	8.9
1990	699.5	2,691	12.2
2000	1,310.0	4,670	13.3
2010	2,600.0	8,417.2	17.4
2011	2,700.7	8,680.0	17.3
2012	2,806.6	8,948.4	17.2
2013	2,914.7	9,216.3	18.0
2014	3,093.2	9,697.3	18.3
2015	3,273.4	10,172.1	18.4
2018	3,889.1	11,771.2	18.5
2022	5,008.8	14,663.8	19.9

* GDP = gross domestic product

SOURCE: Cuckler et al. (2013); Martin et al. (2014).

why so many employers—especially small businesses—are forcing their employees to pay more for insurance, or are dropping their coverage entirely. It's why so many aspiring entrepreneurs cannot afford to open a business in the first place, and why American businesses that compete internationally—like our automakers—are at a huge disadvantage. And it's why those of us with health insurance are also paying a hidden and growing tax for those without it—about $1,000 per year that pays for somebody else's emergency room and charitable care.

Finally, our healthcare system is placing an unsustainable burden on taxpayers. When healthcare costs grow at the rate they have, it puts pressure on programs like Medicare and Medicaid. If we do nothing to slow these skyrocketing costs, we will eventually be spending more on Medicare and Medicaid than every other government program combined. Put simply, our healthcare problem is our deficit problem. Nothing else even comes close. Nothing else.

Increasing political and economic pressure to reduce the deficits and resulting national debt means that the country must reduce the rate of growth of healthcare spending. This will be especially difficult as the baby boomers, who became eligible for Medicare in 2011, demand greater amounts of healthcare as they age for the next 30 years.

Economists believe, and research supports, that as much as 30 percent of all healthcare spending is inappropriate or unnecessary. In 2009, Thomson Reuters (now Truven Health Analytics) attempted to quantify the almost 30 percent ($700 billion on $2.5 trillion in healthcare spending that year) that could be eliminated without harming quality (Kelley 2009):

- ◆ $250 to $325 billion on unwarranted use

- ◆ $125 to $175 billion on fraud and abuse

- ◆ $100 to $150 billion on administrative system inefficiencies

- ◆ $75 to $100 billion on provider inefficiency and error

- ◆ $25 to $50 billion on lack of care coordination

- ◆ $25 to $50 billion on preventable conditions and avoidable care

Research supports the following ten proposals to reduce costs (or bend the cost curve) in healthcare (Moore, Eyestone, and Coddington 2013):

1. Replace fee-for-service reimbursement with value-based contracting.

2. Increase the supply and effective utilization of primary care physicians and physician extenders.

3. Focus more attention on the management of individuals with chronic disease.

4. Pass tort reform.

5. Discourage the use of physician-owned ambulatory surgery centers, imaging centers, and specialty hospitals.

6. Encourage the formation of multispecialty group practices and integrated systems.

7. Reduce administrative complexity.

8. Stop accepting excuses that providers cannot cover their costs under public programs and must shift unreimbursed costs to the private sector.

9. Expect more from the customer.

10. Develop strategies that work for end-of-life decision-making.

EARLY HEALTHCARE REFORM

The discussion regarding healthcare reform and universal health insurance coverage has a long history in the United States, beginning with Teddy Roosevelt in 1910. Until the defeat of President Clinton's healthcare proposal, the American Health Security Act of 1993, it was unclear whether healthcare reform would be market based, legislation based, or both. Healthcare reform prior to 1994 could best be characterized as reactionary, meaning that policy and resulting legislation reacted to each problem without overall guiding principles.

In 1973, Congress passed legislation to facilitate the development and growth of health maintenance organizations (HMOs). In addition to allocating seed money to develop HMOs, the law also required employers of 25 or more employees to offer HMO coverage, if available, as a competitive alternative to traditional indemnity coverage.

Legislation that ended Medicare cost-based reimbursement for hospitals and initiated a competitive environment under prospective payment was passed by Congress in 1983. Eastaugh (1987) compared prospective payment in the healthcare industry to the deregulation in the airline industry. When routes were deregulated in the airline industry, excess capacity diminished and prices fell markedly (and some would say quality improved). By deregulating payment methods in healthcare, or by eliminating the guaranteed return provided by cost-based reimbursement, excess capacity should be diminished and prices should fall as a result of increased competition.[1]

In 1984, Congress passed the Deficit Reduction Act (DEFRA) that limited the amount an employer could deduct for health benefits for employees, and—because costs beyond the limits were absorbed by employees and, through employees, the employers—employers became sensitive to the costs of health benefits. Managed care became an alternative for many employers seeking to reduce health benefit costs.

Congress then passed the Omnibus Reconciliation Act of 1989, which ended Medicare charge-based reimbursement for physicians and initiated a competitive environment under prospective payment in 1992.

UNSUCCESSFUL LEGISLATIVE ATTEMPTS AT REFORM

During the late 1980s and early 1990s, a variety of healthcare reform bills circulated through Congress. While none of these bills was passed into law, reviewing them in broad classifications is useful for better understanding the Clinton plan's demise and subsequent legislation.

Incremental proposals assumed that the current healthcare system was working well and needed only minor changes. The advantages of the incremental proposals were that they attempted to build on the current public/private healthcare system, spent fewer federal dollars, and enjoyed bipartisan support. The disadvantages included the assumption that the private sector would be able to control costs, the continuance of patching healthcare coverage, and the provision of solutions to symptoms of healthcare problems and not to the problems themselves. Examples of incremental proposals included the Affordable Health Care Now Act of 1993 by Senator Robert Michel (R-IL) and the Health Equity and Access Reform Today Act of 1993 by Senator John Chafee (R-RI).

Single-payer proposals assumed that the current healthcare system was broken and needed a radical change—the provision of near-universal coverage from a single payer, presumably the federal government. Advantages of the single-payer proposals included eliminating cost shifting, providing near-universal coverage, reducing administrative costs by billing one payer, and accommodating spending limits through global budgeting. Disadvantages included shifting resources from the relatively efficient private sector to the relatively inefficient public sector, allowing financing and management by the federal government, and forcing waiting periods for elective procedures. Examples of single-payer proposals included the American Health Security Act of 1993 by Representative James McDermott (D-WA) and the Mediplan Health Care Act of 1993 by Representative Pete Stark (D-CA).

Employer-based proposals assumed that businesses were responsible for providing health insurance coverage to their employees. Advantages included building on the current public/private system, providing increased access, and decreasing the government cost burden. Disadvantages included placing an unfair burden on business and encouraging businesses to dump high-risk workers. An example of an employer-based proposal was Health America of 1993 by Senator Elizabeth Mitchell (D-ME).

Managed competition proposals assumed that the advantages of government regulation, including improved access, could be integrated with the advantages of free-market competition, including lower prices. Advantages included the fixing and provision

single-payer proposal
A health reform idea that a single payer, namely the government, should pay for all healthcare.

employer-based proposal
A health reform idea that employers should provide health insurance for their employees.

managed-competition proposal
A health reform idea that blended government regulation with free-market competition.

of community rating of health insurance premiums, which requires that the fortunate healthy subsidize the unfortunate sick; encouraging competition based on quality; providing portable coverage that employees could transfer from one employer to another; and prohibiting insurers from canceling or declining insurance coverage based on illness, preexisting illness, or high risk for illness. Disadvantages included mandating participation, requiring management of the system by the federal government, establishing community rating of premiums that discourages incentives for leading healthy lifestyles, limiting physician and hospital choice, and limiting access to certain procedures. An example of a managed competition proposal was the Managed Competition Act of 1993 by Senator James Cooper (D-TN).

THE CLINTON PLAN

In early 1992, presidential candidate Bill Clinton seemed to be favoring employer-based proposals while promising to lower healthcare costs to win support from businesses.

The Health Security Act of 1993 had two major goals: to achieve universal coverage, making healthcare a right for all Americans, and to curtail rapidly rising healthcare costs. Building on the success of HMOs in improving access while containing costs, the act proposed a choice of private health insurance plans through regional healthcare alliances, with exceptions to those already covered by Medicare or large employers. Clinton's act was a compromise between the liberals, led by Senator Edward Kennedy (who wanted a single-payer plan) and conservatives, who supported market-based reforms to promote voluntary health insurance (Kooijman 1999).

As Clinton's Health Security Act moved from theory to legislation, conservatives attacked the act as the epitome of big government. Although the content of the act was sound, Congress never voted on it because of several mistakes in strategy on Clinton's part: the insurance industry resisted the insurance reform that was necessary; the conservatives characterized the alliances as cooperatives; the goal of universal coverage led to endless rules and legislative demands; in the face of calls for a balanced budget, conservatives characterized the act as an open-ended entitlement; and the act made some sense in theory, but became increasingly difficult to operationalize (Zelman 1996).

AFTER THE CLINTON PLAN

With the failure of the Clinton plan, no one in Congress or the White House was willing to introduce the massive legislation necessary for managed competition, single-payer, or employer-based healthcare reform. In the absence of such legislation, it appeared that the country was willing to let Congress address the access problem with incremental legislation and to let the free market control healthcare costs with competition.

FEDERAL REFORM

The first major piece of health-related legislation enacted by Congress after the Clinton plan defeat was the Health Insurance Portability and Accountability Act (HIPAA) of 1996, which included the following provisions:

◆ Insurance reform to protect currently insured people from losing coverage as a result of job change or family illness and to require insurance companies who offer small-group insurance coverage to make policies available to all small groups[2]

◆ Medical savings accounts (MSAs)

◆ Administrative simplification, which mandated the development of standardized electronic billing, claims, and remittance

◆ Healthcare tax rule changes, which allowed the self-employed to increase their deduction for healthcare costs and insurance premiums from 30 percent in 1996 to 80 percent by 2006 and made long-term care costs and insurance premiums and costs tax deductible

◆ Medicare fraud and abuse changes

The Balanced Budget Act (BBA) of 1997, in addition to cutting Medicare expenditures over a five-year period, included provisions for increasing access. It allowed provider-sponsored organizations to bid on Medicare and Medicaid business and gave states the option to require Medicaid beneficiaries to enroll in managed care plans. The act also adopted Kids Care, a proposal to provide $23.4 billion over five years to expand health coverage for children whose parents' income is too high to qualify for Medicaid but too low to afford private insurance. The act also established the sustainable growth rate (SGR), which calculates the amount of increase physicians would receive each year from Medicare.

After significant evidence that the BBA was cutting more than the projected $115 billion from the budget (some estimate that it cut two to three times more than the $115 billion originally intended), Congress passed and the president signed the Balanced Budget Refinement Act (BBRA) in November 1999. The plan provided an estimated $16 billion in increased Medicare payments to providers over five years.

In December 2000, Congress passed and the president signed the Medicare, Medicaid, and SCHIP Benefits Improvement and Protection Act (BIPA). BIPA provided about $35 billion in Medicare relief over five years and increased Medicare and Medicaid healthcare provider payments; added preventive benefits and reduced beneficiary cost sharing under Medicare; and improved insurance options for low-income children, low-income families, and low-income seniors.

In late November 2003, Congress passed the Medicare Prescription Drug, Improvement, and Modernization Act (MMA), which President Bush signed in early December. Heralded as the most significant expansion of the Medicare program since its inception, the act was a compromise between Republicans who wanted to privatize Medicare and Democrats who wanted to expand Medicare benefits. In addition to the increased payments to healthcare providers, MMA provided a Medicare-endorsed prescription drug discount card, a Medicare prescription drug benefit beginning in 2006, more rapid delivery of generic drugs to market, and other features.

The Deficit Reduction Act (DEFRA) of 2005 was signed into law by President Bush in 2006. DEFRA achieved $8.3 billion in savings from Medicare and $4.7 billion in savings from Medicaid, including SCHIP, over five years. The act provided for the following (HFMA 2006):

◆   Starting in 2008, reduced Medicare payments for services provided as a result of certain hospital-acquired infections

◆   Addressed the calculation of a hospital's Medicare disproportionate-share hospital adjustments

◆   Provided that Medicare-dependent hospitals—hospitals with 100 or fewer beds and a high proportion of Medicare patients—receive special payments

◆   Reduced the reimbursement to ambulatory surgery centers (ASCs) if the ASC payment exceeds the hospital outpatient department fee schedule

President Bush signed into law the Tax Relief and Health Care Act of 2006, which included provisions to prevent a 2007 cut in Medicare physician payments mandated under DEFRA of 2005.

In 2007, President Bush signed into law the Medicare, Medicaid, and SCHIP Extension Act, which included the following provisions to extend funding for the SCHIP program: extended funding for the program through March 31, 2009; a 0.5 percent Medicare payment increase for physicians for six months; and an extension of transitional medical assistance eligibility for Medicaid beneficiaries for six months.

In 2009, President Obama signed into law the American Recovery and Reinvestment Act, which provided $224 billion for education and healthcare as well as entitlement programs (states received $15 billion in Medicaid relief).

On March 23, 2010, President Obama signed into law the Senate version of healthcare reform—the Patient Protection and Affordable Care Act. On March 30, 2010, the president signed into law the House version of healthcare reform, the Health Care and Education Reconciliation Act. Together, the two laws were projected to cost $940 billion over ten years and provide insurance coverage to an additional 32 million Americans, increasing health insurance coverage to 94 percent of the population (Lubell and DoBias

2010). The reform laws include the following provisions that address the three big problems in healthcare: access, quality, and cost (AHA 2010).

◆ Expand coverage to 32 million people through a combination of public program and private-sector insurance expansions, including a mandate for individuals to purchase health insurance; a mandate for employers with 50 or more employees to provide or contribute to health insurance; low-income subsidies to help individuals purchase health insurance; expansion of Medicaid eligibility to 133 percent of the federal poverty level; and the creation of state-based insurance exchanges to provide low-cost health insurance to individuals and small businesses (fewer than 100 employees).

◆ Reduce the rate of increase in Medicare and Medicaid spending through reduced payment updates, decrease disproportionate share hospital payments, and initiate financial penalties for unnecessary hospital readmissions and hospital-acquired infections.

◆ Adopt several delivery system reforms to better align reimbursement with improved coordination of patient care and quality. These reforms include value-based purchasing; pilot projects to test Medicare bundled payments; and voluntary pilots for accountable care organizations (ACOs).

◆ Provide grants and loans to improve workforce education and training on healthcare issues.

◆ Include provisions to reduce waste, fraud, and abuse in Medicare and Medicaid programs.

◆ Impose new reporting requirements for tax-exempt hospitals.

◆ Place significant restrictions on the expansion of physician-owned hospitals and prohibit new facilities.

The constitutionality of the Affordable Care Act was challenged by 26 states, and the Supreme Court ruled on the act in 2012. While articulating the role of the new Roberts Supreme Court, the court ruled on the following (Carlson 2012):

◆ The individual mandate is unconstitutional under the Constitution's commerce clause.

◆ The individual mandate is constitutional under the federal government's authority to tax.

◆ The Medicaid mandate, putting all of a state's federal Medicaid money at risk if the state does not expand Medicaid eligibility, is unconstitutional.

In response to the unconstitutionality of the Medicaid mandate, the federal government asked the states to expand Medicaid eligibility from 100 percent of the federal poverty level to 138 percent of the federal poverty level (providing Medicaid coverage to an additional 17 million low-income adults and children). In order to incentivize the states, the federal government offered to pick up 100 percent of the expansion costs for the first three years and no less than 90 percent of the expansion costs on a permanent basis. As of January 1, 2014 (the date of implementation of the Medicaid expansion), 25 states and the District of Columbia, largely along party lines, had agreed to expand their Medicaid programs.

The Budget Control Act of 2011 was passed in August 2011 in response to President Obama requesting permission to raise the debt ceiling. The act established the Joint Select Committee on Deficit Reduction to identify at least $1.2 trillion in cuts over ten years. In the event the committee could not identify the cuts, an across-the-board cut in the same amount, called *sequestration*, would automatically be enforced. On December 23, 2011, the Joint Select Committee announced that it could not reach agreement on the cuts. Despite the sequestration, the act continued funding for healthcare fraud and abuse investigations.

The American Taxpayer Relief Act was passed on January 1, 2013, and delayed sequestration for two months. The act raised taxes on the wealthy, generating $600 billion over ten years. Regarding healthcare, the act delayed a pending 26.5 percent cut in Medicare reimbursement to physicians based on the SGR established in 1997. Sequestration went into effect on March 1, 2013, and cut $1.2 trillion in federal spending over ten years ($42 billion in cuts during 2013), including a 2 percent cut from Medicare reimbursement to hospitals, or about $10 billion over ten years.

In late 2013, the House and Senate passed and President Obama signed a two-year federal budget, the Bipartisan Budget Act, averting a federal government shutdown. The budget eliminated many automatic spending cuts and delayed for three months pending cuts to physician reimbursement mandated under the SGR. During the fall of 2013, both the House Appropriations Committee and the Senate Finance Committee discussed an elimination of the SGR in a bill called the Medicare Patient Access and Quality Improvement Act of 2013. The bill proposed replacing the pending 24 percent cut in Medicare physician payment with 0.5 percent increases in Medicare physician payment per year for five years and value-based reimbursement after five years. The Medicare Patient Access and Quality Improvement Act of 2013 was replaced in 2014 by the SGR Repeal and Medicare Provider Modernization Act, which proposed replacing the SGR with a merit-based incentive pay system, which combined three existing incentive programs for physicians: Physician Quality Reporting System, Value-Based Payment Modifier, and the meaningful use of electronic health records. Although the act had broad bipartisan support, the parties differed on how to pay for the amount physicians owed to the federal government under the SGR, estimated by the Congressional Budget Office to be $140 billion. Republicans proposed to pay for the act by delaying the individual mandate under ACA for five years, which Democrats would not support.

STATE REFORM

With the growing state and local expense of providing healthcare to the uninsured and with little hope of federal legislation to address the problem, states have been experimenting with reform on their own. Massachusetts was the first state to address healthcare reform with legislation in 2006, but its circumstance was unique given the relatively low number of uninsured, the agreements with major insurers in the state, and the arrangement with the federal government to help pay for uncompensated care (Mantone 2006). The Massachusetts plan included the following:

◆ An individual mandate for individuals to find health insurance coverage or face a $1,069 per year fine

◆ MassHealth (Medicaid) and SCHIP expansion to provide health insurance coverage for individuals earning up to 150 percent of the poverty level

◆ A state plan, Commonwealth Care, to provide subsidized health insurance coverage for those individuals making between 150 and 300 percent of the poverty level

◆ A mandate for employers with 11 or more employees to provide health insurance coverage to their employees or face a $295 per employee per year fine

◆ A state plan, Commonwealth Choice, to provide health insurance coverage at group rates to individuals making more than 300 percent of the poverty level and to small businesses

◆ A waiver based on an affordability standard for families making less than $114,000 who cannot find health insurance coverage

Because of a slow start in enrolling individuals, 2007 actual costs of $133 million came in under budget. However, 2008 actual costs came in significantly over budget at $625 million and 2009 budget requests were $869 million. Facing large budget deficits in the state, MassHealth (Medicaid) payment levels were reduced. Even with the cost problems, the Massachusetts plan still seems to have widespread bipartisan support of the legislature as well as public support (Larkin 2009).

In 2010, a four-year review of the Massachusetts plan was conducted, with mixed reviews. Uninsured numbers improved from 10.9 percent in 2006 to 6.3 percent in 2010, while per capita health spending is 15 percent higher than the national average (KFF 2012b).

In 2007, California governor Arnold Schwarzenegger announced his healthcare initiative. Citing the uninsured as the major problem with healthcare costs, Schwarzenegger said healthcare to the uninsured cost the average insured family about $1,186 in increased insurance costs, or a "hidden tax," each year. Under his initiative, all Californians would be required to have health insurance coverage. Insurers would be required to guarantee coverage. The initiative would encourage personal responsibility for health and wellness by providing incentives and rewards. After passing the California Assembly in December 2007, a California Senate panel rejected Governor Schwarzenegger's proposal in January 2008 as too risky and too expensive (Rau 2008).

FREE MARKET REFORM

After the defeat of the Clinton plan in 1994, managed care began to dominate the marketplace, having evolved on its own in response to economic pressures. Eighty-five percent of all workers were covered by some form of managed care in 1998, up from 50 percent in 1994. Managed care, although still plagued with complaints regarding limited choice, slowed soaring healthcare costs.[3] Although the nation's spending for healthcare reached $1 trillion in 1996, the amount was only $50 billion more than that spent in 1995, for an increase of 4.4 percent, which was the smallest percent increase in 37 years (Kilborn 1998).

Regarding clinical quality, growing evidence suggests that managed care provides better healthcare than the previous fee-for-service plans. For example, HMO patients are 25 percent less likely to endure futile, painful, degrading, unwanted care during the last six months of a terminal illness. Such care accounts for 21 percent of all Medicare spending (Cher and Lenert 1997). Because of the emphasis on prevention and early detection, managed care should detect cancers at an earlier stage than fee-for-service plans and, as a result, reduce the need for surgical intervention. Regarding patient satisfaction, enrollees continue to complain about managed care limiting the number of providers patients can choose and about waiting times for elective procedures.

As employers continue to seek strategies to reduce healthcare costs and as providers continue to consolidate resources in reaction to market forces, the answer may well be direct contracting, which is discussed in Chapter 4. Direct contracting is the practice of large employers contracting directly with integrated delivery systems or systems of healthcare providers capable of accepting a financial risk and delivering a full range of healthcare services. Direct contracting stimulates competition between integrated delivery systems and encourages local control and innovation. It also reduces administrative costs, which in turn reduces employer health plan costs (Burrows and Moravec 1997).

The need for clinical coordination among physicians and between physicians and hospitals is addressed by the ACA, which authorized ACO pilots for Medicare patients beginning in 2012. ACOs can take many forms, but they generally provide high-quality care at the least possible cost by exploring new ways to minimize fragmented care between professionals in an organizational provider and between organizational providers, avoid repetitive services, and improve clinical and service performance. Several successful ACOs exist today, including Kaiser Permanente and Geisinger Health System, whose models of in-house insurance plans (risk taking) and employed physicians have proven effective in improving quality and reducing costs (HFMA 2010).

THE FUTURE OF HEALTHCARE

With the passage of the ACA, national healthcare reform is a reality. However, three "brutal facts" about the US healthcare system exist, according to Kaufman (2011): (1) the healthcare bubble will eventually burst; (2) neither ACOs nor first-generation clinical integration will produce the desired results; and (3) physician autonomy and the organized medical staff will become less relevant.

Supporting the notion that the healthcare bubble is coming to an end, the Bipartisan Debt Reduction Task Force in late 2010 called for immediate steps to reduce the federal debt caused in part by the aging population and rising healthcare costs (Domenici and Rivlin 2010). The Congressional Budget Office has released projections indicating the ACA will not reduce the deficit by the $143 billion originally planned during the first ten years (Daly 2011). And the *Wall Street Journal* has predicted that the states will be unable to absorb the increased healthcare costs passed to them by the ACA in 2014 (Chen 2011). Kaufman predicts that federal and state governments will continue to reduce payments to providers in the current fee-for-service reimbursement environment, and in the future, governments will move to bundled payments and capitated payments to further reduce healthcare costs.

Regarding the "brutal fact" that neither ACOs nor first-generation clinical integration will produce desired results (significant cost savings through improved quality and efficiency), Kaufman (2011) notes that

◆ generating significant savings on Medicare fee-for-service patients is difficult for integrated medical groups; and

◆ when groups receive shared savings payments, the payments are insufficient to cover the increased costs.

Kaufman recommends a second-generation clinical integration characterized by primary care–based medical homes, electronic health records with point-of-care protocols, disease management programs, relationships with post-acute providers, and a culture (and reimbursement environment) committed to improving cost and quality rather than to maintaining provider autonomy and income.

Regarding the prediction that physician autonomy and the organized medical staff will become less relevant, Medicare reimbursement strategies, such as value-based purchasing (VBP), will hold hospitals increasingly responsible, from a financial perspective, for patient care provided by physicians. Under VBP, hospital revenue will be at risk as Medicare and other insurers reduce payments for hospital-acquired infections and unnecessary readmissions, for example. According to Kaufman, hospitals can no longer afford to delegate the authority for the quality or cost of patient care to autonomous physicians practicing a highly variable model of care. Hospitals will need to work with medical staffs to

◆ modify medical staff bylaws to require conformance to patient safety, patient satisfaction, process, and quality metrics as a condition of hospital privileges; and

◆ develop a medical staff organization in which medical leaders have authority over cost, quality, and patient satisfaction decisions of physicians.

The next reform that will have an important effect on the healthcare industry is entitlement reform (Nowicki 1996b). As president-elect, Obama pledged entitlement reform, saying that the nation's long-term economic recovery was dependent on controlling America's most costly entitlement programs: Medicare and Social Security (Sheer 2009).

The government funds the vast majority of entitlement payments through current tax revenues and the hope for future tax revenues (deficit spending that increases the national debt).[4] Peterson (1996) argues that much of the economic burden for funding current entitlements will fall to future generations. The national debt based on future promised and funded benefits is $62.3 trillion, which represents an additional tax burden of $200,000 for every man, woman, and child in America today (Peterson Foundation 2008).

The deficit commission established by President Obama agreed with many of the entitlement reforms proposed by Peterson. In late 2010, co-chairmen Erskine Bowles, chief of staff in the Clinton White House, and former Republican Senator Alan Simpson presented a draft plan that identifies $200 billion in discretionary-spending cuts by 2015. The cuts include limits on federal spending on healthcare, a gradual increase of the Social Security retirement age, and a reduction in defense spending and federal government spending. On the tax side, the plan lowers the corporate tax rate, increases the gasoline tax, limits tax breaks on second-home mortgages, and increases taxes on social benefits for wealthy seniors (Boles and Vaughan 2010).

CHAPTER KEY POINTS

➤ Healthcare reform attempts to improve quality, lower cost, and increase access.

➤ Healthcare reform during the last 20 years has been incremental in nature, in that it attempted to improve quality or lower cost or increase access.

➤ The Affordable Care Act of 2010 attempted to improve quality, lower cost, and increase access.

➤ In the absence of meaningful healthcare reform from the federal government before 2010, some states attempted healthcare reform.

➤ The free market has attempted reform through managed care movements and direct contracting.

➤ With the passage of healthcare reform, entitlement reform to guarantee the sustainability of federal entitlement programs will be a legislative priority.

➤ Healthcare and the nation's economy will be interdependent in future decades.

DISCUSSION QUESTIONS

1. Discuss the history of healthcare reform.

2. Identify the key provisions of the Affordable Care Act of 2010.

3. Identify the key provisions of the Massachusetts health plan.

4. Discuss why the California health plan failed to gain legislative support.

5. Discuss the two major free market initiatives and their impact on quality, cost, and access.

6. Discuss the need for entitlement reform and what entitlement reform might look like in the future.

NOTES

1. Growth in the number of physicians in relation to the population should increase competition and lower prices. However, the federal government did not take into account the effects of supplier-induced demand, which is the degree to which physicians can control the demand for their services. Several studies during the 1970s reported that higher physician density had little effect on physician income. Three hypotheses have been forwarded to explain this contradiction to the law of supply and demand. The first suggests that an increase in physician density results

in an increase in service to previously unserved populations and stable physician incomes. The second suggests that new demand is physician generated. The third suggests that in the face of increasing competition, physicians simply increase fees in a fee-for-service environment.

2. The law attempts to make insurance coverage more accessible to the self-employed and small businesses by forcing insurance companies that offer such coverage to be less selective.

3. The patient's freedom of choice for providers may be more of an emotional issue than an economic one. The Rand Health Insurance Experiment concluded that patient loyalty to their physicians had a minimal price—patients were willing to change physicians for a small reduction in premiums (patient loyalty to OB/GYN physicians had a somewhat high price). In point-of-service managed care plans, only 16 percent of the enrollees use the out-of-network option, reflecting a relatively high satisfaction level with network physicians (Gabel 1994, in Zelman 1996).

4. While President Bush and legislative leaders argued the best ways to spend the budget surplus, most economists warned that the budget surplus was illusory. Virtually the entire surplus involves the Social Security retirement and disability funds—funds that are earmarked for future retirees and should be accounted for separately from the general fund. When those surpluses were added, the fiscal 1997 budget deficit was only $22.6 billion; when subtracted those surpluses result in a fiscal 1997 budget deficit of $103.9 billion (Sloan 1998).

RECOMMENDED READINGS—PART VI

Brownlee, S. 2007. *Overtreated: Why Too Much Medicine Is Making Us Sicker and Poorer.* New York: Bloomsbury.

Coile, R. C. 2000. *New Century Healthcare: Strategies for Providers, Purchasers, and Plans.* Chicago: Health Administration Press.

Creador, P. 2008. *IOUSA: Part 4 of 5.* www.youtube.com/watch?v=9ain_VXnUhs.

Davidson, S. M. 2013. *A New Era in US Health Care: Critical Next Steps Under the Affordable Care Act.* Stanford: Stanford Briefs.

Dorsey, J. R. 2010. *Y-Size Your Business: How Gen Y Employees Can Save You Money and Grow Your Business.* Hoboken: John Wiley & Sons.

Dychtwald, K. 2000. *Age Power: How the 21st Century Will Be Ruled by the New Old.* New York: J. P. Tarcher.

———. 1989. *Age Wave.* New York: St. Martin's Press.

Eastaugh, S. R. 1994. *Facing Tough Choices: Balancing Fiscal and Social Deficits*. Westport, CT: Praeger Press.

Eberstadt, N. 2012. *A Nation of Takers: America's Entitlement Epidemic*. West Conshohocken: Templeton Press.

Healthcare Financial Management Association. 2001. "Healthcare Financial Management's Healthcare Outlook." *2001 Resource Guide*. Chicago: HFMA.

Helms, R. B. (ed.). 1993. *American Health Policy: Critical Issues for Reform*. Washington, DC: AEI Press.

Herzlinger, R. E. 1997. *Market-Driven Healthcare: Who Wins, Who Loses in the Transformation of America's Largest Service Industry*. New York: Perseus Books.

———. (ed.). 2004. *Consumer-Driven Health Care: Implications for Providers, Payers, and Policy Makers*. San Francisco: Jossey-Bass.

Holland, D., and D. Rohe. 2012. *Surviving and Thriving in Waves of Change: For Healthcare Leaders*. Bloomington: Xlibris Corporation.

Institute of Medicine. 1999. *To Err Is Human: Building a Safer Health System*. Washington, DC: National Academies Press.

Institute of Medicine. 2001. *Crossing the Quality Chasm: A New Health System for the 21st Century*. Washington, DC: National Academies Press.

Kaiser Family Foundation. 2012. "Massachusetts Health Care Reform: Six Years Later." http://kaiserfamilyfoundation.files.wordpress.com/2013/01/8311.pdf.

Kaufman, N. S. 2011. "Three 'Brutal Facts' That Provide Strategic Direction for Healthcare Delivery Systems: Preparing for the End of the Healthcare Bubble." *Journal of Healthcare Management* 56 (3): 163–168.

Kelley, R. 2009. "Where Can $700 Billion In Waste Be Cut Annually from the US Healthcare System?" Thomson Reuters. www.ncrponline.org/PDFs/2009/Thomson_Reuters_White_Paper_on_Healthcare_Waste.pdf.

Kooijman, J. 1999. *The Incremental Strategy Toward National Health Insurance in the United States of America*. Amsterdam: Rodopi.

Kotlikoff, L. J. 1993. *Generational Accounting: Knowing Who Pays, and When, for What We Spend*. New York: Free Press.

Koitz, D. 2012. *Entitlement Spending: Our Coming Fiscal Tsunami*. Stanford: Hoover Institution Press.

Kotlikoff, L. J., and S. Burns. 2005. *The Coming Generational Storm: What You Need to Know About America's Economic Future*. Cambridge: MIT Press.

Modern Healthcare. 2007. "Labor and Delivery: The Connection Between Hospital Performance and Labor Costs." A supplement to *Modern Healthcare* 37 (19): 1–24.

———. 1999. "Bringing the Future into Focus: Envisioning Healthcare 20 Years into the New Millennium." A supplement to *Modern Healthcare* 29 (39): 1–32.

Obama, B. H. 2009. "Remarks by the President to a Joint Session of Congress on Healthcare." www.whitehouse.gov/the_press_office/Remarks-by-the-President-to-a-Joint-Session-of-Congress-on-Health-Care.

Peterson, P. G. 2004. *How the Democratic and Republican Parties Are Bankrupting Our Future and What Americans Can Do About It.* New York: Farrar, Straus, and Giroux.

———. 2004. *Running on Empty.* New York: Farrar, Straus, and Giroux.

———. 1996. *Will America Grow Up Before It Grows Old?* New York: Random House.

Society for Healthcare Strategy and Market Development. 2014. *Futurescan: Healthcare Trends and Implications 2014–2019.* Chicago: Health Administration Press.

Walker, D. M. 2010. *Comeback America: Turning the Country Around and Restoring Fiscal Responsibility.* New York: Random House.

Zelman, W. A. 1996. *The Changing Health Care Marketplace.* San Francisco: Jossey-Bass Publishers.

Zuckerman, A. M., and R. C. Coile. 2003. *Competing on Excellence: Healthcare Strategies for a Consumer-Driven Market.* Chicago: Health Administration Press.

APPENDIX

ANSWERS TO SELF-QUIZZES

Cost Shifting/Cost Cutting (p. 95)

Charge per patient to recover cost = $3,731

Amount of costs to cut = $54,650

Differential Cost Analysis (p. 156)

The sleep disorder program should be kept, showing a gain of $1.2 million.

Job-Order Costing (p. 160)

	RVU	Cost ($)
Amylase	18	69.30
Bleeding time	14	53.90
Uric acid	12	46.20
Platelet count	10	38.50
Hematocrit	9	34.65

Activity-Based Costing (p. 165)

	Total Cost ($)
Evaluation	64.96
Education	77.54
Exercise	53.99

Breakeven Analysis (p. 168)

125 units
Breakeven point = $12,500
80%
Contribution margin = $80

RVU Rate-Setting (p. 189)

	Charge ($)
Amylase	76.23
Bleeding time	59.29
Uric acid	50.82
Platelet count	42.35
Hematocrit	38.12

RVU Rate Setting (p. 189)

Evaluation	69.51
Education	82.97
Exercise	57.77

Hourly Rate-Setting (p. 192)

Rate to break even = $48.00

Surcharge Rate-Setting (p. 195)

Rate to break even = $8.40

Effective Annual Interest Rate on Short-Term Loans (p. 215)

7.25%

Effective Annual Interest Rate on Trade Credit (p. 218)

Annual interest rate of 1,216.67% on day 16
Annual interest rate of 81.10% on day 30

Future Value (p. 220)

Value of investment = $1,643,619

Inventory Valuation (p. 254)

Ending cost of inventory:
FIFO = $3,975
LIFO = $3,850
Weighted average = $3,906

Economic Order Quantity (p. 257)

EOQ = 447.21 units
TC = $100,894

$$\frac{20,000}{447.21} = 44.72 \text{ orders per year}$$

$$\frac{20,000}{365} \times 5 = 273.97 \text{ units on the shelf}$$

$$\frac{365}{44.72} = 8.16 \text{ days between orders}$$

Carrying cost = $447.21
Opportunity cost = $111.80
Cost of average inventory = $1,118.02
Volume of average inventory = 223.61 units
New price to be negotiated = $4.46

Reorder Point Under Conditions of Uncertainty (p. 259)

Low-cost reorder point = 103 units

Payback Period (p. 318)

Payback period = 1.667 years

Present Value (p. 321)

Present value = $22,549

Net Present Value/Internal Rate of Return (p. 324)

–$1,571 NPV (formula solution)

8.642% IRR (formula solution)

–$1,566 NPV (calculator solution)

8.144% IRR (calculator solution)

Ratio Analysis (p. 353)

Current ratio = 2.116—better, good to benchmark

Collection period ratio = 165.427—better, poor to benchmark

Days cash on hand, short-term sources, ratio = 7.547—worse, poor to benchmark

Days cash on hand, all sources, ratio = 11.790—worse, poor to benchmark

Average payment period ratio = 82.547—better, good to benchmark as long as credit is not affected

Operating margin ratio = –0.023%—better, poor to benchmark

Excess margin ratio = 1.076%—better, poor to benchmark

Return on net assets ratio = 2.097—better, poor to benchmark

Total asset turnover ratio = 0.884—better, poor to benchmark

Age of plant ratio = 3.673—worse, good to benchmark

Fixed asset turnover ratio = 1.664—better, poor to benchmark

Current asset turnover ratio = 2.233—better, poor to benchmark

Inventory ratio = 49.926—worse, poor to benchmark

Net asset financing ratio = 44.870—worse, poor to benchmark, though nondirectional

Long-term debt to capitalization ratio = 44.804—worse, poor to benchmark

Debt service coverage ratio = 2.279—better, poor to benchmark

Cash flow to debt ratio = 10.351—better, poor to benchmark

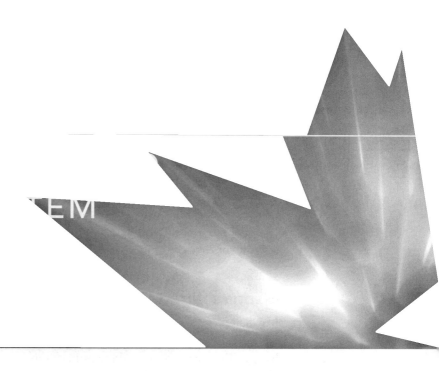

Your IDS

It is December 2014, and you have just accepted the CFO position at Bobcat Integrated Delivery System (IDS). You will be reporting to Mr. Salter, Bobcat IDS chief executive officer, a retired schoolteacher who was hired last year. Also reporting to Mr. Salter are Mr. Wannabe, Bobcat IDS chief operating officer; Dr. Spok, Bobcat IDS medical director; and Ms. Care, Bobcat IDS director of nursing. When announcing your appointment, Mr. Salter stated that your primary objective in the coming year (2015) would be to reverse the ominous financial trend that began in 2013 with an operating loss and continued in 2014. Previous operating losses were funded with investment income (however, investment income was only $200,000 in 2014 because of weakening market conditions). Moreover, your board recently passed a resolution discontinuing that practice and restricting investment income to capital expenditures.

Bobcat IDS is a not-for-profit corporation and includes a 120-bed acute care hospital, a 25-bed skilled nursing facility (SNF), a 15-bed rehab facility, a home health care agency, and an outpatient clinic. The hospital, Bobcat Community Hospital (BCH), is the only hospital in Bobcat, a rural community of 50,000 in your state.

To acquire background information, you decide to meet with each member of the executive team first, then with selected members of senior management.

Meeting with Dr. Spok

Dr. Spok, hospital medical director, told you, "Most doctors have been on the medical staff for at least ten years. There is little loyalty to the hospital, and most doctors also have admitting privileges at County Hospital, a newer public hospital with better facilities 30 miles away. While it is a hassle for the doctors to drive to County Hospital to make rounds, there are few good reasons for the doctors to admit their patients to Bobcat Community Hospital. County Hospital has a hospitalist and pays physicians large amounts of money for menial service assignments like committee work (a practice that Bobcat has refused to participate in)."

Meeting with Mr. Salter

Mr. Salter, CEO, stated, "I just don't understand why we are losing money. I spent a considerable amount of time recruiting new doctors while keeping the existing doctors happy. The new, younger doctors just don't seem to have a sense of loyalty to Bobcat Community Hospital. Furthermore, I've tried to establish a 'family atmosphere' for our employees, which stresses getting along well with others in return for job security. Everyone seems happy. Everyone except Ms. Fi Nance Myway, whom you'll be replacing. She and I both started in January 2013, and she seemed increasingly frustrated with the way I do things here—she just didn't fit in. I tried to accommodate her by implementing some of her recommendations, even though they were against my better judgment—like charging visitors for parking [generating $100,000 in other operating revenue for 2010]. And when I announced that I was bringing in more business to the hospital by entering into a two-year capitated managed care agreement with the city (it expires this month)—we get $250 per month per family for taking care of the 300 city employees and their families, whether they're sick or not—Ms. Myway threw a fit at an executive team meeting. She claimed that my decisions were driving Bobcat IDS deeper into the red. I finally had to show Ms. Myway the highway for insubordination. That happened in November 2014."

Each of the following 20 numbered assignments should be addressed in a one-page memo to the person(s) giving you the assignment. The memo should include a brief summary of the assignment and the results of the assignment, including your specific recommendation(s). You may include relevant attachments to your memo, but only to provide additional detail to your results and recommendations.

1. During the interview, the board made it clear that you will be reporting to it as well as to Mr. Salter. The board has asked you for a confidential report to them on (1) the medical staff and what the board can do to keep them satisfied and (2) the financial job performance of Mr. Salter. (Reflection— what kind of organizational issues does the board create in making this request?)

Mr. Salter has asked you to do the following:

2. Develop a 2014 statement of operations and a 2014 balance sheet (you can assume the format and numbers are correct on the 2013 balance sheet, and you can further assume that all balances carry forward to the 2014 balance sheet, with the exception of accounting for the 2014 loss from the statement of operations).

3. Analyze the Scruggs lawsuit (page 53). I would like your analysis of what we would need to do to avoid a class-action suit similar to Scruggs. Also tell me what the Affordable Care Act (ACA) does for/to nonprofit hospitals.

4. Many of our physicians are now admitting patients at County Hospital because County pays them for service assignments, such as committee work. County also provides physicians with a hospitalist. What can we do for our physicians, and how much will it cost us? Please make sure you explain the typical financial arrangements with hospitalists, whether or not you recommend one.

5. Analyze the ACA as it relates to accountable care organizations (ACOs). Should we become an ACO? What are the advantages and disadvantages?

6. Under the ACA, bad debt expense and charity care expense are projected to decline. Can you give me the rationale for this projection and give me an estimate on expense savings for our hospital?

7. I have received a letter from the Office of Civil Rights informing me that we are under investigation for privacy violations related to HIPAA. What could they be looking at, and how much financial exposure (fines) is possible?

8. US attorneys are reviewing our billing practices and physician relationships. Explain to me what they're looking for and whether you think we have any liability. What actions have been brought against hospitals like ours during the last two years? Do we need a corporate compliance plan and, if so, what should it include? Do rural hospitals get any breaks in dealing with physicians?

9. I need your analysis of three Medicare initiatives. First, Medicare keeps threatening to cut physician payments. Give me the history of this threat; the likelihood this cut will happen and how you think physicians will be reimbursed by Medicare in the future; and what you think physicians will do in reaction, including the possible effect on our hospital. Second, is it true that Medicare will no longer pay for healthcare-associated infections and readmissions? How much revenue will we lose and what should we be doing now in preparation? And third, how much have hospitals, and our hospital in particular, lost in Medicare reimbursement since 2010?

10. Analyze my capitated managed care agreement with the city. Using differential cost analysis for 2014 data, tell me the full cost profit/loss and the differential cost profit/loss. Should we renew the contract for next year at present rates, or should we ask for a rate increase and if so, how much rate increase do we need to cover our full cost? To cover our differential cost?

11. Our radiology department is in violation of antitrust statutes because it created a fee schedule using relative value units (RVUs) developed by the radiologist's professional society. You must establish a new RVU system before we can set FY 2015 rates. The radiology manager has already completed some of the work and I'll send it over to you (see Table V). Please develop a hospital-specific RVU schedule and assign FY 2015 radiology department rates using job-order costing (total radiology expenses for FY 2010 are projected to be $6.5 million).

12. How close is our state to requiring hospitals to release their prices under some consumer-driven or transparent pricing legislation? Should we begin releasing pricing now in anticipation of the legislation? What should we do in preparation of either a mandated release or a voluntary release?

13. I also need your assistance in calculating the following economic order quantity (EOQ) given new data for 2014. Our inventory generally follows Pareto's Law; therefore, I have emphasized controlling those items representing the majority of our inventory activity. One of those items is IV setups. Our current situation is as follows:

    2014 price   = $50
    2015 projected demand = 50,000
    2014 ordering cost   = $25
    2014 interest   = 6.25 percent
    2014 holding cost   = $0.50

The IV distributor would like to distribute a new model setup in 2015 at the same price, but is willing to reduce our carrying costs by making equal monthly deliveries. After discussing the proposal with Ms. Care, I discovered that in-service training will be required for the new model. I believe that each RN will be required to attend a two-hour seminar. I'm not quite sure where to put this training cost in the EOQ formula. Ms. Care also tells me that there are significant quality advantages with the new model, and she thinks we should order and stock the new model. What do you think? If we lose money on the new model, what price can we negotiate with the IV distributor to cover our loss?

14. Develop a five-year strategic financial plan for Bobcat IDS, including benchmarked financial metrics. Our strategic plan calls for a replacement facility about the same size, but at about twice the capital cost as our present facility.

15. For 2015, develop a statistical budget; then develop a revenue budget (using a financial model, determine whether to increase rates and if so, how much) and an expense budget in statement of operations format including detailed footnotes explaining any changes in the numbers.

I would like to see at least five different expense scenarios:

    i. maintain expenses at 2014 levels after adjusting for volumes and mandated expenditures identified in earlier steps;

    ii. maintain expenses at 2014 levels after adjusting for volumes and mandated expenditures identified in earlier steps and honoring all requests (i.e., raises, additional personnel, etc.);

    iii. cut expenses (from expense scenario #1) to break even in 2015; and

    iv. cut expenses (from expense scenario #1) to break even in 2015 and recover FY 2014 losses

    v. cut expenses (from expense scenario #1) assuming Medicare payment levels for all payers

16. Calculate the financial impact of buying a CT unit that would cost $3 million, would have a five-year useful life, would have a 10 percent salvage value, would have a profit per procedure of $400, and would generate an estimated volume of 450 procedures per year. The bank tells me the discount rate should be 10 percent. If the project loses money, let me know how many procedures in addition to the 450 projected per year we would need to generate in order to break even.

17. Our long-term debt represents the remaining balance on a 30-year loan taken out in 1994 at 13 percent with options to refinance every 10 years. If we refinance for the remaining 10 years at 7 percent, how much interest expense will we save over the remainder of the loan?

18. Analyze 2014's financial statements using ratio analysis and identify strengths, weaknesses, and recommendations for improvement.

Meeting with Mr. Operator

Mr. Operator, chief operating officer and a recent graduate from a program in healthcare administration, expressed the following concerns regarding the hospital: "It's easy to understand how we lost money last year—Mr. Salter just won't say no to the doctors... or the nurses, for that matter. Our revenue is down for a variety of reasons and our expenses continue to increase. I don't know why the board ever picked a schoolteacher to run a healthcare system."

Meeting with Ms. Pincher

Ms. Penny Pincher, Bobcat IDS controller, in answer to your question regarding last year's loss, believes the following: "While acute care days are flat and SNF and rehab days and outpatient visits are up, our real financial problems involve our patient mix by financial class—commercial and self-pay continue to decline, and fixed payment and capitation continue to increase, and our board won't approve more than a 2 percent rate increase for 2015 (which affects collections for only commercial and managed care with discount— you need to make assumptions regarding Medicare and Medicaid collections)."

2014 Collections/Discharge

	Acute	SNF	Rehab	Home	ER	Out
Medicare	6,400	4,000	8,000	140	350	190
Medicaid	6,200	4,300	8,300	120	480	180
Commercial	9,600	5,200	10,000	250	800	200

Meeting with Ms. Care

Ms. Patty Care, director of nursing, seeks your support in the following proposal: "While our financial loss is serious, most of it is attributable to low rates—we need to increase our rates to reflect our quality services. Our nurses are overworked and underpaid. I've been working on two solutions that I would like your support on. First, I believe strongly in primary care nursing and as a result, 90 percent of the nursing staff is RNs. RNs can perform more tasks than LPNs and nursing assistants, and therefore are more efficient. This can be further justified by the acuity of our patients. Using the DRG scale as a severity index, our patients are sicker than those in the average hospital. However, I am having some difficulty getting the RNs to administer meds, empty bed pans, and feed patients. Therefore, I have developed a total quality management (TQM) program designed to convince the RNs that all their tasks are important. All RNs are required to attend five hours of TQM training each week. Even though patient days are down, I would like to hire ten more RNs to help cover the floors when the other RNs are in training. In order to recruit these RNs in light of the nursing shortage, we need to increase their average hourly rate to $50, which is competitive with County Hospital (see Table VI-A). This, of course, would be in addition to the cost-of-living raises already announced by the personnel director (Assignment #19 is to calculate the possible nurses' compensation packages). I also would like for you to include a doctorally prepared entry-level nurse in our strategic plan for ten years from now. If physical therapy can require a doctorate for entry level, so should we!"

MEETING WITH MS. PERSONAL

Ms. Personal, personnel director, reluctantly admits the following to you. "Hospital practice in the past has been to give the employees a cost-of-living raise equal to the previous year's percentage increase in the Consumer Price Index. Also, historically, we have allocated 5 percent of total wages to a merit pool to be awarded to meritorious employees based on their annual evaluations. Because Mr. Salter treats the employees like family, virtually everyone gets the raise. Because of shortages in nursing, I am recommending a market raise of 3 percent, in addition to the above raises, to keep us competitive.

"Here is a wage comparison to the facilities that we compete with for new hires (see Table VI-A). Mr. Salter asked us not to announce raises until your financial analysis is complete. In the event we can't give the expected raises, I need an explanation from you giving the reason (Assignment #20)."

MEETING WITH MR. MATERIALS

Mr. Materials, materials manager, reports the following: "I am projecting a 5 percent increase in supply and food prices for 2015 and a 10 percent increase in drug prices. All other prices should remain constant."

TABLE 1

Bobcat IDS Balance Sheet as of December 31, 2013: Assets

	2013
Current Assets	
Cash and cash equivalents	$178,750
Marketable securities	1,100,500
Accounts receivable less allowances	11,250,000
Inventories at cost	3,368,000
Other current assets	992,500
Total Current Assets	16,889,750
Land and improvements	3,250,000
Buildings	36,485,750
Fixed equipment	8,063,250
Moveable equipment	4,466,750
Property, Plant & Equipment	52,265,750
Less accumulated depreciation	(18,080,750)
Total Property, Plant & Equipment	34,185,000
TOTAL ASSETS	**$51,074,750**
Liabilities and Net Assets	
Current Liabilities	
Current portion of long-term debt	$ 2,151,000
Accounts payable & accrued expenses	5,400,000
Estimated amounts due to third-party payers	1,423,750
Other current liabilities	1,500,000
Total Current Liabilities	10,474,750
Long-term debt, net of current portion	37,000,000
TOTAL LIABILITIES	**47,474,750**
Net Assets	
Unrestricted	2,100,000
Temporarily restricted	1,000,000
Permanently restricted	500,000
TOTAL NET ASSETS	**3,600,000**
TOTAL LIABILITIES AND NET ASSETS	**$ 51,074,750**

TABLE II

Bobcat IDS Actual Expenses Through December 31, 2014

Wages, Taxes, Benefits	$ 42,000,000
Professional Fees & Commissions	3,000,000
Drugs	4,000,000
Medical and Other Supplies	4,000,000
Food	2,000,000
Purchased Services	2,000,000
Repairs & Maintenance	4,000,000
Utilities	2,000,000
Interest	4,019,000
Depreciation	6,500,000
TOTAL EXPENSES	**$ 73,519,000**

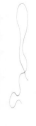

Table III

Selected Industry Financial & Productivity Ratios

Financial Ratios	Benchmark for Your Region*
Liquidity Ratios	
Current ratio	
Collection period ratio	
Days cash-on-hand, short-term sources	
Days cash-on-hand, all sources	
Capital Structure Ratios	
Net asset financing ratio	
Debt service coverage ratio	
Efficiency Ratios	
Total asset turnover ratio	
Age of plant ratio	
Fixed asset turnover ratio	
Current asset turnover ratio	
Inventory turnover ratio	
Profitability Ratios	
Excess margin	
Operating margin	
Return on net assets	
Operating Indicators	
Length of stay	
Occupancy rate	

Productivity Ratios	
Cost per adjusted discharge	$8,100
Nursing Service	
Nursing hours per adjusted discharge	50.00
RNs as a percent of total nursing	32.20
LPNs as a percent of total nursing	21.70
Nursing salary expense per adjusted discharge	$313
Full-Time Equivalent Employees	
Per occupied bed	6.02
Per bed	3.31
Total hours per adjusted discharge	**85**
Compensation per discharge	**$2,000**

*Find a reasonable benchmark for your region. Possible sources include Standard & Poor's, Moody's, Fitch, or Ingenix's *Almanac of Hospital Financial and Operating Indicators*.

TABLE IV-A

Discharges

Service (LOS)	2010	2011	2012	2013	2014
Acute (4)	8,000	7,500	7,000	7,000	7,000
SNF (13)	130	132	134	136	138
Rehab (20)	138	140	142	144	146
Home Health	30,000	25,000	20,000	15,000	15,000
Emergency	32,500	35,000	37,500	40,000	42,500
Outpatient	27,500	30,000	32,500	37,500	42,500

TABLE IV-B

Percentage of Discharges by Payer

	2010	2011	2012	2013	2014
Medicare	43	44	45	45	46
Medicaid	23	24	25	25	26
Commercial	9	7	5	3	2
MC—dis	19	19	19	15	15
MC—cap	0	0	0	6	6
Bad Debt	3	3	3	4	2
Charity	3	3	3	2	3

TABLE IV-C

2010 Charges per Discharge

Per Discharge/Visit	Bobcat	County Hospital
Acute	$9,600	$9,500
SNF	5,200	5,200
Rehab	10,000	9,500
Home Health	250	240
Emergency	800	750
Outpatient	200	180

Table V

Radiology Department Procedures

Procedure	Tech Minutes	Supply Expense	Machine Minutes	2010 Volume
Radiology				
Chest 2-view	14	10	10	20,000
Chest 4-view	28	20	10	15,000
Hand	05	05	05	7,000
Arm	10	10	05	4,000
Foot	05	05	05	1,000
Leg	10	10	05	6,000
Fluoroscopy	30	30	15	3,000
Ultrasound				
Abdomen	15	10	10	5,000
Other	10	10	10	5,622
Nuclear Medicine				
Scan	60	30	30	2,000
CT				
Head w/o contrast	30	50	30	200
Head w/ contrast	60	75	45	300
Body w/o contrast	30	75	30	400
Body w/ contrast	60	100	45	500

TABLE VI-A

Salary Survey of Area Hospitals
Average Hourly Rates (without benefits), December 2014

Position	Bobcat	County Hospital
Head Nurse	$38.00	$35.00
Staff RN	33.50	32.00
Staff LPN	26.00	25.00
Nursing Assistant	20.70	18.00
Lab Tech	32.00	30.00
Rad Tech	28.00	25.00
Food Server	18.40	15.00
Housekeeper	18.40	15.00
Accountant	30.00	15.00
Clerk	21.00	10.50

TABLE VI-B

Bobcat Staffing as of December 31, 2014

Department	FTEs
Administration	50
Medical Records	9
Dietary	35
Housekeeping	25
Laundry	*
Physical Plant	9
Nursing**	365
Laboratory	16
Radiology	9
Respiratory Therapy	5
Physical Therapy	*
Emergency Department Physicians	*
KG/EEG	

*contract

**90 percent RNs, 10 percent clerks

TABLE VII*

Bobcat City and County Ad Valorem/Property Tax Schedule per $100 Assessed Value

Aquifer	.00981
County	.35510
City	.47000
ISD	1.23554
Special Roads Project	.06010
Upper Bobcat River Watershed	.02000

State sales tax   **8.25 percent**

*This table is used only if your state requires nonprofit hospitals to provide community benefits in relation to their potential state and local tax liabilities.

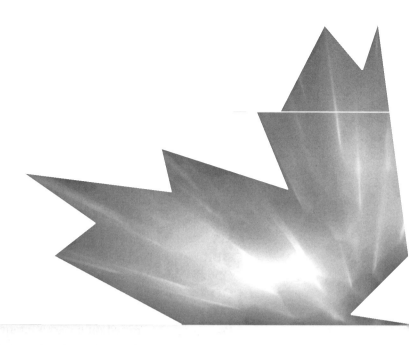

ACA	Affordable Care Act
ACHE	American College of Healthcare Executives
ACO	accountable care organization
AHA	American Hospital Association
AHBE	American Health Benefit Exchange
AHERF	Allegheny Health, Education and Research Foundation
AHIMA	American Health Information Management Association
AICPA	American Institute of Certified Public Accountants
ALOS	average length of stay
AMA	American Medical Association
APC	ambulatory payment classification
ASC	ambulatory surgical center
AUPHA	Association of University Programs in Health Administration
BBA	Balanced Budget Act of 1997
BBRA	Balanced Budget Refinement Act of 1999
BH	Basic Health program
BIPA	Medicare, Medicaid, and SCHIP Benefits Improvement & Protection Act of 2000
CAH	critical access hospital
CBO	Congressional Budget Office
CCO	corporate compliance officer
CDC	Centers for Disease Control and Prevention
CEO	chief executive officer
CEP	coordinated examination program
CFO	chief financial officer

CHIP	Children's Health Insurance Program
CHIPS	Center for Healthcare Industry Performance Studies
CHSO	cooperative hospital service organization
CIA	Corporate Integrity Agreement (also CI)
CIO	chief information officer
CLASS	Community Living Assistance Services and Supports
CMMI	Center for Medicare and Medicaid Innovation
CMP	civil monetary penalty
CMS	Centers for Medicare & Medicaid Services
COBRA	Consolidated Omnibus Budget Reconciliation Act
CON	certificate of need
COO	chief operating officer
CO-OP	Cooperative Health Plan
CPA	certified public accountant
CPT	current procedural terminology
CT	computed tomography
DEFRA	Deficit Reduction Act
DGME	direct graduate medical education
DME	durable medical equipment
DOJ	U.S. Department of Justice
DRG	diagnosis-related group
DSH	disproportionate share hospital
EDI	electronic data interchange
EFT	electronic funds transfer
EHP	essential health benefits program
EIN	Employer Identification Number
EMR	electronic medical record
EMTALA	Emergency Medical Treatment and Active Labor Act
EOQ	economic order quantity (also Q_e)
EPSDTS	early and periodic screening, diagnosis, and treatment services
ERISA	Employee Retirement Income Security Act of 1974
FASB	Financial Accounting Standards Board
FICA	Federal Insurance Contribution Act
FIFO	first-in, first-out
FMAP	federal medical assistance percentage
FMR	focused medical review
FPL	federal poverty level

FQHC	federally qualified health center
FSA	flexible spending account
FTE	full-time equivalent personnel
FV	future value
GAAP	generally accepted accounting principles
GAO	Government Accountability Office
GCD	greatest common denominator
GME	graduate medical education
GNP	gross national product
HAC	hospital-acquired condition
HCBS	home and community-based services
HCCA	Health Care Compliance Association
HCERA	Health Care and Education Reconciliation Act of 2010
HCFA	Health Care Financing Administration
HCFAC	Health Care Fraud and Abuse Control
HFMA	Healthcare Financial Management Association
HHA	home health agency
HHS	U.S. Department of Health and Human Services
HI	hospital insurance
HIM	health information management
HIPAA	Health Insurance Portability and Accountability Act
HIT	health information technology
HMO	health maintenance organization
HRP	high-risk pool
HPSA	health professional shortage area
HRSA	Health Resources and Services Administration
HSA	health savings accounts
HVBP	hospital value-based purchasing
ICF	intermediate care facility
IDFS	integrated delivery and financing system
IFR	interim final rule
IME	indirect medical education
IOM	Institute of Medicine
IPA	independent practice association
IPAB	independent payment advisory board
IPPS	inpatient prospective payment system
IRC	Insurance Research Council

IRR	internal rate of return
IRS	Internal Revenue Service
JIT	just-in-time inventory
LHI	leading health indicator
LIFO	last-in, first-out
LOS	length of stay
LTSS	long-term services and supports
MA	Medicare Advantage
MAAC	maximum allowable actual charge
MAC	Medicare administrative contractor
MACPAC	Medicaid and CHIP Payment Access Commission
MAGI	modified adjusted gross income
MBO	management by objectives
MCO	managed care organization
MEDPAC	Medicare Payment Advisory Commission
Med-Mal	medical malpractice
MDH	Medicare-dependent hospital
MIP	Medicare Integrity Program
MLR	medical loss ratio
MMA	Medicare Prescription Drug, Improvement, and Modernization Act of 2003
MMSA	Medicare medical savings account
MOS	measures of success
MRI	magnetic resonance imaging
MRS	medical record system
MSA	medical savings account
NAIC	National Association of Insurance Commissioners
NPSG	national patient safety goals
NPV	net present value
NR	departments that do not generate revenue
OASIS	Outcome and Assessment Information Set
OB/GYN	obstetrician/gynecologist
OBRA	Omnibus Budget Reconciliation Act
OIG	Office of Inspector General
ODS	organized delivery system

OPPS	outpatient prospective payment system
P4P	pay for performance
PCORI	Patient-Centered Outcomes Research Institute
PERT	program evaluation and review technique
PHI	protected health information
PHO	physician-hospital organization
PHR	personal health record
PI	program integrity
PILOT	payment in lieu of taxes
POS	point-of-service plan
PPO	preferred provider organization
PPS	prospective payment system
PQRI	Physician Quality Reporting Initiative
PRO	Peer Review Organization
PSO	patient safety organization
PSO	provider-sponsored organization
PSRO	Professional Standards Review Organization
PV	present value
Q_e	economic order quantity (also EOQ)
QHP	qualified health plan
RAC	recovery audit contractor
RBRVS	Resource-Based Relative Value System
RCC	ratio of cost to charges
ROI	return on investment
RUG	resource utilization group
RVU	relative value unit
SAS	Statement on Auditing Standards
SCH	sole community hospital
SCHIP	State Children's Health Insurance Program
SEC	Securities and Exchange Commission
SGR	sustainable growth rate
SHOP	Small Business Health Option Program (a type of insurance exchange)
SMI	supplemental medical insurance
SNF	skilled nursing facility
SOI	severity of illness
SNP	special needs plan

SSDI	Social Security Disability Insurance
SSI	Supplemental Security Income
SWOT	strengths, weaknesses, opportunities, and threats
TEFRA	Tax Equity and Fiscal Responsibility Act of 1982
THA	Texas Hospital Association
TQM	total quality management
UPL	upper payment limit
VPB	value-based purchasing

GLOSSARY

Abuse. An unintentional misrepresentation of fact.

Accountable care organization (ACO). An organization that coordinates care among healthcare organizations and physicians. A key element of an ACO is that some portion of its reimbursement is tied to accountability.

Accounts payable. Amounts the hospital owes to suppliers and other trade creditors for merchandise and services purchased from them, but for which the hospital has not paid.

Accrued expenses payable. Liabilities for expenses that have been incurred by the hospital, but for which the hospital has not yet paid, such as compensation to employees.

Activity-based costing. A method of determining product cost by using cost drivers to assign indirect costs to products.

Actual costs. Historic costs incurred.

Allocate. Assign costs to a department.

Asset efficiency ratios. Ratios that measure efficiency by comparing revenue to assets.

Assets. Economic resources that provide or are expected to provide benefit to the organization.

Average collection period. A financial ratio that shows the average time a healthcare organization takes to collect money owed to it.

Average costs. Full costs divided by the number of products or services.

Bad debt. A healthcare organization's unpaid patient bills.

Book overdraft. Process of transferring money from an interest-bearing account to the checking account as the money is drawn.

Capital analysis. A process to determine how much a capital expenditure will cost and what return it will generate.

Capital expenditures. Purchases of land, buildings, and equipment used for operations.

Capital structure ratios. Ratios that measure an organization's long-term liquidity by measuring a variety of relationships to capital.

Capitated price, capitation. A healthcare payment system in which an organization accepts a monthly payment from a third-party payer for each individual covered by that payer's plan, regardless of whether a given individual is treated in a given month. Capitation provides a financial incentive to a healthcare organization to keep its population from using more healthcare services than necessary because the organization only profits if the total cost of treating the specified population falls below the total capitation provided by the third-party payer.

Carrying cost. The cost incurred by the organization for extending credit to the patient after the organization has provided services; the cost of carrying an inventory of items, such as the opportunity cost of the money invested in the inventory.

Cash budget. Predicts the timing and amount of cash flows and systematically examines the cost implications with each alternative.

Cash conversion cycle. The process of converting resources into products or services.

Charge. The amount patients are charged for services; also called *prices* or *rates*.

Charge capture assessment. A comparison of medical records to patient invoices to make sure the organization is not missing billable items.

Charge masters. List of items providers charge for.

Charge master enrichment. An analysis of charges to make sure every item is recognized by third-party payers as a legitimate charge.

Charging analysis. An examination of charges to make sure maximum reimbursement is being received.

Charitable organization. An organization that provides community benefit or serves the public interest. In the case of healthcare, a hospital is a charitable organization if it provides care to people who cannot pay for their care or provides community health benefits.

Charity care. Care provided to patients who the organization knows cannot pay for the care.

Closed-panel HMO. An HMO that contracts with or employs physicians to treat enrollees exclusively (i.e., the physicians do not treat other patients).

Collection period. The number of days between the time of service and the time of payment.

Commercial indemnity plan. An arrangement whereby an employer pays an insurance company, which in turn reimburses hospitals and physicians chosen by the employees.

Common stock. Money invested in the organization by its owners.

Community rating. A premium-setting method in which all groups covered by an insurance company pay essentially the same premiums, regardless of their health risks.

Compounding. The action of adding interest to interest on an investment.

Compulsory health insurance. A requirement that everyone have health insurance.

Consumer-driven plan. A health plan that provides information and incentives to encourage enrollees to make wise healthcare choices.

Controllable costs. Costs that management can control.

Controller. The chief accounting officer of an organization.

Coordination of benefits. Step in the billing process during which the order of insurance company liability is identified for accounts that have multiple insurance companies.

Corporate restructuring. A legal strategy involving the establishment of subsidiaries or related corporations in order to maximize the economic position of a healthcare organization.

Cost center. A department; from an accounting standpoint, a department that consumes money.

Cost-led pricing. Setting prices after costs have been projected.

Cost shifting. Practice of shifting costs to some payers to offset losses from other payers.

Credit-and-collection cost. The cost incurred by the organization for billing and collecting during the organization's average payment cycle.

Current assets. Economic resources that the organization expects to consume in less than one year.

Current liabilities. Economic obligations, or debts, that are due in less than one year.

Debt. Money that is borrowed by an organization.

Deferred revenue. Revenue received by the hospital but not yet earned by the hospital, such as premium revenue from managed care organizations.

Defined-benefit plan. A health plan in which the employer pays the premium, or an established part of the premium, regardless of the cost.

Defined-contribution plan. A health plan in which the employer pays a set amount toward the cost of the premium and the employee pays the rest. Thus if an employee chooses an expensive plan, he pays more than if he chose a less expensive plan.

Delinquency cost. The cost incurred by the organization for the patient not paying on time. These costs can include the costs associated with turning the account over to a collection agency or with writing off the account to bad debt.

Depreciation and amortization. The expensing of long-term assets over time to show their declining value.

Diagnosis-related group. A grouping of similar healthcare cases that should require similar resource consumption. DRGs are used by Medicare to calculate prospective payments.

Differential costing. A method of assembling costs and sometimes revenues to alternative decisions.

Differential costs. The difference in costs between two or more alternatives.

Direct apportionment. A cost allocation method that moves costs from departments that do not generate revenue to departments that do generate revenue.

Direct contracting. The practice of contracting directly with an integrated health organization to service the health needs of a large employer.

Direct costs. Costs that can be traced directly to a department, product, or service.

Directionality. Statistical property for numbers that always improve in one direction and always worsen in the other direction.

Direct service plan. An arrangement whereby an employer prepays specific hospitals and physicians to take care of employees.

Discontinuities. Disruptions to the inventory process, such as the introduction of a new version of a product.

Disproportionate share hospital. Hospitals that qualify for increased payments from Medicare because they treat a high percentage of low-income patients and patients on Medicare, early Medicare on disability, and Medicaid.

Double apportionment. A method that allocates costs from non–revenue-generating cost centers to other non–revenue-generating cost centers (as appropriate), then allocates costs from revenue-generating cost centers to other revenue-generating cost centers (as appropriate), and then allocates costs from non–revenue-generating cost centers to revenue-generating cost centers.

Economic order quantity. The quantity of items that should be ordered each time to result in the minimum total inventory costs.

Electronic data interchange. A method of payment in which the payer, such as Medicare, wires payment to the healthcare organization's bank, and transmits related information to the organization.

Employer-based proposal. A health reform idea that employers should provide health insurance for their employees.

Equity. Money that comes into an organization from investors.

Excess of revenues over expenses. Operating income plus the other income minus total expenses.

Executive committee. A committee of the governing body of an organization that monitors all the other committees.

Experience rating. A premium-setting method in which different groups covered by an insurance company pay different premiums based on their risk.

Factoring receivables. The practice of selling accounts receivable to a third party at a discount. The third party attempts to collect the accounts and keeps the money.

Fiduciary. A person, or governing body, in a position of great trust and confidence. The term is typically used to describe the duty of an entity to be loyal and responsible.

Finance committee. A committee of the governing body of an organization that monitors the CEO's performance in financial affairs.

Financial accounting costs, or accounting costs. The amount of money used for a certain purpose.

Financial analysis. Methods used by investors, creditors, and management to evaluate past, present, and future financial performance.

First-in, first out (FIFO). An inventory valuation system that assumes that the first items put into inventory will be the first taken out. Thus, the value of the remaining inventory is based on the cost of the latest additions to inventory.

Fixed costs. Costs that remain constant in relation to changes in volume.

Float period. The time between when a check is written and when it is presented for payment.

Foundation. A not-for-profit corporation, usually a subsidiary of a for-profit organization, that facilitates education and research or otherwise undertakes charitable projects.

Fraud. An intentional misrepresentation of fact designed to induce reliance by another.

Full costing. A method of assembling direct and indirect costs to a product or service to determine its profitability.

Future value. The future value of an investment, taking into account factors such as interest rate, time, and the frequency of compounding.

Gross patient services revenue. The total amount of charges for patients utilizing the hospital, regardless of the amount actually paid.

Gross receivable. The full amount a healthcare organization charges.

Healthcare Financial Management Association (HFMA). Association of healthcare financial managers; confers four certifications: certified revenue cycle representative, certified technical specialist, certified healthcare financial professional, and fellow of the Healthcare Financial Management Association.

Health Insurance Portability and Accountability Act of 1996 (HIPAA). Legislation that mandated privacy and security regulations for the healthcare industry.

Health maintenance organization. An organization that integrates the financing and delivery of healthcare into one organization.

Horizontal analysis. An evaluation of the trend in a line item that examines the percentage change of that line item over time.

Incremental budgeting. Budgeting only for changes, such as new equipment. The assumption in incremental budgeting is that current budget is already optimal.

Incremental planning. Planning only for changes, such as new equipment. The assumption in incremental planning is that current operations are already optimal.

Indirect costs. Costs that cannot be traced directly to a department, product, or service.

Integrated delivery system. A system of healthcare providers capable of accepting financial responsibility for and delivering a full range of clinical services.

Interest. The expense incurred with borrowed money.

Internal auditor. Staff member who monitors the effectiveness of an accounting system by verifying the system's internal control.

Internal control. Accounting systems and procedures that protect the integrity of an organization's accounting information.

Internal rate of return. The necessary net present value of an investment that, when added to the final market value of the investment, equals the current cost of the investment. In other words, the IRR is the minimum return one needs to break even on an investment.

Inurement. Providing an employee benefit, such as salary, that is greater than the value of the employee's work.

Inventory. The cost of food, fuel, drugs, and other supplies purchased by the hospital but not yet consumed.

Inventory management. The management and control of items that have an expected useful life of less than 12 months.

Inventory turnover. A ratio that measures how many times an organization turns over its inventory relative to its operating revenue.

Investment policy. Directs the chief financial officer or controller in making short-term investment decisions.

Job-order costing. A method of determining product cost by sampling the product's actual direct costs and developing a relative value unit (RVU)—a measure of resources consumed by each product—in varying amounts for each product.

The Joint Commission. The primary accrediting body for healthcare organizations.

Joint venture. A relationship between two business entities entered into for a specific purpose and period of time.

Just-in-time inventory method. Inventory method in which supply items are delivered immediately prior to use.

Last-in, first-out (LIFO). An inventory valuation system that assumes that the last items put into inventory will be the first taken out. Thus, the value of the remaining inventory is based on the cost of the earliest additions to inventory.

Liabilities. Economic obligations, or debts, of the organization.

Liquidity. A characteristic of an investment that pertains to how quickly it can be converted to cash.

Liquidity ratio. Ratio that measures an organization's ability to meet short-term obligations.

Lock box. A system in which payments from patients are mailed directly to a bank, which credits the healthcare organization's account more quickly than if the check had been mailed to the organization.

Long-term debt, net of current portion. A debt that is due in more than one year, minus the amount that is due within one year.

Long-term investments. Economic resources that the hospital owns, such as corporate bonds and government securities, and intends to hold for more than one year.

Long-term liabilities. Economic obligations, or debts, that are due in more than one year.

Loss-leader pricing. Practice of pricing products and services low to attract customers to complementary products and services.

Managed care organization. An organization that manages the cost and quality of and access to healthcare.

Managed-competition proposal. A health reform idea that blended government regulation with free-market competition.

Management connective processes. Management functions that connect elements of the healthcare organization, including communicating, coordinating, and decision making.

Management functions. The key functions of a manager, including planning, organizing, staffing, directing, and controlling.

Managerial accounting costs, or financial costs. Costs that help management make better decisions.

Marginal costs. The cost of producing one more unit of something.

Materials management. The management and control of inventory, services, and equipment from acquisition to disposition.

Medicaid. A program created by the federal government, funded by the federal and state government, and administered by the state government, to provide free or low-cost healthcare to low-income recipients.

Medicare. A federally funded program that provides health insurance to Americans at age 65.

Multiple apportionment. A two-step cost allocation method that makes multiple, simultaneous apportionments during the first step.

National Patient Safety Goals. A set of goals established by The Joint Commission to address safety areas of special concern for hospitals.

Net assets. The difference between assets and liabilities in a not-for-profit organization.

Net assets released from restrictions used for operations. Money previously restricted by donors that has become available for operations.

Net patient services revenue. Patient services revenue minus the amount the organization will not collect as a result of bad debt.

Net present value. The present value of the future cash flow of an investment. NPV takes into account the fact that future cash flows are "discounted" to determine their present value.

Net receivable. The gross receivable minus any negotiated discounts.

Network HMO. An HMO that contracts with physician groups to provide care for enrollees. A network HMO may be either open or closed panel.

Nonoperating costs. Costs associated with supporting the production of a product or service.

Nonoperating or other income. Money earned from non–patient care services, such as investment income.

Open-panel HMO. An HMO that exerts moderate control over physicians by contracting with them to provide care for enrollees. However, these physicians can see other patients.

Operating costs. Costs associated with producing a product or service.

Operating expenses. Money spent on operations to generate revenue.

Operating income. Money earned from providing patient care services; includes the total revenue, gains, and other support minus the total expenses.

Operational planning. The process of translating the strategic plan into a year's objectives.

Opportunity costs. The cost of potential revenue forgone when an alternative is rejected.

Other operating expenses. Miscellaneous expenses that have not been reported elsewhere.

Other operating revenue. Money generated from services other than health services to patients and enrollees.

Overstock cost. The cost of carrying more inventory than demand calls for.

Patient services revenue. Money generated by providing patient care minus the amount the organization will not collect as a result of discounting charges per contractual agreement and providing charity care.

Payback period. The number of years necessary for cash flows to recover the original investment.

Peer review organization. An organization that ensures that providers give appropriate care to Medicare recipients.

Per diagnosis rate. A method of paying for healthcare in which the hospital is paid a flat fee for each given diagnosis, regardless of the actual service provided.

Per diem rate. A method of paying for healthcare in which the hospital is paid a flat fee per day, regardless of the service delivered on any given day.

Permanently restricted net assets. Donor-restricted net assets with restrictions that never expire, such as endowment funds.

Physician–hospital organization. Joint venture between healthcare organizations and physicians that is capable of contracting with managed care organizations.

Planning horizon. The length of time management is looking into the future.

Plant and equipment, net. Economic resources, such as land, buildings, and equipment, minus the amount that has been depreciated over the life of the buildings and equipment.

Pledging receivables. The practice of using accounts receivable as collateral for a loan.

Preferred provider organization. An organization that provides discounted healthcare services to insurance carriers and employers.

Premium revenue. Money generated from capitation arrangements that must be reported separately from patient services revenue.

Prepaid expense. Money paid in one accounting period for something that will be consumed in a later period.

Present value. The current value of an investment.

Price-led costing. Reducing costs after prices, or effective prices meaning collections, have been determined by the payers.

Process costing. A method of determining product cost by dividing the full costs of the organization or department during a given accounting period by the number of products or services produced during the given accounting period.

Production units. The best measures of what an entity is producing. For example, patient days and admissions are both considered production units for a hospital.

Profitability ratios. Ratios that measure an organization's ability to exist and grow.

Prospective payment. A payment system in which a healthcare organization accepts a fixed, predetermined amount to treat a patient, regardless of the true ultimate cost of that treatment. Diagnosis-related groups (DRGs) are one type of prospective payment; Medicare pays hospitals a fixed amount for an episode of treatment based on that treatment's DRG.

Rate-based indicator. Measures a process of lesser importance; a manager initiates an individual case review only after a certain rate is exceeded. For example, a pharmacy manager might initiate case reviews if the expected medication error rate of 5 percent is exceeded.

Ratio. A comparison between two or more financial facts, such as income to assets or assets to liabilities.

Ratio analysis. Evaluation of an organization's performance by computing the relationships of important line items in the financial statements.

Ratio of costs to charges. A method of determining product cost by relating its cost to its charge. This ratio is usually calculated by dividing an organization's total operating expenses by the gross patient revenue. The resulting percentage is then applied to any product's charge in the organization to calculate the product's cost.

Receivables, net. Money due to the organization from patients and third parties for services already provided.

Recovery audit contractor. A private business that detects and recovers improper Medicare payments to providers.

Relevant costs. Costs that are important to a decision at hand.

Resource-based relative value system. A Medicare reimbursement system that provides a flat, per-visit fee to physicians rather than reimbursing them according to their customary charges.

Responsibility costing. A method of assembling costs by cost center or department.

Retained earnings. Income earned by the organization from operations minus dividends.

Revenue center. A cost center (department) that generates revenue.

Revenue cycle. A multidisciplinary approach to reducing the amount in accounts receivable by effectively managing the production and payment cycles.

RVU schedule. A list of charges, such as procedures performed by the radiology department, based on relative value units (RVUs).

Second-party payment. Payment for healthcare that comes from the person receiving the service (i.e., patients paying their own bills).

Semivariable costs. Costs that vary incrementally with changes in volume.

Sentinel indicator. Measures a process so important that every time the indicator occurs, the manager initiates an individual case review. For example, an ICU manager would initiate a review for each patient that dies in ICU.

Shareholders' equity. The difference between assets and liabilities in for-profit healthcare organizations; it represents the ownership interest of stockholders in the organization.

Single-payer proposal. A health reform idea that a single payer, namely the government, should pay for all healthcare.

Skill mix. The mix of different skilled positions in a department.

Skiptracing. Provision of the Fair Debt Collections Practices Act that governs whom collection agencies can communicate with other than the consumer owing the debt and how the agency can communicate with those people.

Specific identification. An inventory valuation system that determines the actual value of each inventory item.

Staffing mix. The mix of full-time, part-time, and temporary employees in a department.

Standard costs. Estimated costs used for comparison.

Strategic planning. Long-range planning that anticipates where an organization will be in three to ten years.

Strategic thrusts. Broad statements of significant results that an organization wants to achieve related to its vision. Also called *goals*.

Step-down apportionment. A cost allocation method that allocates costs from non-revenue-generating cost centers to other non-revenue-generating cost centers (as appropriate) and then to revenue-generating cost centers.

Stock-out cost. The cost of running out of inventory on an item, such as the cost of making a rush order.

Sunk costs. Costs that have already been incurred and thus will not play a role in future decisions.

Tax-exempt. The status that allows an organization to pay no taxes, including sales tax, income tax, and property tax. Tax-exempt organizations may also raise capital by selling tax-exempt bonds, for which they can pay lower interest than comparable taxable bonds.

Temporarily restricted net assets. Donor-restricted net assets that the organization can use for the donor's specific purpose once the organization has met the donor's restriction, such as the passage of time or an action by the organization.

Third-party payer. An agent of the patient (the first party) who contracts with providers (the second party) to pay all or a portion of the bill to the patient.

Trade credit. Credit extended to an organization by vendors.

Treasurer. The person responsible for managing the capital of an organization.

True costs. Hypothetical costs that are the most accurate representation of full costs that can be determined by management.

Uncontrollable costs. Costs that management cannot control.

Unrestricted net assets. Net assets that have not been externally restricted by donors or grantors, such as the excess of revenues to expenses from operations.

Variable costs. Costs that vary proportionately to volume.

Variance analysis. An examination of the differences (variances) between budgeted and actual amounts; variance analysis requires managers to explain why budgeted and actual amounts do not match.

Vertical analysis. Evaluation of the internal structure of an organization by focusing on a base number and showing percentages of important line items in relation to the base number.

Weighted average. An inventory valuation system that uses an average of the costs of inventory items to determine the value of inventory.

Working capital. An organization's current assets; the assets available to run the organization in the short term.

Working capital policy. Sources and methods used to finance working capital, as well as the quantity of working capital to be maintained.

Zero-base budgeting. Budgeting that requires all operations to be justified anew; nothing in the current budget is assumed to be already optimal.

Zero-base planning. Planning that requires all operations to be justified anew; nothing is assumed to be already optimal.

REFERENCES

ABC News. 1991. "The Humana Cost." *Prime Time Live*, August 8.

American College of Healthcare Executives (ACHE). 2013. "ACHE 2013 Members and Fellows Profile." www.ache.org/abt_ache/member_demographics.cfm.

American Hospital Association (AHA). 2014a. "Uncompensated Hospital Care Cost Fact Sheet, 2014 Update." www.aha.org/content/14/14uncompensatedcare.pdf/.

———. 2014b. "Underpayment by Medicare and Medicaid Fact Sheet, 2014 Update." www.aha.org/content/14/2012-medicare-med-underpay.pdf.

———. 2013. "TrendWatch Chartbook 2012." www.aha.org/aha/research/reports/tw/chartbook.html.

———. 2012. "Hospital Capital Financing." www.aha.org/content/12/12-ip-hosp-cap-finance.pdf.

———. 2010. "Healthcare Reform Implementation." *Hospitals in Pursuit of Excellence: A Compendium of Implementation Guides*. Chicago: AHA.

———. 2006. "Bush Signs Tax-Health Care Bill." www.ahanews.com/ahanews/jsp/display.jsp?dcrpath=AHANEWS/AHANewsNowArticle/data/ann_061221_Bush&domain=AHANEWS.

———. 1985. *American Hospital Association Hospital Statistics: 1985 Edition.* Chicago: AHA.

American Institute of Certified Public Accountants (AICPA). 2012. *AICPA Audit and Accounting Guide for Health Care Entities.* New York: AICPA.

———. 2010. *AICPA Audit and Accounting Guide for Health Care Entities.* New York: AICPA.

———. 1996. *AICPA Audit and Accounting Guide for Health Care Organizations.* New York: AICPA.

Arrington, B., and C. C. Haddock. 1990. "Who Really Profits from Nonprofits?" *Health Services Research* 25 (2): 291–304.

Austin, C. J., and S. B. Boxerman. 2008. *Information Systems for Health Services Administration*, 5th ed. Chicago: Health Administration Press.

Barry, D., and C. L. Keough. 2005. "Ready for Prime Time? Make Your Financial Assistance Policy a Class Act." *Healthcare Financial Management* 59 (3): 48–55.

Becker, C. 2006. "Charitable Obligations." *Modern Healthcare* 36 (32): 6–7, 16.

Bellandi, D. 2001. "IHC Must Show It's Tax-Exempt." *Modern Healthcare* 31 (20): 16.

Benko, L. 2006. "California Governor Signs Pricing Bill." *Modern Healthcare* 36 (40): 10.

Berger, S. 2007. *Fundamentals of Healthcare Financial Management*, 3rd ed. San Francisco: Jossey-Bass.

Berman, H. J., S. F. Kukla, and L. E. Weeks. 1994. *The Financial Management of Hospitals*, 8th ed. Chicago: Health Administration Press.

Betbeze, P. 2013. "Compounding the Uncompensated Care Problem." *Health Leaders* 16 (4): 34–37.

Biesch, G. 2009. "Kyphoplasty Cacophony." www.modernhealthcare.com/article/20091005/SUB/910029988/.

Bittel, L. R., and M. A. Bittel. 1978. "Forecasting Business Conditions." *Encyclopedia of Professional Management*. New York: McGraw-Hill.

Blankenau, R. 1994. "Measuring Up: Congress Reconsiders Tax-Exemption Standards Under Reform." *Hospitals & Health Networks* 68 (1): 14.

Boles, C., and M. Vaughan. 2010. "Deficit Advisors Back Sweeping Cuts." Published November 8. http://online.wsj.com/article/SB10001424052748703805004575606643067587042.html.

Brigham, E. F. 1992. *Fundamentals of Financial Management*, 6th ed. New York: Dryden Press.

Bromberg, M. D. 1983. "The Medical-Industrial Complex: Our National Defense." *New England Journal of Medicine* 309 (21): 1314–16.

Burrows, S. N., and R. C. Moravec. 1997. "Direct Contracting: A Minnesota Case Study." *Healthcare Financial Management* 51 (8): 50–55.

Bush, H. 2012. "Health Care's Costliest 1%." *Hospitals and Health Networks* 86 (9): 30–36.

Carlson, J. 2012. "Clarity at Last." *Modern Healthcare*, 42 (27): 2–6.

Centers for Medicare & Medicaid Services (CMS). 2014. "National Health Expenditures by Type of Service and Source of Funds." www.cms.gov/Research-Statistics-Data-and-Systems/Statistics-Trends-and-Reports/NationalHealthExpendData/NationalHealthAccountsHistorical.html.

———. 2013. "2014 Medicare Costs." www.medicare.gov/Pubs/pdf/11579.pdf.

————. 2012a. "National Health Expenditures Projections 2012–2022." www.cms.gov/Research-Statistics-Data-and-Systems/Statistics-Trends-and-Reports/NationalHealthExpendData/Downloads/Proj2012.pdf.

————. 2012b. "National Health Expenditures by Type of Service and Source of Funds, CY 1960–2012." .www.cms.gov/Research-Statistics-Data-and-Systems/Statistics-Trends-and-Reports/NationalHealthExpendData/NationalHealthAccountsHistorical.html.

————. 2009. "Health and Healthcare of the Medicare Population. Table 4:1 Personal Health Care Expenditures for Medicare Beneficiaries, by Source of Payment and Type of Service, 2009." www.cms.gov/Research-Statistics-Data-and-Systems/Research/MCBS/Data-Tables.html.

————. 2004. "The Health Insurance Portability and Accountability Act (HIPAA) of 1996." www.cms.gov/Regulations-and-Guidance/HIPAA-Administrative-Simplification/HIPAAGenInfo/Downloads/HIPAALaw.pdf.

Chazin, S., I. Friedenzohn, E. Martinez-Vidal, and S. A. Somers. 2010. "The Future of U.S. Charity Care Programs: Implications of Health Reform." Center for Health Strategies, Academy of Health. www.academyhealth.org/files/publications/FutureofCharityCare-Programs.pdf.

Chen, L. 2011. "How Obamacare Burdens Already Strained State Budgets." *Wall Street Journal*, November 16.

Cher, D. J., and L. A. Lenert. 1997. "Method of Medicare Reimbursement and the Rate of Potentially Ineffective Care of Critically Ill Patients." *Journal of the American Medical Association* 278 (12): 1001–7.

Childs v. Weiss, 440 S.W.2d 104. 1969. Tex. Civ. App.

Clarke, R. 2006. "The Real Price of Transparency." *Modern Healthcare* 36 (25): 34.

————. 2000. "Beyond Managed Care" *Healthcare Financial Management* 54 (7): 16.

Cleverley, W. O. 2010. *Essentials of Health Care Finance*, 7th ed. Boston: Jones & Bartlett.

Congressional Budget Office (CBO). 2014. "Medicare Baseline." Published April 14. www. cbo.gov/sites/default/files/cbofiles/attachments/44205-2014-04-Medicare.pdf.

————. 2013a. "CBO's Estimate of the Net Budgetary Impact of the Affordable Care Act's Health Insurance Coverage Provisions Has Not Changed Much Over Time." www.cbo.gov/ publication/44176.

————. 2013b. "H.R. 2810: Medicare Patient Access and Quality Improvement Act of 2013." www.cbo.gov/sites/default/files/cbofiles/attachments/hr2810.pdf.

————. 2013c. "Medicare Baseline." www.cbo.gov/sites/default/files/cbofiles/ attachments/4A205_Medicare_O.pdf.

————. 2006. *Nonprofit Hospitals and the Provision of Community Benefits.* Washington, DC: CBO.

Conn, J. 2006. "Hospitals' Dirty Secret." *Modern Healthcare* 36 (47): 6–7.

Conrad, C. F., and R. T. Blackburn. 1985. "Program Quality in Higher Education: A Review and Critique of Literature and Research." In *Higher Education: Handbook of Theory and Research*, vol. I, edited by J. Smart. New York: Agathon Press.

Cross, R. G. 1997. *Revenue Management: Hardcore Tactics for Market Domination.* New York: Broadway.

Cuckler, A. M., S. P. Sisko, S. D. Smith, A. J. Madison, J. A. Poisal, C. J. Wolfe, J. M. Lizonitz, and D. A. Stone. 2013. "National Health Expenditure Projections, 2012–22: Slow Growth Until Coverage Expands and Economy Improves." *Health Affairs* web exclusive, http:// content.healthaffairs.org/content/32/10/1820.

Daly, R. 2011. "CMS Actuary Affirms Spending Projections." *Modern Healthcare*, January 26.

Darr, K. 2011. *Ethics in Health Services Management*, 5th ed. Baltimore, MD: Health Professions Press.

DeLuca, M., and C. Smith. 2010. "Impacting Patient Care Through Cost-Effective Solutions." *Healthcare Financial Management* 64 (3).

DeNavas-Walt, C., D. Proctor, and J. C. Smith. 2013. US Census Bureau Current Population Report P60-245, *Income, Poverty, and Health Insurance Coverage in the United States, 2012*. Washington, DC: US Government Printing Office.

Dennis, J. C. 2001. "The New Privacy Officer's Game Plan." *Journal of AHIMA* 72 (2): 33–37.

Dobson, A., J. DaVanzo, and S. Namrata. 2006. "The Cost-Shift Payment 'Hydraulic': Foundation, History, and Implications." *Health Affairs* 25 (1): 22–33.

Domenici, P., and A. Rivlin. 2010. "Restoring America's Future: Reviving the Economy, Cutting Spending and Debt, and Creating a Simple, Pro-Growth Tax System." Report. Washington DC: Bipartisan Policy Center.

Doody, M. F. 2000. "Broader Range of Skills Distinguishes Successful CFOs." *Healthcare Financial Management* 54 (9): 52–57.

———. 1998. "Corporate Compliance Officer Role Is Emerging." *Healthcare Financial Management* 52 (5): 78.

Dunn, R. 2010. *Dunn and Haimann's Healthcare Management*, 9th ed. Chicago: Health Administration Press.

Dutton, A. 2013. "Idaho Hospital Systems Exempt from Millions in Taxes." *Idaho Statesman*, March 12. www.idahostatesman.com/2013/03/12/2487493/hospital-systems-exempt-from-millions.html.

Eastaugh, S. R. 1992. *Health Care Finance: Economic Incentives and Productivity Enhancement*. Westport, CT: Auburn House.

———. 1987. *Financing Health Care: Economic Efficiency and Equity*. Dover, MA: Auburn House.

Eiland, G. W. 1996. "The Scary New World of Fraud and Abuse: Recent Medicare Settlements." Paper presented to the South Texas Chapter of the Healthcare Financial Management Association, Corpus Christi, TX.

Emery, J. D. 2001. "The Defined-Contribution Plan: The Next Generation of Healthcare Financing." *Healthcare Financial Management* 55 (1): 37–39.

Ernst & Young. 1997. *Just Another Day in Healthcare*. Washington, DC: Ernst & Young.

Federal Register. 1998. "Publication of the OIG Compliance Program Guidance for Hospitals" *Federal Register* 63 (35) February 23: 8987–98.

Finkler, S. A. 2003. *Finance and Accounting for Nonfinancial Managers*, 3rd ed. Englewood Cliffs, NJ: Prentice Hall.

———. 1982. "The Distinction Between Costs and Charges." *Annals of Internal Medicine* 96 (1): 102–10.

Fisher, E. S., D. O. Staiger, J. P. W. Bynum, and D. J. Gottlieb. 2007. "Creating Accountable Care Organizations: The Extended Hospital Medical Staff." *Health Affairs* 26 (1): 44–57.

Forney, S. W., and W. T. Phillips. 2011. "RAC Attack: How to Prepare and Defend Your Hospital." Paper presented at the American College of Healthcare Executives' Congress on Healthcare Leadership, March 22.

Glasser, D. L., and D. E. Bloomquist. 2000. "New and Clarified Safe Harbors May Ease Certain Provider Transactions." *Healthcare Financial Management* 54 (2): 42–47.

Grassley, C. 2010. "Grassley's Provisions for Tax-Exempt Hospital Accountability Included in New Health Care Law." www.grassley.senate.gov/news/Article.cfm?customel_dataPageID_1502=25912.

Grauman, D. M., J. M. Harris, and C. Martin. 2010. "Access to Capital: Implications for Hospital Consolidation." *Healthcare Financial Management* 64 (4): 62–70.

Gundling, R. L. 1998. "Hospital Transfers and Discharges Defined." *Healthcare Financial Management* 52 (11): 72–73.

Gurny, P., D. K. Baugh, and F. A. Davis. 1992. "A Description of Medicaid Eligibility." *Health Care Financing Review: Medicare and Medicaid Statistical Supplement 1992*: 207–26.

Guyton, E. M., and C. Lund. 2003. "Transforming the Revenue Cycle." *Healthcare Financial Management* 57 (3): 72–78.

Hammer, M., and J. Champy. 2001. *Reengineering the Corporation: A Manifesto for Business Revolution*. New York: HarperBusiness.

Harris, S. E. 1975. *The Economics of Health Care: Finance and Delivery*. Berkeley, CA: McCutchan.

Hartman, M., A. Catlin, D. Lassman, J. Cylus, and S. Heffler. 2008. "US Health Spending by Age, Selected Years Through 2004." *Health Affairs* 27 (1): w1–w12.

Health Care Compliance Association (HCAA). 2013. "Healthcare Compliance Staff Salary Survey." www.hcca-info.org/Resources/View/ArticleId/4478/2013-Healthcare-Compliance-Staff-Salary-Survey.aspx.

Healthcare Financial Management Association (HFMA). 2014. E-mail correspondence with Shirley Heavlin, January 20.

———. 2013. "Compensation Surveys." www.hfma.org/Content.aspx?id=1084.

———. 2010. "Hospital Strategies to Support Accountable Care." *Leadership* (Fall/Winter): 1–6.

———. 2007. *2007 Compensation Survey. Healthcare Financial Management* 61 (8): special section, page 1.

———. 2006. "President Asks for Another $36 Billion in Medicare Cuts: Signs Deficit Reduction Act." *Healthcare Financial Management* 60 (3): 18.

———. 2005. "HFMA's Biennial Career and Compensation Guide." *Healthcare Financial Management* 59 (7, suppl.): CS12–CS24.

———. 2004. *Financing the Future Report 6: How Are Hospitals Financing the Future? Where the Industry Will Go from Here.* www.hfma.org/WorkArea/linkit.aspx?LinkIdentifier=id&ItemID=3168.

———. 2000. "Industry Scan." *Healthcare Financial Management* 54 (7): 20.

———. 1999. "Industry Scan." *Healthcare Financial Management* 53 (9): 18.

———. 1998. *HFMA Core Certification Exam Self-Study Manual.* White Plains, NY: The MGI Management Institute.

———. 1997. "HFMA News." *Healthcare Financial Management* 51 (12): 24.

———. 1992. "Updata." *Healthcare Financial Management* 46 (6): 6.

Health Care Financing Administration (HCFA). 1996. "Overview of the Medicaid Program." *Health Care Financing Review: Medicare and Medicaid Statistical Supplement 1996*, 144–87. Baltimore, MD: HHS.

Helbing, M. 1993. "Medicare Program Expenditures." *Health Care Financing Review: Medicare and Medicaid Statistical Supplement 1992.* Baltimore, MD: HHS.

Hepner, J. O., and D. M. Hepner. 1973. *The Health Strategy Game: A Challenge for Reorganization and Management.* St. Louis, MO: C. V. Mosby.

Herkimer, A. G. 1988a. "Capital Expenditure Planning." In *Understanding Health Care Budgeting.* Rockville, MD: Aspen.

———. 1988b. *Understanding Health Care Budgeting.* Rockville, MD: Aspen.

———. 1993. *Patient Financial Services.* Chicago: HFMA/Probus Press.

Herman, B. 2013. "Moody's: Hospital Downgrades Have Surpassed Upgrades Every Quarter This Year." *Becker's Hospital Review.* www.beckershospitalreview.com/finance/moody-s-hospital-downgrades-have-surpassed-upgrades-every-quarter-this-year.html.

Herzlinger, R. E. (ed.). 2004. *Consumer-Driven Healthcare: Implications for Providers, Payers, and Policymakers.* San Francisco: Jossey-Bass.

Herzlinger, R., and W. Krasker. 1987. "Who Profits from Nonprofits?" *Harvard Business Review* 65 (1): 93–105.

Holder, A. R. 1973. "Law & Medicine." *Journal of the American Medical Association* 225 (9): 1157–58.

House Committee on Ways and Means. 2012. "Boustany Announces Hearing on Tax Exempt Organizations." May 16. http://waysandmeans.house.gov/news/documentsingle.aspx?DocumentID=294777.

Institute of Medicine (IOM). 2001. *Crossing the Quality Chasm: A New Health System for the 21st Century.* www.iom.edu/Reports/2001/Crossing-the-Quality-Chasm-A-New-Health-System-for-the-21st-Century.aspx.

———. 1999. *To Err Is Human: Building a Safer Health System.* Washington, DC: National Academies Press. www.nap.edu/openbook.php?isbn=0309068371.

Internal Revenue Service (IRS). 2012. *Additional Requirements for Charitable Hospitals.* www.irs.gov/pub/irs-drop/reg-130266-11.pdf.

———. 2009. *IRS Nonprofit Hospital Project—Final Report.* www.irs.gov/Charities-&-Non-Profits/Charitable-Organizations/IRS-Nonprofit-Hospital-Project---Final-Report.

Ivancevich, J. M., J. H. Donnelly, and J. L. Gibson. 1989. *Management Principles and Functions,* 4th ed. Homewood, IL: Irwin. Cited in Rakich, J. S., B. Longest, and K. Darr. 1992. *Managing Health Services Organizations,* 3rd ed. Baltimore, MD: Health Professions Press.

Joint Commission. 2014. *National Patient Safety Goals.* www.jointcommission.org/standards_information/npsgs.aspx.

———. 2013. *2013 Hospital Accreditation Standards.* Oakbrook Terrace, IL: Joint Commission.

———. 2009. *2009 Hospital Accreditation Standards.* Oakbrook Terrace, IL: Joint Commission.

———. 2001. Accessed January 21, 2001. www.jcaho.org/news/nb300.html.

———. 1996. *1997 Hospital Accreditation Standards.* Oakbrook Terrace, IL: Joint Commission.

Kaiser Commission on Medicaid and the Uninsured. 2010. "Health Coverage for Children; the Role of Medicaid and CHIP." http://kaiserfamilyfoundation.files.wordpress.com/2013/01/7698-06.pdf.

Kaiser Family Foundation. 2013a. "2013 Employer Health Benefits Survey, Exhibit E." kff.org/report-section/2013-summary-of-findings/.

———. 2013b. "Health Reform Implementation Timeline." www.kff.org/interactive/implementation-timeline/.

———. 2013c. "Medicaid and CHIP." http://kff.org/state-category/medicaid-chip/.

———. 2012a. "Medicare Benefit Payments by Type of Service, 2012." http://kff.org/health-costs/slide/medicare-benefit-payments-by-type-of-service-2012/.

———. 2012b. "Massachusetts Health Care Reform: Six Years Later." *Focus on Health Reform.* http://kaiserfamilyfoundation.files.wordpress.com/2013/01/8311.pdf.

———. 2010. "Summary of the Affordable Care Act." *Focus on Health Reform.* http://kaiserfamilyfoundation.files.wordpress.com/2011/04/8061-021.pdf.

Kaissi, A. A., and J. W. Begun. 2008. "Strategic Planning Processes and Hospital Financial Performance." *Journal of Healthcare Management* 53 (3): 197–208.

Kaufman, N. 2011. "Three 'Brutal Facts' That Provide Strategic Direction for Health Delivery Systems: Preparing for the End of the Healthcare Bubble." *Journal of Healthcare Management* 56 (3): 163–68.

Kelley, R. 2009. "Where Can $700 Billion in Waste Be Cut Annually from the US Healthcare System?" Ann Arbor, MI: Thomson Reuters. www.ncrponline.org/PDFs/2009/Thomson_Reuters_White_Paper_on_Healthcare_Waste.pdf.

Kilborn, P. T. 1998. "Managed Care: Looking Back at Jackson Hole." *New York Times*, March 22.

Kongstvedt, P. R. 2013. *Essentials of Managed Health Care*, 6th ed. Boston: Jones & Bartlett.

Kooijman, J. 1999. *The Incremental Strategy Toward National Health Insurance in the United States of America*. Amsterdam: Rodopi.

Kuchler, J. A. 1992. "Tax-Exempt Yardstick: Defining the Measurements." *Healthcare Financial Management* 46 (2): 21–31.

Kutscher, B. 2013. "Record Number of Debt Downgrades for Not-for-Profits in 2012: Moody's." *Modern Healthcare*. February 12. www.modernhealthcare.com/article/20130212/NEWS/302129860/record-number-of-debt-downgrades-for-not-for-profits-in-2012-moodys.

Laforge, R. W., and J. S. Tureaud. 2003. "Revenue-Cycle Redesign: Honing the Details." *Healthcare Financial Management* 57 (1): 64–71.

Larkin, H. D. 2009. "Mass. Appeal?" *Hospitals & Health Networks* 83 (5): 26–29.

Laribee, S. 1994. "The Psychology Types of College Accounting Students." *Journal of Psychology Type* 28: 37–42.

Lovern, E. 2001. "JCAHO's New Tell-All." *Modern Healthcare* 31 (1): 2, 15.

Lubell, J. 2009. "A Stimulating Conversation." *Modern Healthcare* 39 (8): 6–7, 14.

Lubell, J., and M. DoBias. 2010. "This Is It." *Modern Healthcare* 40 (13): 6–7.

Lutz, S., and E. P. Gee. 1998. *Columbia/HCA: Healthcare on Overdrive.* New York: McGraw-Hill.

Mantone, J. 2006. "Stating the Case for Coverage." *Modern Healthcare* 36 (18): 6–7, 16.

Martin, A., D. Lassman, L. Whittle, and A. Catlin. 2014. "Recession Contributes to Slowest Annual Rate of Increase in Health Spending in Five Decades." *Health Affairs* 33 (1): 67–77.

Marx, K. 1998 [1848]. *Communist Manifesto.* New York: Signet Classic.

Millenson, M. (moderator). 2003. "Healthcare's Challenge: Rising Consumer Expectations." *HealthLeaders* 6 (1): RT1–RT15.

Modern Healthcare. 2006. "Community-Benefits Debate." *Modern Healthcare* (30 Trends/ Innovations to Watch suppl.): 60.

———. 2003. "They 'Just Do It Better.'" *Modern Healthcare* 33 (39, suppl.): 6–12.

Moore, K. D., K. Eyestone, and D. C. Coddington. 2013. "The Healthcare Cost Curve Can Be Bent." *Healthcare Financial Management* 67 (3): 78–84.

Murray, B. P., R. B. Dwore, R. J. Parsons, P. M. Smith, and L. H. Vorderer. 1994. "Methods of Optimizing Revenue in Rural Hospitals." *Healthcare Financial Management* 48 (3): 52–60.

National Center for Health Statistics. 2013. *Health, United States,* 2012. www.cdc.gov/nchs/ data/hus/hus12.pdf.

National Conference of State Legislators (NCSL). 2009. "Transparency and Disclosure of Health Costs and Provider Payments: State Actions." www.ncsl.org/default. aspx?tabid=14512

Nowicki, M. 2004. "Key Indicators in Hospital Financial Statements." Presentation to governing board chairs at American Hospital Association meeting, Washington, DC, May 3.

———. "Evolving Role of the Healthcare CFO." Presentation to Healthcare Financial Management Association CFO Exchange, San Francisco, March 10.

———. 1995. "Conflicts of Interest." *Journal of Healthcare Resource Management* 13 (10): 34–35.

Nowicki, M., and J. Summers. 2001. "Managing Impossible Missions: Ethical Quandaries and Ethical Solutions." *Healthcare Financial Management* 55 (6): 62–67.

Obama, B. 2010. "Presidential Proclamation—45th Anniversary of Medicare and Medicaid." www.whitehouse.gov/the-press-office/presidential-proclamation-45th-anniversary-medicare-and-medicaid.

Office of Inspector General (OIG). 2013. *Semiannual Report to Congress*. http://oig.hhs.gov/reports-and-publications/archives/semiannual/2013/SAR-F13-OS.pdf.

———. 2010a. *Fall 2010 Semiannual Report*. http://oig.hhs.gov/reports-and-publications/archives/semiannual/2010fall.asp.

———. 2010b. "Archive: Safe Harbor Regulations." http://oig.hhs.gov/reports-and-publications/archives/safe-harbor-regulations/index.asp.

———. 2009. *Semiannual Report to Congress*. http://oig.hhs.gov/publications/docs/semiannual/2009/semiannual_fall2009.pdf.

———. 1995. *Medicare and Medicaid Guide*. Report A-03-94-00021. Washington, DC: OIG.

Optum. 2014. *2014 Almanac of Hospital Financial and Operating Indicators: A Comprehensive Benchmark of the Nation's Hospitals*. Salt Lake City, UT: Optum.

Pallarito, K. 1997a. "Getting in Harmony: As Markets Change, Hospitals Struggle with Pricing." *Modern Healthcare* 27 (26): 100–11.

————. 1997b. "Indiana Hospital Sticks to Guns on 'Fair' Pricing." *Modern Healthcare* 27 (26): 106.

Pearce, J. A., and F. David. 1987. "Corporate Mission Statements and the Bottom Line." *Academy of Management Executives* 1 (2): 109–16.

Person, M. W. 1997. *The Zero-Base Hospital: Survival and Success in America's Evolving Healthcare System*. Chicago: Health Administration Press.

Peter G. Peterson Foundation. 2008. *I.O.U.S.A.* www.iousathemovie.com.

Peters, T. 1988. *Thriving on Chaos*. New York: Alfred A. Knopf.

Peterson, P. G. 1996. *Will America Grow Up Before It Grows Old?* New York: Random House.

Piotrowski, J. 2003a. "HealthSouth's Most Wanted." *Modern Healthcare* 33 (45): 6–7, 16.

————. 2003b. "Yale–New Haven Sued." *Modern Healthcare* 33 (8): 16.

Pirsig, R. 1974. *Zen and the Art of Motorcycle Maintenance*. New York: William Morrow.

Porter, M. 1980. *Competitive Strategy: Techniques for Analyzing Industries and Competitors*. New York: Free Press.

Pressey, D. 2010. "Timeline of Major Developments in Provena Covenant's Property Tax Case." *Champaign-Urbana News-Gazette*. www.news-gazette.com/news/politics-and-government/2010-03-19/timeline-major-developments-provena-covenants-property-tax-c.

Rau, J. 2008. "State Health Plan Killed; Calling It 'Fundamentally Flawed,' Senators Reject Gov's Proposal." *Los Angeles Times* January 29, A1.

Rauber, C. 2003. "The New Face of Health Plans." *HealthLeaders* 6 (1): 37–43.

Reeves, P. N., D. F. Bergwall, and N. B. Woodside. 1979. *Introduction to Health Planning*, 2nd ed. Arlington, VA: Information Resources Press.

Reinstein, A., and R. J. Dery. 1999. "AICPA Standard Aids in Detecting Risk Factors for Fraud." *Healthcare Financial Management* 53 (10): 48–50.

Relman, A. S. 1980. "The New Medical-Industrial Complex." *New England Journal of Medicine* 303: 963–70.

Reserve Life Insurance Company v. Salter. 1957. 152 F. Supp. 868.

Roberts, M., and J. Rhoades. 2010. "The Uninsured in America, First Half of 2009: Estimates for the US Civilian Noninstitutionalized Population Under Age 65." Statistical Brief #291. Rockville, MD: Agency for Healthcare Research and Quality.

Romano, M. 2006. "Looking for Volunteers." *Modern Healthcare* 36 (13): 6–7, 16.

———. 2001. "Less Stark, More Clarity." *Modern Healthcare* 31 (2): 2–3, 9.

Rosenthal, E. 2013. "Benefits Questioned in Tax Breaks for Nonprofit Hospitals." *New York Times*, December 16. www.nytimes.com/2013/12/17/us/benefits-questioned-in-tax-breaks-for-nonprofit-hospitals.html?_r=0.

Rosenthal, M., C. Hsuan, and A. Milstein. 2005. "A Report Card on the Freshman Class of Consumer-Directed Health Plans." *Health Affairs* 24 (6): 1592–1600.

Runy, L. 2004. "Managing Revenue, Reducing Debt." *Hospitals & Health Networks* 78 (2): 30.

Russo, J. J. 1997. "Health Care Fraud/Abuse: Recent Developments." Presentation to Healthcare Financial Management Association Annual National Institute, Orlando, FL, July 1.

Russo, R., and J. Russo. 1998. "Healthcare Compliance Plans: Good Business Practice for the New Millennium." *Journal of the American Health Information Management Association* 69 (1): 24–31.

Salb, D. 2008. "Doctor's Orders: Health Coverage for Everyone." *Yes Magazine.* http://yesmagazine.org/issues/purple-america/doctors-orders-health-coverage-for-everyone.

Scalise, D., and T. H. Thrall. 2002. "American's Uninsured: Rethinking the Problem That Won't Go Away." *Hospitals & Health Networks* 76 (11): 31–40.

Scruggs, R. 2004. "First Two Class Action Lawsuits in Northwest by Uninsured Patients Against Nonprofit Hospital Systems and Hospitals Filed in Federal Courts in the States of Oregon and Washington." *PR Newswire*. www.prnewswire.com/news-releases/first-two-class-action-lawsuits-in-northwest-by-uninsured-patients-against-nonprofit-hospital-systems-and-hospitals-filed-in-federal-courts-in-the-states-of-oregon-and-washington-73986762.html.

Selivanoff, P. 2011. "The Impact of Healthcare Reform on Hospital Costing Systems." *Healthcare Financial Management* 65 (5): 110–16.

Siegel, J. G., and J. K. Shim. 2006. *Accounting Handbook*, 4th ed. Hauppauge, NY: Barron's Educational Series.

Showalter, J. S. 2011. *The Law of Healthcare Administration*, 6th ed. Chicago: Health Administration Press.

Society of Actuaries. 2010. *The Economic Measurement of Medical Errors*. www.soa.org/files/research/projects/research-econ-measurement.pdf.

Social Security and Medicare Trustees. 2011. *2011 Annual Report of the Boards of Trustees of the Federal Hospital Insurance and Federal Supplementary Medical Insurance Trust Funds*. www.cms.gov/reportstrustfunds/downloads/tr2011.pdf.

Somerville, M. H., G. D. Nelson, and C. H. Mueller. 2013. "Hospital Community Benefits after the ACA: The State Law Landscape." *The Hilltop Institute*. www.hilltopinstitute.org/publications/HospitalCommunityBenefitsAfterTheACA-StateLawLandscapeIssueBrief6-March2013.pdf.

St. Mary's Honor Center v. Hicks. 1993. No. 92-602.

Standard & Poor's. 2013. *The Outlook for U.S. Not-For-Profit Health Care Providers Is Negative from Increasing Pressures*. www.standardandpoors.com/spf/upload/Events_US/article5_dec112013.pdf.

Starr, P. 1982. *The Social Transformation of American Medicine*. New York: Basic.

Stromberg, R. E. 1982. "Legal Issues for Diversification and Divestiture." In *The Financial Management of Hospitals*, 5th ed., by H. J. Berman and L. E. Weeks. Chicago: Health Administration Press.

Sturn, W. C. 1995. "Must Insurance Payment Made in Error Be Returned?" *Healthcare Financial Management* 49 (5): 27–30.

Suver, J. D., B. R. Neumann, and K. E. Boles. 1995. "Pricing Strategies." In *Management Accounting for Healthcare Organizations*, 4th ed. Chicago: Pluribus Press.

Taylor, M. 2003. "Exemption Denied." *Modern Healthcare* 33 (50): 16.

———. 2001. "End to Legal Odyssey." *Modern Healthcare* 31 (20): 16.

Texas Tax Code. 1993. "Charity Care and Community Benefits Requirements for Charitable Hospital." §11.1801. http://codes.lp.findlaw.com/txstatutes/TX/1/C/11/B/11.1801.

Thompson Powers LLC. 1999. *The Politics of Exemption: Tax Revenue vs. Community Benefit—Not-for-Profit Hospitals Under Pressure*. Irving, Texas: VHA Inc.

Tieger, P., and B. Barron-Tieger. 2001. *Do What You Are: Discover the Perfect Career for You Through the Secrets of Personality Type*, 3rd ed. New York: Little, Brown.

Tuma, L. 2010. "Accountable Care Organizations: Bending the Cost Curve Toward More Efficient Care." *Texas Hospitals* 8 (4): 18–21.

United States Sentencing Commission (USSC). 1991. *United States Sentencing Guidelines*. 8A1.2. Washington, DC: USSC.

US Chamber of Commerce. 2010. "Health Care." www.uschamber.com/issues/health.

US Department of Health and Human Services (HHS). 2013a. "Health Information Privacy: Enforcement Highlights." www.hhs.gov/ocr/privacy/hipaa/enforcement/highlights/index.html.

———. 2013b. "Health Information Privacy: HHS Announces First HIPAA Breach Settlement Involving Less Than 500 Patients." www.hhs.gov/ocr/privacy/hipaa/enforcement/examples/honi-agreement.html.

———. 2013c. "Wellpoint Pays HHS $1.7 Million for Leaving Information Accessible over Internet." www.hhs.gov/ocr/privacy/hippa/enforcement/examples/wellpoint-agreement.html.

———. 2010a. "Rite Aid Agrees to Pay $1 Million to Settle HIPAA Privacy Case." News Release. www.hhs.gov/ocr/privacy/hipaa/enforcement/examples/riteaidresagr.html.

———. 2010b. Healthy People 2020 brochure. www.healthypeople.gov/2020/topicsobjectives2020/default.aspx.

———. 2009. News Release. http://www.hhs.gov/news/press/2009pres/02/20090218a.html.

Utah State Tax Commission. 1990. *Non-profit Hospital and Nursing Home Charitable Property Tax Exemption Standard*. Salt Lake City: Utah State Tax Commission.

Wang, T., and J. R. Wambsganns. 1997. "Is Your Organization's Tax-Exempt Status at Risk?" *1997 Resource Guide*. Chicago: HFMA.

Watnik, R. 2000. "Antikickback Versus Stark: What's the Difference?" *Healthcare Financial Management* 54 (3): 66–67.

Weidenbaum, M. L., and R. DeFina. 1981. *The Rising Cost of Government Regulations*. St. Louis, MO: Center for the Study of American Business.

William, J., and J. Rakich. 1973. "Investment Evaluation in Hospitals." *Hospital Financial Management* 23 (2): 30–35.

Winslow, R., and J. Goldstein. 2009. "Cutting Repeat Hospital Trips—Simple Idea, Hard to Pull Off." *Wall Street Journal*, July 28, A1, A4.

Witek, J. E., D. L. Milligan, and J. B. Ryan. 1993. "Managing Charitable Purpose: Issues and Answers." Presentation to American College of Healthcare Executives Congress on Healthcare Leadership, Chicago, March 4.

Young, G. L., C. Dhou, J. Alexander, S. D. Lee, and E. Rover. 2013. "Provisions of Community Benefits by Tax-Exempt U.S. Hospitals." *New England Journal of Medicine* 368 (16): 1519–27.

Zelman, W. A. 1996. *The Changing Health Care Marketplace: Private Ventures, Public Interests*. San Francisco: Jossey-Bass.

Zelman, W. N., M. J. McCue, N. D. Glick, and M. S. Thomas. 2014. *Financial Management of Health Care Organizations,* 4th ed. San Francisco: Jossey-Bass Publishers.

Zigmond, J. 2014. "U.S. Chamber Looks to Fix, Not Repeal Obamacare." *Modern Healthcare* January 8. www.modernhealthcare.com/article/20140108/NEWS/301089973.

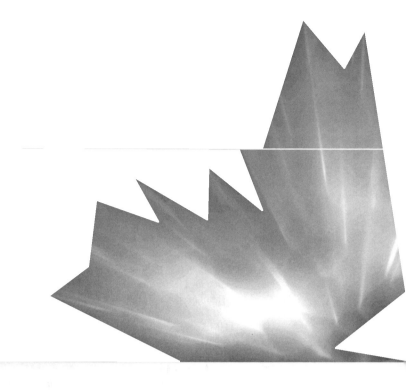

ABOUT THE AUTHOR

Dr. Michael Nowicki is a professor of health administration at Texas State University, where his teaching, research, and service have been recognized with several university awards, including teacher of the year.

Prior to joining academe, Dr. Nowicki was director of process management in the Hospital Division of Humana for six years. Dr. Nowicki has also held a variety of administrative positions at Valley Medical Center in Fresno, Hutzel Hospital in Detroit, Georgetown University Medical Center, and Lubbock Medical Center. Dr. Nowicki has provided recent training support to such organizations as University Health in Indianapolis, Cardinal Health, Kaiser Permanente, University Hospitals in Cleveland, HCA, Mercy Hospitals of Northern Ohio, Baylor Healthcare System, and Howard University Hospital.

Dr. Nowicki received his doctorate in educational policy studies and evaluation from the University of Kentucky, his master's in healthcare administration from The George Washington University, and his bachelor's in political science from Texas Tech University. Dr. Nowicki is board-certified in healthcare management and a Fellow in the American College of Healthcare Executives (ACHE). Related to ACHE, he has served as founder and advisor of student chapters, founder and president of the Central Texas Chapter, and chair of the national Book-of-the-Year Committee. Dr. Nowicki is also board-certified in healthcare financial management and is a Fellow in the Healthcare Financial Management Association (HFMA). Dr. Nowicki has served as president of the South Texas Chapter of HFMA and regional executive for HFMA Region 9. He also has served on the national HFMA board of directors as chair of the Chapter Services Council and the Council of Forums. He was also the chair of the HFMA board of examiners in 2001.

Dr. Nowicki has presented financial management seminars to audiences worldwide, including the Russian Ministry of Health in Moscow, Russian hospital executives in Golitsyno, Estonian hospital executives in Tallin, Indonesian hospital executives visiting the University of Massachusetts, and numerous other audiences in the United States. Dr. Nowicki is a frequent speaker at national meetings of the American Hospital Association, the Healthcare Financial Management Association, the American College of Healthcare Executives, and Voluntary Hospitals of America. He has written dozens of articles on leadership in financial management. In addition to *Introduction to the Financial Management of Healthcare Organizations*, Dr. Nowicki authored the fifth edition of *HFMA's Introduction to Hospital Accounting* in 2006.

Other Books in the *Gateway* to Healthcare Management Series

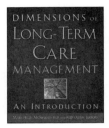

Dimensions of Long-Term Care Management: An Introduction
Mary Helen McSweeney-Feld, PhD, and Reid Oetjen, PhD, Editors

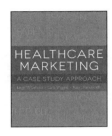

Healthcare Marketing: A Case Study Approach
Leigh W. Cellucci, PhD, Carla Wiggins, PhD, and Tracy J. Farnsworth, EdD

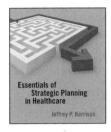

Essentials of Strategic Planning in Healthcare
Jeffrey P. Harrison, PhD, FACHE

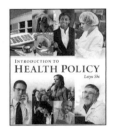

Introduction to Health Policy
Leiyu Shi, DrPH

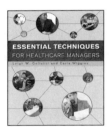

Essential Techniques for Healthcare Managers
Leigh W. Cellucci, PhD, and Carla Wiggins, PhD

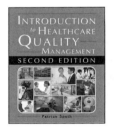

Introduction to Healthcare Quality Management, Second Edition
Patrice L. Spath, RHIT

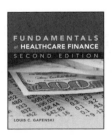

Fundamentals of Healthcare Finance, Second Edition
Louis C. Gapenski, PhD

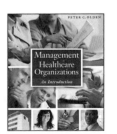

Management of Healthcare Organizations: An Introduction
Peter C. Olden, PhD

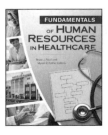

Fundamentals of Human Resources in Healthcare
Bruce J. Fried, PhD, and Myron D. Fottler, PhD, Editors

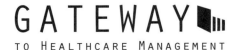
GATEWAY
TO HEALTHCARE MANAGEMENT